HIPAA Plain & Simple

Second Edition

A Health Care Professionals Guide to Achieve HIPAA and HITECH Compliance

By Carolyn P. Hartley, MLA, and
Edward D. Jones, III

With Forewords by Louis W. Sullivan, MD, and
David J. Brailer, MD, PhD

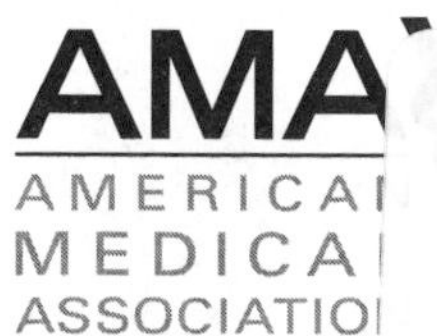

Executive Vice President, Chief Executive Officer: Michael D. Maves, MD, MBA

Chief Operating Officer: Bernard L. Hengesbaugh

Senior Vice President, Publishing and Business Services: Robert A. Musacchio, PhD

Vice President, Business Operations: Vanessa Hayden

Publisher, AMA Publications and Clinical Solutions: Mary Lou White

Senior Acquisitions Editor: Elise Schumacher

Manager, Book and Product Development and Production: Nancy Baker

Senior Developmental Editor: Lisa Chin-Johnson

Production Specialist: Mary Ann Albanese

Director of Sales, Business Products: Mark Daniels

Marketing Manager: Lauren Jones

Reviewers: Barney Cohen, Health Law; Catherine Hanson, VP, Private Sector Advocacy

www.ama-assn.org

Additional copies of this book may be ordered by calling 800 621-8335 or from the secure AMA bookstore Web site at *www.amabookstore.org*. Refer to product number OP320710.

Library of Congress Cataloging-in-Publication Data

Hartley, Carolyn P.

HIPAA plain & simple: a compliance guide for health care professionals by Carolyn P. Hartley and Edward D. Jones III; with forewords by Louis W. Sullivan and David J. Brailer.— 2nd ed.

p. ; cm.

Other title: HIPAA plain and simple

Includes bibliographical references and index.

Summary: This book is for nurses, billing and insurance specialists, business associates, physicians and office managers. A resource for help understanding risk analysis, security implementation process, HIPAA and HITECH strategies

ISBN 978-1-60359-205-5 (alk. paper)

1. Medicine—Practice—United States. I. Jones, Ed (Edward Douglass) II. American Medical Association. III. Title. IV. Title: HIPAA plain and simple.

[DNLM: 1. United States. Health Insurance Portability and Accountability Act of 1996. 2. Medical Records Systems, Computerized—United States. 3. Confidentiality—United States. 4. Practice Management, Medical—organization & administration—United States. WX 173 H332h 2010]

R728.H3628 2010
610'.68—dc22

2010017438

ISBN 978-1-60359-205-5
BP02:10-P-033:10/10

Dedications

To Caitlyn, Keegan, Nathaniel, Abigail, and Andrew, in expectation of a more efficient health care system for your generation.

To Michyla, Logan, Jackson, Brooks, and Emily and their parents, already HIPAA-aware, wise health care consumers.

Table of Contents

Foreword

It gives me great pleasure to write the foreword for the second edition of *HIPAA Plain and Simple: A Health Care Professionals Guide to Achieve HIPAA and HITECH Compliance*. During my tenure as Secretary of the US Department of Health and Human Services (HHS) from 1989 to 1993, I recognized that the federal government had to address the problem of rapidly rising health care costs.

In 1991, I asked leaders in the health care industry, from both business and government, to come together in a collaborative effort to examine ways to lower administrative costs, particularly those associated with paper transactions, and to ascertain how electronic technology could help. This collaborative effort was the genesis of the Workgroup for Electronic Data Interchange (WEDI). The work of WEDI in the early 1990s provided the framework for the Administrative Simplification provisions that were enacted as part of the Health Insurance Portability and Accountability Act of 1996 (HIPAA). WEDI was one of four organizations to serve as advisors to the Secretary of HHS on HIPAA implementation issues. Those regulations are the subject of *HIPAA Plain and Simple*.

To facilitate its advisory role, WEDI created the Strategic National Implementation Process (SNIP) initiative in 2000 as a forum for health care industry participants to collaborate on addressing and resolving business and technical issues associated with implementing the HIPAA Administrative Simplification standards. Many of these standards and implementation specifications are detailed and complex.

Fortunately, the authors of *HIPAA Plain and Simple* have taken these details and complexities and turned them into understandable explanations of actions health care providers, particularly physician practices, must take to become "HIPAA compliant." As you read through the chapters on HIPAA Administrative Simplification transactions, Privacy Rules and Security Rules, I think that you will find the following sections (with examples) particularly useful:

- What to do
- How to do it
- Critical points.

As you move toward HIPAA compliance, I would like you to keep in mind the original objectives of Administrative Simplification, which were to:

- attain more efficient and effective health care system exchange of administrative and financial information using electronic transaction standards;
- realize increased protection of such information and patients' medical records; and
- reduce costs of health care transactions.

I am as certain today as I was in 1991 that in the years ahead the health care industry in the United States will realize these objectives. Further, with a more efficient and less costly administrative structure, the health care industry can devote more of its resources to improving the quality of health care delivered.

Access to health care and improving the quality of health care are significant focal points of my career as a physician, as US Secretary of HHS, and as founding dean and president of Morehouse School of Medicine (MSM) in Atlanta, Georgia. The mission of MSM, an historically black institution, is to recruit and train minority and other students as physicians, biomedical scientists, and public health professionals committed to the health care needs of the underserved in our society. Enhancing that mission is MSM's new National Center for Primary Care (NCPC), directed by Dr David Satcher, the former Surgeon General of the US Public Health Service. The Center's focus is on "improving health care and healthcare access for low-income, minority, and other underserved populations using a number of strategies—research, health policy alternatives, cost-effective programs, professional training, and supporting collaborative efforts."

For clinical staff, like those at MSM, *HIPAA Plain and Simple* presents a set of understandable explanations, tools, examples, and references that will help health care providers become compliant with HIPAA Administrative Simplification standards. Many underserved provider communities will gain by having access to the information presented in the book, including references to additional sources of information that can be accessed through the Internet.

HIPAA compliance opens up new possibilities for improving access to and delivery of quality health care in all medical practices. The electronic standards and accompanying privacy and security mandates discussed in *HIPAA Plain and Simple* are the beginning of the electronic revolution in health care. Electronic methods of communicating data, including e-mail, facilitate collaboration. This opens new ways for patients to communicate with medical staff and physicians. It also supports an easier way for physicians, specialty organizations, and academic medical centers to communicate with one another and with remote health care facilities. The development of electronic medical records will provide greater access to health care resources and the delivery of quality health care to all of our citizens.

Those are goals that we all strive for as we go into the future.

I recommend *HIPAA Plain and Simple* and wish you successful compliance with HIPAA Administrative Simplification standards.

Louis W. Sullivan, MD
President Emeritus, Morehouse School of Medicine
Former Secretary, US Department of Health and Human Services

Foreword

In 2004 President George W. Bush launched an initiative, which I had the privilege of leading, to advance the health care industry into the digital era. We knew then—as we all do now—that it was time for physicians, hospitals, and patients to move into the information age. State and federal policies were not being mindful of the future, and hospitals and physicians were falling behind the information curve. We outlined four strategic goals:

1. *Inform clinicians*: Get information to physicians by investing in electronic records and other information tools that support clinical decision making.
2. *Build a community of sharing*: Develop a health information infrastructure so that health care information follows the patient.
3. *Personalize care*: Give patients more access to information about their own and their family's care and give them more control over their information.
4. *Advance public health and research*: Expand public health monitoring and research by enabling data to be collected and analyzed without compromising privacy.

We laid the groundwork for an ongoing, evolutionary shift toward an information-rich health care system. The federal government had to lead this effort, but the health care industry's professionals and institutions had to be the ones to make it happen. The Obama Administration has built momentum and brought substantial funding to health information technology, but the underlying goals remain the same and the importance of what physicians and hospitals do for their patients is unchanged.

The physician's office has not been able to keep pace with the tremendous changes in technology, services, and management. It is a site that is about to go through major change in how medical practice is conceptualized, organized, and delivered. Physicians are beginning to take responsibility for their patients far beyond when they are in front of them during a visit. Physicians are becoming advocates for wellness and prevention: not just for their patients, but also within society. The changes happening in a physician's office have several important characteristics. First, a physician has to be able to assimilate information regarding a patient's medical history in order to treat the patient. Second, physicians have to keep up with constant changes and apply that up-to-date knowledge to their patient's care—*and* get it right every time. Third, a physician has to share information when the patient is treated elsewhere. Fourth, a physician has to monitor the patient throughout the patient's experience outside of the physician's office. Finally, physicians have to communicate in real time with many other caregivers—including patients themselves and their families—in order to manage the complexity of care. Information technology will realize all of these changes, and in so doing, it will reinvent care delivery as we know it.

The Decade of Health Information Technology was the name that we gave to the 2004 initiative. We are halfway into that decade, which has seen unprecedented progress. When President Obama was elected, he chose to build upon that progress making health information technology one of the few bipartisan health care issues. The next five years will be about moving from the big picture to the small picture: the small changes shaping the physician's office, the patient's life, and the way hospitals, pharmacies, and laboratories work. The experience of a physician, a nurse, a secretary, or a patient in a typical physician's office five years ago and five years from now will be fundamentally different. For example, a patient should not be handed a clipboard and be expected to provide the same information over and over again. Their information should already be known. If laboratory tests are ordered or if medication is prescribed, the patient will not have to come back in order to follow-up, instead the patient can e-mail his or her physician. It will be a very different experience, which will be more like what Americans experience in other parts of their daily lives. It will be much more customer friendly, much more tailor-made, much more able to respond to a patient's needs.

Electronic record technology and thoughtful policy are important pieces of our progress, but we can only realize this future through widespread adoption of clear and unambiguous information standards. Standards require an agreement on how we store, share, and communicate health information. Physicians have to possess the mechanisms for connecting their information tools to hospital systems, to tools in patients' homes, and to devices in or on patients' bodies, as well as the ability to link into health plans and into other physicians' systems. This shift relies upon interoperability—true multilateral movement of health information in a timely manner.

The promise of health information technology will be realized only through physician leadership. If today's physicians do their part, future physicians will see health information tools, databases, and information standards as tools in their practices just like antibiotics and surgical procedures.

David J. Brailer, MD, PhD
America's first National Coordinator for Health Information Technology, appointed by President George W. Bush

About the Authors

Carolyn P. Hartley, MLA

Carolyn is President, CEO of Physicians EHR, Inc, a rapid growth company that serves as provider/clinic advocate, managing the EHR selection, training, negotiating, and implementation processes. She also is VP of HIPAA, LLC, where she serves as content management advisor for the organization.

She and her EHR project management team oversee the complex paper to paperless migration, including implementing the privacy and security infrastructure for clinics in 17 states, and also serve as EHR technical advisor to national and state medical societies and quality improvement organizations. She also served on the Technical Advisory Panel for the Health Information Security and Privacy Collaborative (HISPC) funded by the Office of the National Coordinator (ONC).

Carolyn readily shares her health IT knowledge in day-to-day EHR implementations, project management in small to multisite installs, vendor management, and with clinical and administrative audiences nationwide. She is the author of 15 textbooks published by the American Medical Association, the American Dental Association, the American Society of Clinical Oncology, and the American Gastroenterological Association on HIPAA Privacy, Security, and EHR Implementation.

Prior to founding Physicians EHR, Carolyn was VP, Fleishman Hillard International Communications, and led clients to receive the distinguished Silver Anvil award. She also is a recipient of the Points of Light Foundation Leadership Award.

She holds a Master of Liberal Arts degree from Baker University with an emphasis in medical anthropology.

Edward D. Jones III

Ed Jones is managing member and CEO of three Cornichon Healthcare companies in Seabrook Island, South Carolina, and president of HIPAA, LLC, located in Beaufort, South Carolina.

Ed and his colleagues at Cornichon consult with health care stakeholders on enabling regulations and electronic business strategies related to the Health Insurance Portability and Accountability Act (HIPAA), the Health Information Technology for Economic and Clinical Health Act (HITECH Act), and the Patient Protection and Affordable Care Act. In addition, they consult with electronic health record (EHR) systems vendors on certification requirements and with health care providers on implementation of EHR and practice management systems, management of the revenue cycle, and evaluation of gaps in HIPAA privacy and security compliance. Cornichon's HIPAA√*RMS*™ software provides health care covered entities and business associates with online risk assessment, sample policy and procedure, and documentation management solutions for achieving HIPAA privacy and security compliance.

Ed and his colleagues at HIPAA, LLC, offer federal health care legislative and regulatory information source material and commentary at HIPAA, LLC's, Web site, www.hipaa.com, and offer online HIPAA and HITECH Act privacy and security training for covered entities and business associates at www.HIPAASchool.com. In partnership with the American Medical Association, HIPAA, LLC, has tailored these privacy and security courses for AMA members and nonmembers at http://AMA.HIPAASchool.com.

Ed brings considerable health care industry and business leadership to these companies. He was elected for two terms as the 2003–2004 chair of the board of directors of the Workgroup for Electronic Data Interchange (WEDI), an association of more than 300 corporate and government members that was founded by former secretary of Health and Human Services (HHS) Louis W. Sullivan, MD. WEDI is an advisor to the secretary of HHS and National Committee on Vital and Health Statistics (NCVHS) on design and implementation of HIPAA administrative simplification standards and on electronic business and clinical tools in health care. Ed also was a founding commissioner of the Electronic Healthcare Network Accreditation Commission (EHNAC) and an architect of its accreditation criteria, serving from 1994 to 2003.

Until it was acquired in December 1999, Ed served as senior vice-president and member of the CEO's Executive Operations Committee of the NYSE-company, The Centris Group, Inc, which comprised seven subsidiary companies with a core focus on underwriting and reinsuring self-funded health plans for US employers. Before joining Centris in 1993, Ed was executive vice-president and a member of the board of directors of Medical Review Systems, a firm that he cofounded in 1990, which was later acquired in 1995 by Equifax. Before that, he served as a consultant to the National Research Council of the National Academy of Sciences, the US Sentencing Commission, and firms in insurance and other industries, and held senior positions in the US Department of Justice and Central Intelligence Agency.

Ed holds degrees in economics from the University of Chicago and Washington University in St. Louis. This is the eighth book he has cowritten with Carolyn Hartley. Ed can be reached at edj3@me.com.

Introduction

Physicians and their workforce members aren't new to regulations, and most of them knew HIPAA would get bolder with the announcement that physicians could receive investment funding for adopting electronic health records.

In their initial versions, HIPAA Privacy and Security Rules were complex. Both are even more complex now with the Breach Notification Rule added to privacy and security standards. Between the three rules, you'll find 143 implementation specifications, any one of which can send you running for cover. Add meaningful use reporting into the mix, with accompanying risk management documentation, and you've got a legitimate reason to throw up your hands and cry, "Why me?"

But if you peel back the layers of convoluted legalese and complex technical interdependencies and tackle HIPAA one bite at a time, it actually starts looking like some of the processes you already have, or have wanted to put in place, as you transition into an electronic environment. If you're the one in the practice that says, "I hate HIPAA," then *HIPAA Plain and Simple* is for you.

HIPAA still makes good business sense. You wouldn't want a hacker to reach up into your bank account and snag a few thousand dollars just because he's a snappy programmer. Similarly, you don't want your patients with whom you've spent years building trust, to find out that their identity has been compromised for lack of a $29 password recovery software to access your user IDs and passwords. In moving to an automated health care system, though, security must be assessed and managed.

The American health care system has delivered some distinguished as well as compassionate clinical minds. Caregivers are the rock foundation that manages our population's health. But you also know all too well that the physician's time is too often diluted to manage bloated and unbalanced administrative processes. Health care has to follow the path of other industries and automate many of its redundant and costly processes while eliminating wasteful workflows. This is not news to those of us who have been in health care for decades. What *is* news is that something is finally being done to blow out the waste.

The federal government, under the leadership of President Obama, is pouring tens of billions of dollars to help you make the transition into an electronic environment. The accountability factor of using taxpayer dollars is to build consumer confidence in the electronic system, and that puts you squarely in the hands of robust privacy and security rules.

HIPAA 2010 and beyond has a lot of teeth in it. The Office for Civil Rights (OCR) of the Department of Health and Human Services (HHS), the enforcement agency for privacy and security, has been criticized for being flaccid and underfunded. The agency has funding now and an empowered force of audit compliance officers are headed to a facility near you. Compliance with HIPAA is no longer just complaint driven, but compliance audit driven as well.

The Breach Notification Rule issued by the Federal Trade Commission (FTC) requires certain Web-based businesses, such as personal health records, blood pressure cuffs, and pedometers, to notify consumers when the security of their electronic protected health information (ePHI) is breached.[1] These businesses are not subject to HIPAA Privacy and Security, but consumers can upload personal health information into their online personal health records. In consultation with FTC, the US Department of Health and Human Services, as required by the HITECH Rule, issued its own Breach Notification Rule to be enforced by the HHS Office for Civil Rights. In that rule, covered entities and through them, their business associates, are required to notify consumers if the privacy or security of their health information is breached.[2]

Most likely you've seen a news story about a bank or federal agency having to announce the loss of hundreds of thousands of electronic records that contain confidential and potentially damaging information. Or, you may have received a notice from your bank that records have been compromised and that you will soon be receiving a new debit or credit card.

Imagine your embarrassment for a friend or colleague being interviewed in the practice's parking lot, explaining to a news reporter how the confidentiality of 500 or more medical records was compromised when he lost his tablet computer. It's bad enough to have lost the tablet, but even worse to admit the potential privacy threat to the media while also posting the infraction on your Web site; then sending a letter to patients; and reporting the breach to HHS and having it publicly posted on the OCR web site. Fortunately, there's a safe harbor built into the new HIPAA regulations discussed in the Security chapter of this book, and the key to the safe harbor is encryption software that *secures* protected health information.

In an effort to fast-track health information technology (health IT) adoption, HIPAA experienced two significant changes; the first relates to

1. "Final Breach Notification Rule for Electronic Health Information" news release, August 17, 2009. Available at: www.ftc.gov/opa/2009/08/hbn.shtm.

2. Department of Health and Human Services, Office of the Secretary, 45 CFR Parts 160 and 164, Breach Notification for Unsecured Protected Health Information; Interim Final Rule, Federal Register, v.74, n.162, August 24, 2009, pp. 42739–42770.

HIPAA transactions and code sets, the second provides reimbursement incentives to providers that implement health IT.

1. HIPAA transactions will be modified from Version 4010 to Version 5010 (compliance by Covered Entities on January 1, 2012), and a code set from ICD-9 to ICD-10 (compliance by Covered Entities on October 1, 2013).
2. The Health Information Technology for Economic and Clinical Health Act (HITECH Act) provisions were enacted as part the American Recovery and Reinvestment Act of 2009 (ARRA)[3]—the "stimulus bill." Health care providers that file Medicare claims are eligible to receive $44,000 per provider[4] if they meet eligibility criteria. Providers that file Medicaid claims are eligible to receive up to 85 percent of $75,000 eligible expenses.[5]

The transition to health IT comes with updated privacy and security responsibilities. These enhanced privacy and security measures apply to all covered entities, regardless of whether an "eligible professional" as a covered entity applies for and/or receives reimbursement funds made available through ARRA's HITECH Act.[6]

We discuss privacy and security updates in Chapter 1, which provides an overview of HIPAA, HITECH Act, and Breach Notification requirements. These updates provide details on:

- The new Breach Notification Rule, the enforcement of which began on February 22, 2010, for breaches occurring on or after that date;
- Significantly higher civil fines for violations of HIPAA standards on or after February 18, 2009; and

---

3. ARRA is available online at: www.ignet.gov/pande/leg/PL1115.pdf. The HITECH Act is comprised of two titles in ARRA: Title XIII (Health Information Technology) in Division A (Appropriations Provisions), pages 226–279; and Title IV (Medicare and Medicaid Health Information Technology; Miscellaneous Medicare Provisions) in Division B (Tax, Unemployment, Health, State Fiscal Relief, and Other Provisions), pages 467–496. Further references to the HITECH Act in this book are in the format: *HITECH Act* <page(s)>. For example, privacy is discussed in Subtitle D of Title XIII: *HITECH Act* 258–279.
4. On June 21, 2010, the Centers for Medicare & Medicaid Services (CMS) launched the official Web site for the Medicare & Medicaid EHR incentive programs. This Web site has the most up-to-date information about those programs, and can be accessed at www.cms.gov/EHRIncentivePrograms. We recommend that you visit this site often in 2010 for updated information on the Medicare & Medicaid EHR incentive programs that are scheduled to begin in January 2011. The final rules for the EHR Incentive and Certification Criteria were published in the Federal Register on July 28, 2010, with references appearing in Table 1.1 in Chapter 1.
5. Ibid.
6. We discuss these privacy and security obligations throughout this book.

- Statutory compliance by Business Associates with standards and implementation specifications of the Security Rule, beginning February 17, 2010.[7]

In addition, in Chapter 1, we outline a summary of a final breach notification rule under review at the Office of Management and Budget (OMB) as this book goes to press. Readers should pay particular attention to this final rule when it is published in the *Federal Register*.

In Chapter 2, we discuss the requirements for the transition from transaction Version 4010 to Version 5010, and the code set from ICD-9 to ICD-10. In addition, we outline statutory financial and administrative simplification standards provisions of the Patient Protection and Affordable Care Act (H.R. 3590), which President Obama signed into law on March 23, 2010, as Public Law 111–148.

In Chapter 3, we provide updates to HIPAA's Privacy Rule, which has required compliance since April 14, 2003, and forever changed the way health care providers create, use, store, transmit, and otherwise disclose protected health information (PHI).

Today, the Privacy Rule is one of several rules that sets the stage for electronic exchange of confidential health information and reimbursement, including new enforcement activities that increase reporting requirements and penalties.

Chapter 4 discusses HIPAA's Security Rule and the April 24, 2009, *Guidance Specifying Technologies and Methodologies that Render Protected Health Information Unusable, Unreadable, or Indecipherable to Unauthorized Individuals* that was included in the August 24, 2009 Breach Notification Interim Final Rule.

Early and mid-term adopters of health IT have demonstrated the transition and provided current adopters with a roadmap that also builds on early regulations. Today, 48 states report that they have successfully and securely exchanged health information between providers, payers, and patients and put at least one formal health information exchange in place.[8]

This second edition and updated *HIPAA Plain and Simple: A Health Care Professionals Guide* to Achieve HIPAA and HITECH Compliance is designed to uncomplicate "HIPAA heavy." It is not "HIPAA light" but rather "HIPAA easy to understand."

---

7. On July 14, 2010, HHS published in the Federal Register a Notice of Proposed Rulemaking (NPRM) related to "modifications to the HIPAA Privacy, Security, and Enforcement Rules under the [HITECH Act], which includes new privacy and security obligations of business associates." The references to the NPRM appear in Table 1.1 and are summarized in Chapter 1.

8. See eHealth Initiative, "National Forum on Health Information Exchange Presentation," July 22, 2010, Washington, DC. Available at: www.ehealthinitiative.org/uploads/file/2010_HIE_Forum_Presentations.pdf.

It is your reference tool when the legal dossier seems a little over the top. HIPAA and the HITECH Act require a certain levels of legal and documentation accuracy, so we didn't substitute a simplified approach for necessary legal advice. The practice's management team should be consulting a health-law attorney to implement HIPAA with or without the plain and simple advice in this book.

This book is for nurses who spend the majority of their time in clinical and personal patient interaction—and are likely to field privacy and security questions for the physician. It's also for the vulnerable receptionist and scheduler—workforce members frequently confronted by patients with near-impossible questions even as they keep the office running smoothly.

To the billing and insurance specialists—hats off for staying current with the new transactions and code sets. You are desperately needed to guide the practice through the detailed workflow redesigns and data capture as we transition from ICD-9 to ICD-10 and from 4010 to 5010.

Business associates must now comply with the HIPAA Security Rule, Breach Notification Rule, and portions of the Privacy Rule; so an amendment to your existing business associate agreement or execution of an updated agreement reflecting new statutory privacy, security, and breach notification obligations may be required to protect you.

HIPAA Plain and Simple, second edition, also is designed for people taking on new responsibilities within the medical practice and new workforce members as they join the practice. Physicians and office managers may use this book as a resource as they integrate complicated HIPAA and HITECH Act strategies. Most importantly, you do not have to go hunting through copies of the *Federal Register* or the *Code of Federal Regulations*, but we tell you where in those documents you can find additional information if you are of a mind to do so.

You have been on our minds throughout the entire development process. In writing this book, we spoke with many of our friends and business colleagues, who like you, are in the trenches making HIPAA happen. We've guided health care providers through the risk analysis, security implementation process, and transition to electronic health record software and supported them when a problem arose.

Each chapter contains **What to do** and **How to do it** directions. The book is chock-full of checklists, charts, quick reference guides, time lines, training plans, and communications plans to make HIPAA easier for you to understand.

In each chapter, you'll find **Critical Points**, in which we highlight the key learning point(s) in that discussion.

Finally, with the help of a dynamic team of publisher, editors, and marketers, we fully engaged in the earlier "HIPAA heavy" products so that we could confidently bring you this plain and simple version. We are better authors for knowing the professionals at AMA, and we're sure you'll find that they had you in mind when publishing this valuable addition to your compliance library.

Warmest wishes as you continue your HIPAA journey. We hope you'll let us know how you're doing.

Carolyn Hartley
Ed Jones

chapter 1

HIPAA, HITECH, and Breach Notification Overview

In the early 1990s, health care leaders came to then Secretary of Health and Human Services (HHS), Louis W. Sullivan, MD, and asked for help to simplify the health care industry's complex and costly administrative mess. The biggest problem at the time was that the administrative process to manage health information, including the billing and claims process, had become out-of-sync with the clinical process and burdensome to health care practitioners. For example, let's say a Blue Cross/Blue Shield (BCBS) health plan indicated that it would pay for a physician to conduct chest percussion therapy on a 60-year-old male patient, but to get paid for the treatment, the physician would need to use a special procedure number that only BCBS recognized. Those numbers were called *local codes*. But if the physician ordered the same procedure for a CIGNA patient, the physician would need to search for the CIGNA number because the BCBS local code would not apply. If you multiply this example by the number of payers, then by the number of diagnoses and procedures, and again by the number of physicians, you definitely have a complex and administrative mess.

Physicians wanted to provide care to patients and get paid for the service, but they faced a language barrier in that few payers spoke the same language of conducting business. Language barriers in an industry where national health expenditure in 1990 was $714.1 billion, or 12.3% of gross domestic product (GDP), and today is $2.34 trillion (2008 data), or 16.2% of GDP,[1] can create significant inefficiencies, processing errors, and large administrative costs. The result: wasted time and effort; repeated filings, denied claims; payment collection debates between payers, providers, and

1. Hartman, M, et al. "Health spending growth at a historic low in 2008." *Health Affairs*. January 2010, 29:1, p. 148.

patients; distrust and anxiety; confusion over the status of claims; excessive postage; and overall heartache.

At that meeting of the minds with Dr Sullivan, health care leaders expressed their exasperation with the clumsy fragmented system, and nearly everyone agreed that the administrative management process needed a major overhaul. Leaders also agreed that the health care industry couldn't come to an agreement on standard language formats by itself; rather, it needed a regulatory body to unravel proprietary, state, and federal codes, and, as we shall see, this is very much a work in progress nearly 20 years later in mid-2010.

Dr Sullivan assigned the following four agencies and organizations to work together and come to an agreement on how to simplify the administrative process:

- The National Committee on Vital and Health Statistics (NCVHS)
- Centers for Disease Control and Prevention (CDC)
- National Institutes of Health (NIH)
- Workgroup for Electronic Data Interchange (WEDI)[2].

The specific challenge to WEDI, a collaboration of government and private industry, was to find a way to decrease administrative costs, eliminate software adaptations for multiple formats, agree on one standard for sending and receiving electronic data, and still allow room for electronic commerce to flourish in the health care industry—a huge undertaking!

To begin, WEDI examined the effect of electronic technology in minimizing administrative costs of health care transactions. WEDI's findings, published in a 1993 report,[3] indicated that the savings from using electronic technology to process health care transactions would be substantial. This report became the foundation of the Administrative Simplification provisions in the Health Insurance Portability and Accountability Act of 1996 (HIPAA), which President Clinton signed on August 21, 1996.[4]

The word *portability* in the title of the law represented the part of the law that guaranteed that an employee could obtain health insurance if he or she changed jobs. The word *accountability* in the title of the law began

2. Today, WEDI is a vibrant organization of more than 300 members that continues to work through these issues to further adoption of electronic technology. You can find the organization online at www.wedi.org.

3. WEDI's 1993 report. Available at: www.wedi.org/public/articles/Full1993report.doc.

4. When we refer to HIPAA in this book, we are referring to the relatively short 14-page Subtitle F—Administrative Simplification, of Title II Of Public Law 104-191, enacted on August 21, 1996, which is available online in portable document format (pdf) at www.hhs.gov/ocr/privacy/hipaa/administrative/statute/hipaastatutepdf.pdf.

FIGURE 1.1

Structure of Administrative Simplification

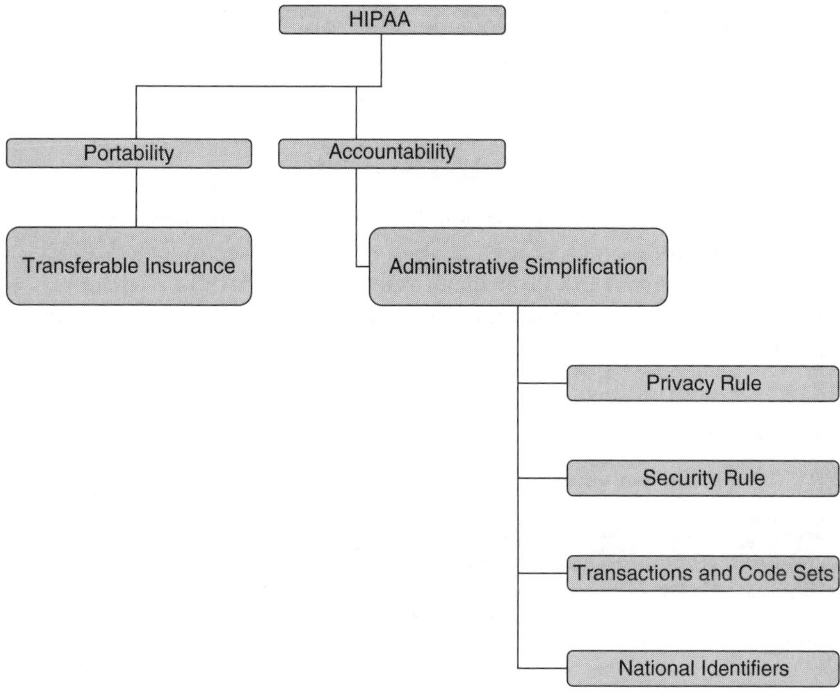

to identify *who*, *what*, *when*, and *how* for specific health care activities and assigned specific job roles for accountability for compliance. One part of accountability is Administrative Simplification, which was designed to address the messy administrative systems in health care. Figure 1.1 gives you a quick overview of the Structure of Administrative Simplification and how it fits into the HIPAA statute. Our focus in this book is on the Transactions and Code Sets (Chapter 2), Privacy Rule (Chapter 3), and Security Rule (Chapter 4). We will briefly outline National Identifiers later in this chapter.

The overall objectives of HIPAA Administrative Simplification are to:

- Improve efficiency and effectiveness of the health care system via electronic exchange of administrative and financial information
- Protect the security and privacy of transmitted and stored administrative and financial information
- Reduce high transaction costs in health care, which include, but are not limited to:
  - Paper-based transaction systems
  - Multiple, nonstandard health care data formats
  - Misuse of, errors related to, and loss of health care records.

Reduced to these objectives, HIPAA Administrative Simplification appears manageable; that is, simplify transactions so that all entities filing electronic transactions use the same set of codes, and keep patient information safe and secure while doing it. Easier said than done, as the past 14 years since the enactment of HIPAA Administrative Simplification have shown.[5]

BUILDING THE INFRASTRUCTURE

The procedural mechanisms for building the HIPAA Administrative Simplification infrastructure are enabling regulations promulgated under the federal Administrative Procedures Act. Table 1.1 provides a HIPAA Administrative Simplification Timeline of the status of enabling regulations through mid-June 2010.

TABLE 1.1

HIPAA Administrative Simplification Timeline

HIPAA Administrative Simplification Rule	Status	Federal Register Publication Date	Compliance Date for Covered Entities	Compliance Date: Other, If Applicable
Transactions and Code Sets	Final	August 17, 2000[i]; Modifications: February 20, 2003[ii]	October 16, 2003	N/A
Privacy	Final	December 28, 2000[iii]; Modifications: August 14, 2002[iv]	April 14, 2003	April 14, 2004 (Small Health Plans)
National Employer Identifier	Final	May 31, 2002[v]	July 30, 2004	August 1, 2005 (Small Health Plans)
Security	Final	February 20, 2003[vi]	April 20, 2005	April 20, 2006 (Small Health Plans); February 17, 2010 (Business Associates of Covered Entities)

5. Please see the discussion in Chapter 2 about enhanced objectives and new provisions regarding administrative simplification that were included in the Patient Protection and Affordable Care Act, enacted on March 23, 2010, as Public Law 111-148 (H.R. 3590).

TABLE 1.1 (continued)

HIPAA Administrative Simplification Timeline

HIPAA Administrative Simplification Rule	Status	Federal Register Publication Date	Compliance Date for Covered Entities	Compliance Date: Other, If Applicable
National Provider Identifier	Final	January 23, 2004[vii]	May 23, 2007	May 23, 2008 (Small Health Plans)
Claim Attachment	Notice of Proposed Rule-making	September 23, 2005[viii]		Withdrawn, January 25, 2010[ix]
Enforcement	Final	February 16, 2006[x]	March 16, 2006	N/A
Modification to Transactions and Code Sets: Version 5010	Final	January 16, 2009[xi]	January 1, 2012	January 1, 2013 (Only for new Medicaid Pharmacy Subrogation Standard Transaction)
Modification to Transactions and Code Sets: ICD-10	Final	January 16, 2009[xii]	October 1, 2013	N/A
HHS Secretary's Delegation of Authority to HHS's Office of Civil Rights (OCR) to Enforce HIPAA Security Rule	Notice	August 4, 2009[xiii]	July 27, 2009	N/A
Breach Notification for Unsecured Protected Health Information	Interim Final Rule	August 24, 2009[xiv]	September 23, 2009 (Effective date for breaches of protected health information occurring on or after this date, with enforcement commencing for breaches occurring on or after February 22, 2010)	N/A

(continued)

TABLE 1.1 (continued)

HIPAA Administrative Simplification Timeline

HIPAA Administrative Simplification Rule	Status	Federal Register Publication Date	Compliance Date for Covered Entities	Compliance Date: Other, If Applicable
Enforcement	Interim Final Rule	October 30, 2009[xv]	November 30, 2009 (Effective date for violations occurring on or after February 18, 2009)	N/A
Modifications to the HIPAA Privacy, Security, and Enforcement Rules Under the [HITECH Act] National Plan Identifier	Notice of Proposed Rule-making Under Develop-ment[xvii]	July 14, 2010[xvi]		Comments to HHS on or before September 13, 2010
National Individual Identifier	Congress-ional Hold on Develop-ment			

[i]HHS, Office of the Secretary, "45 CFR Parts 160 and 162—Health Insurance Reform: Standards for Electronic Transactions; Final Rule," *Federal Register*, v.65, n.160, August 17, 2000, pp. 50311–50372. Available at: www.cms.hhs.gov/TransactionCodeSetsStands/Downloads/txfinal.pdf; and "45 CFR Parts 160 and 162—Health Insurance Reform: Standards for Electronic Transactions; Corrections," *Federal Register*, v.65, n.227, November 24, 2000, p. 70507. Available at: www.cms.hhs.gov/TransactionCodeSetsStands/Downloads/StandardsForElectronicTransactions-Corrections.pdf.

[ii]HHS, Office of the Secretary, "45 CFR Part 162—Health Insurance Reform: Modifications to Electronic Data Transaction Standards and Code Sets; Final Rule," *Federal Register*, v.68, n.34, February 20, 2003, pp. 8381–8399. Available at: http://edocket.access.gpo.gov/2003/pdf/03-3876.pdf.

[iii]HHS, Office of the Secretary, "45 CFR Parts 160 and 164—Standards for Privacy of Individually Identifiable Health Information; Final Rule," *Federal Register*, v.65, n.250, December 28, 2000, pp. 82461–82829. Available at: www.hhs.gov/ocr/privacy/hipaa/administrative/privacyrule/prdecember2000all8parts.pdf.

[iv]HHS, Office of the Secretary, "45 CFR Parts 160 and 164—Standards for Privacy of Individually Identifiable Health Information; Final Rule," *Federal Register*, v.67, n.157, August 14, 2002, pp. 53181–53273. Available at: www.hhs.gov/ocr/privacy/hipaa/administrative/privacyrule/privrulepd.pdf.

[v]HHS, Office of the Secretary, "45 CFR Parts 160 and 162—Health Insurance Reform: Standard Unique Employer Identifier; Final Rule," *Federal Register*, v.67, n.105, May 31, 2002, pp. 38009–38020. Available at: www.cms.hhs.gov/EmployerIdentifierStand/Downloads/emplDfinal.pdf.

[vi]HHS, Office of the Secretary, "45 CFR Parts 160, 162, and 164—Health Insurance Reform: Security Standards; Final Rule," *Federal Register*, v.68, n.34, February 20, 2003, pp. 8333–8381. Available at: www.cms.hhs.gov/SecurityStandard/Downloads/securityfinalrule.pdf.

[vii]HHS, Office of the Secretary, "45 CFR Part 162—HIPAA Administrative Simplification: Standard Unique Health Identifier for Health Care Providers; Final Rule," *Federal Register*, v.69, n.15, January 23, 2004, pp. 3433–3469. Available at: www.cms.hhs.gov/NationalProvIdentStand/Downloads/NPIfinalrule.pdf.

As we go through the chapters of this book, we shall explore the content of these enabling regulations. Note in the table that it was almost 7 years after enactment of HIPAA Administrative Simplification, in April 2003, that the first standard requiring health care industry compliance—privacy—was in place. The Administrative Procedures Act is a relatively slow process, and the health care industry is complex. Yet, as we pass the 14th anniversary of enactment of HIPAA Administrative Simplification, we are still wrestling with proposals for and implementation of HIPAA Administrative Simplification standards, well beyond the timeframes for implementation that Congress envisioned. Given rapid change in electronic technologies—the growth of Internet sourcing of information and as a vehicle for transactions, and the increasing switch of financial transactions from cash and check to debit and credit cards and online payments—since the enactment of HIPAA Administrative Simplification, can relatively slow federal initiative processes

---

(continued)

[viii]HHS, Office of the Secretary, "45 CFR Part 162—HIPAA Administrative Simplification: Standards for Electronic Health Care Claims Attachments; Proposed Rule," *Federal Register*, v.70, n.184, September 23, 2005, pp. 55989–56025. Available at: http://edocket.access.gpo.gov/2005/pdf/05-18927.pdf.

[ix]HHS, Office of the Secretary, "Semiannual Regulatory Agenda," *Federal Register*, v.75, n.79, April 26, 2010, p. 21804. Available at: http://frwebgate.access.gpo.gov/cgi-bin/getdoc.cgi?dbname=2010_unified_agenda_&docid=f:ua100407.pdf. Please see the discussion in Chapter 2 about administrative simplification provisions of the Patient Protection and Affordable Care Act, which was enacted on March 23, 2010, for the new statutory adoption date deadline of January 1, 2014, and effective date deadline of January 1, 2016, for *health claims attachment standard*.

[x]HHS, Office of the Secretary, "45 CFR Parts 160 and 164—HIPAA Administrative Simplification: Enforcement; Final Rule," *Federal Register*, v.71, n.32, February 16, 2006, pp. 8389–8433. Available at: www.hhs.gov/ocr/privacy/hipaa/administrative/privacyrule/finalenforcementrule06.pdf.

[xi]HHS, Office of the Secretary, "45 CFR Part 162—Health Insurance Reform; Modifications to the Health Insurance Portability and Accountability Act (HIPAA); Final Rules," *Federal Register*, v.74, n.11, January 16, 2009, pp. 3295–3328. Available at: http://edocket.access.gpo.gov/2009/pdf/E9-740.pdf.

[xii]HHS, Office of the Secretary, "45 CFR Part 162—HIPAA Administrative Simplification: Modifications to Medical Data Code Set Standards to Adopt ICD-10-CM and ICD-10-PCS; Final Rule," *Federal Register*, v.74, n.11, January 16, 2009, pp. 3328–3362. Available at: http://edocket.access.gpo.gov/2009/pdf/E9-743.pdf.

[xiii]HHS, Office of the Secretary, "Office for Civil Rights; Delegation of Authority: Notice," *Federal Register*, v.74, n.148, August 4, 2009, p. 38630.

[xiv]HHS, Office of the Secretary, "45 CFR Parts 160 and 164—Breach Notification for Unsecured Protected Health Information; Interim Final Rule," *Federal Register*, v.74, n.162, pp. 42739–42770. Available at: http://edocket.access.gpo.gov/2009/pdf/E9-20169.pdf.

[xv]HHS, Office of the Secretary, "45 CFR Part 160—HIPAA Administrative Simplification: Enforcement; Interim Final Rule," *Federal Register*, v.74, n.209, October 30, 2009, pp. 56123–56131. Available at: http://edocket.access.gpo.gov/2009/pdf/E9-26203.pdf.

[xvi]HHS, Office of the Secretary, "45 CFR Parts 160 and 164: Modifications to the HIPAA Privacy, Security, and Enforcement Rules Under the Health Information Technology for Economic and Clinical Health Act; Proposed Rule," Federal Register, v.75, n.134, July 14, 2010, pp. 40867–40924. Available at: http://edocket.access.gpo.gov/2010/pdf/2010-16718.pdf.

[xvii]Please see the discussion in Chapter 2 about administrative simplification provisions of the Patient Protection and Affordable Care Act, which was enacted on March 23, 2010, for the new statutory effective date deadline of October 1, 2012, for *the unique health plan identifier*.

keep up with market developments, or do they impede them?[6] You be the judge as we explore HIPAA Administrative Simplification standards and their implementation specifications as we go through the book.

FOUR SETS OF STANDARDS[7]

In this section, we outline the characteristics of each of the four sets of standards: transactions and code sets, privacy, security, and identifiers.

Transactions and Code Sets

The Transaction and Code Sets (TCS) Rule required compliance on October 16, 2003, by covered entities: health plans, health care clearinghouses, and health care providers. A modified version of the transaction standards—from ASC X12[8] Version 4010 to 5010—will require compliance on January 1, 2012. See Appendix C for additional resources and information on TCS from the AMA.

A *transaction* refers to the electronic transmission of information between two parties to carry out financial or administrative activities. *Code sets* are data sets that identify diagnoses, treatment procedures, drug codes, equipment codes, financial codes, location codes, and other codes necessary to effect a transaction by identifying a value that will populate a specified data element in a transaction. The change in code set—from ICD-9 to ICD-10—will require compliance on October 1, 2013.

We identify and discuss transaction standards and code sets in detail in Chapter 2.

The importance of codes to the physician practice is this: when the diagnostics match a complicated set of health plan payer-approved procedure codes, then the payers understand how the provider intends to

---

6. Since passage of the HITECH Act, enacted on February 17, 2009, as part of the American Recovery and Reinvestment Act—the "stimulus bill"—the federal government has relied more on Interim Final Rules in an effort to enable privacy and security provisions of the HITECH Act more quickly than the typical Notice of Proposed Rulemaking and Final Rule procedures of the federal Administrative Procedures Act.

7. A standard is a requirement, and a rule is a document that includes the standards in the context of HIPAA Administrative Simplification.

8. ASC X12 means Accredited Standards Committee X12. The ASC X12N Insurance Subcommittee prepared documentation on the transaction standards. We identify the documentation currently in use (Version 4010/4010A1 Implementation Guides) and the documentation that is required for transaction standards compliance on January 1, 2012 (Version 5010 Technical Reports Type 3), in Chapter 2. Washington Publishing Company (WPC) is the source of each type of documentation and can be accessed at www.wpc-edi.com.

treat the patient, and payers reimburse the provider for services rendered. If the codes are accurate and properly inserted as data element values in a transaction, then appropriate claim information moves from the provider to the payer and cash moves from the payer to the provider with few interruptions or disruptions.

In past decades, a very complicated network of billing and software companies was retained by physician practices to facilitate payment on claims. Prior to the promulgation of the HIPAA Administrative Simplification transaction rules, most of the companies used different formats, which sometimes made it difficult for payers to understand the connection between treatment and payment. Also, each payer required different information about the treatment or the individual. The result was a proliferation of nonstandard transaction formats and data-content requirements that complicated and slowed the claim-reimbursement process. Each side blamed the other for these complications, but one thing was certain: everyone was unhappy with the process, including the patient. So HHS, through HIPAA, said: health plan payers, health care providers, and health care clearinghouses—HIPAA's covered entities—must send or receive transactions using standard formats and data content.

As you will see in Chapter 2, use of situational variables and companion guides continues to frustrate the transaction process, but, we hope, the ASC X12 Version 5010 of the standards, which requires compliance by January 1, 2012, and addresses those uses, will help to expedite the transaction process.

Achieving agreement on standards formats for electronic transactions is a challenge, but the standards development process allows all parties—vendors, payers, providers, clearinghouses, and government—to come together to make their business cases for what should be reflected in the standards. Each of the parties has an opportunity to identify information that it needs to complete a transaction. Then, the parties as a group negotiate a common set of requirements that they would use to transact business. That process is ongoing because the parties continue to meet to discuss new or revised data requirements in response to innovations in technologies that may further improve business processing in the health care industry.

CRITICAL POINT

Your practice must ensure that your software vendor as a business associate can send and receive electronic health care (EHR) information using required transaction standard data formats and data content.

HIPAA provides for a designated standard-maintenance organization (DSMO)[9] process to handle industry recommended modifications to the standards that may enhance Administrative Simplification. Health care

9. To learn more about the DSMO process, visit www.hipaa-dsmo.org/.

stakeholders have expended considerable resources of time and money not only in the development of standards, but also in the implementation process, including the capability of testing transactions amongst trading partners. While health plan payers and health care providers use the electronic transactions process as a business tool, ultimately it is the responsibility of their system vendors and health care clearinghouses to make the process as seamless as possible. You also will see in Chapter 2, in the discussion of the background relating to ASC X12 Version 5010 and in the new administrative simplification provisions of the Patient Protection and Affordable Care Act, that the *adoption and implementation* of the transactions standards is still very much a work in progress.

Privacy Standards

The US Department of Health and Human Services (HHS) recognized that if it required covered entities to use a standard set of formats and data content to transmit files electronically, consumers would expect their medical files to be kept confidential. That is why HHS also developed standards that protect patients' rights, including unauthorized use and disclosure of their health information. The HIPAA Privacy Rule has garnered considerable attention because it is nontechnical—mainly policies and procedures—and is an important issue to users of the health care system. Compliance with the Privacy Rule was required on April 14, 2003, with small health plans having an additional year to comply.

Table 1.2 outlines the HIPAA Privacy Rule standards, which cover requirements related to protected health information (PHI): use and disclosure, notice of privacy practices, access, restrictions, amendment, accounting, and administrative safeguards. Later in this chapter and in Chapter 3, we cover these requirements, as well as how HITECH Act provisions related to breach notification and marketing are affecting HIPAA Privacy in mid-year 2010.

TABLE 1.2

HIPAA Privacy Rule Standards

Subpart E—Privacy of Individually Identifiable Health Information
164.502 Uses and disclosures of protected health information: General rules
Standard: A covered entity may not use or disclose PHI, except as permitted or required.
Permitted uses and disclosures
Required disclosures
Standard: Minimum necessary
Standard: Uses and disclosures of protected health information subject to an agreed upon restriction
Standard: Uses and disclosures of de-identified PHI
Standard: Disclosures to business associates

TABLE 1.2 (continued)

HIPAA Privacy Rule Standards

Standard: Deceased individuals

Standard: Personal representatives

Standard: Confidential communications

Standard: Uses and disclosures consistent with notice

Standard: Disclosures by whistleblowers and workforce member crime victims

164.504 Uses and disclosures: Organizational requirements

Standard: Business associate contracts

Standard: Requirements for group health plans

Standard: Requirements for a covered entity with multiple covered functions

164.506 Uses and disclosures to carry out treatment, payment, or health care operations

Standard: Permitted uses and disclosures

Standard: Consent for uses and disclosures permitted

164.508 Uses and disclosures for which an authorization is required

Standard: Authorizations for uses and disclosures

164.510 Uses and disclosures requiring an opportunity for the individual to agree or to object

Standard: Use and disclosure for facility directories

Standard: Uses and disclosures for involvement in the individual's care and notification purposes

164.512 Uses and disclosures for which an authorization or opportunity to agree or object is not required

Standard: Uses and disclosures for which an authorization or opportunity to agree or object is not required

Standard: Uses and disclosures for public health activities

Standard: Disclosures about victims of abuse, neglect or domestic violence

Standard: Uses and disclosures for health oversight activities

Standard: Disclosures for judicial and administrative proceedings

Standard: Disclosures for law enforcement purposes

Standard: Uses and disclosures about decedents

Standard: Uses and disclosures for cadaveric organ, eye or tissue donation purposes

Standard: Uses and disclosures for research purposes

Standard: Uses and disclosures to avert a serious threat to health or safety

Standard: Uses and disclosures for specialized government functions

Standard: Disclosures for workers' compensation

164.514 Other requirements relating to uses and disclosures of protected health information

Standard: De-identification of protected health information

Standard: Minimum necessary requirements

Standard: Limited data set

Standard: Uses and disclosures for fundraising

(continued)

TABLE 1.2 (continued)

HIPAA Privacy Rule Standards

Standard: Uses and disclosures for underwriting and related purposes

Standard: Verification requirements

164.520 Notice of privacy practices for protected health information

Standard: Notice of privacy practices

164.522 Rights to request privacy protection for protected health information

Standard: Right of an individual to request restriction of uses and disclosures

Standard: Confidential communications requirements

164.524 Access of individuals to protected health information

Standard: Access to PHI

164.526 Amendment of protected health information

Standard: Right to amend

164.528 Accounting of disclosures of protected health information

Standard: Right to an accounting of disclosures of PHI

164.530 Administrative requirements

Standard: Personnel designations

Standard: Training

Standard: Safeguards

Standard: Complaints to the covered entity

Standard: Sanctions

Standard: Mitigation

Standard: Refraining from intimidating or retaliatory acts

Standard: Waiver of rights

Standard: Policies and procedures

Standard: Changes to policies and procedures

Standard: Documentation

Standard: Group health plans

The Privacy Rule requires that you change some of your day-to-day tasks so that information used to identify a patient is protected and that this PHI is safeguarded to prevent unauthorized use or disclosure. PHI is information that is in use during creation, retrieval, revision, or deletion; at rest in a database; in motion during a transmission; and in oral, hard copy, or electronic form.

Security Standards

Security standards go hand in hand with privacy standards. The Security Rule is about controlling access to electronic protected health information (ePHI) only, while the Privacy Rule, as just indicated above, covers oral, hard copy, and ePHI.

CRITICAL POINT

Security is about controlling access to ePHI. Privacy is about controlling how oral, hard copy, and ePHI is used and disclosed.

The Security Rule required compliance by covered entities on April 20, 2005, with small health plans having an additional year to comply. Under the HITECH Act, discussed later in this chapter, business associates of covered entities were required by statute to comply with the Security Rule on February 17, 2010, and business associate agreements between a covered entity and its business associates had to be updated or amended to incorporate that compliance specifically, in addition to the other satisfactory assurances that the business associate agrees to about safeguarding the covered entity's ePHI.

In Chapter 4, we examine each of the security standards and implementation specifications in detail. It is important to note the 10 key attributes of the Security Rule. Each workforce member in your practice should have a working knowledge of these attributes because they are key components of your policies, procedures, actions, and assessments that will underpin your practice's security strategy and successful compliance efforts.

1. The Security Rule is a set of standards and implementation specifications that your practice, as a covered entity, must comply with by federal law.
2. The Security Rule standards are always required for compliance by your practice, while implementation specifications can be either *required* or *addressable.*
3. The Security Rule is scalable, ie, taking into consideration the size of your practice, and flexible, ie, taking into consideration the structure of the practice, costs of security measures, and probability and criticality of potential risks (threats and vulnerabilities).
4. The Security Rule is reasonable and permits your practice to implement security safeguards that are appropriate.
5. The Security Rule is built on key principles of availability, confidentiality, and integrity of patients' health information.
6. The Security Rule is technology neutral, with one exception,[10] ie, the choice of protection measures (inputs) is up to your practice, as long as the safeguard performance measures (outputs) are achieved.

---

10. The one exception is, if your practice chooses to secure its electronic protected health information (ePHI) through encryption, that it must use the encryption technologies and methodologies specified in the Guidance issued by HHS in the August 24, 2009, Interim Final Rule pertaining to Breach Notification published in the *Federal Register*. We discuss this further later in this chapter and, with respect to two Technical Safeguard encryption implementation specifications, in Chapter 4.

7. The Security Rule is based on risk analysis and mitigation of risk, ie, identifying potential vulnerabilities in and threats to the practice, and taking risk avoidance measures.
8. The Security Rule is built on a foundation of safeguarding ePHI, so maintaining the availability of electricity is a key factor.
9. The Security Rule formalizes many of the policies, procedures, actions, assessments, and documentation requirements that you likely use in your practice today.
10. The Security Rule is an investment in the future of your practice, ie, as a successful business.

Identifiers

Four identifiers are specified as HIPAA Administrative Simplification standards:

- The National Employer Identifier[11]
  - Compliance required July 30, 2004.[12]
- The National Provider Identifier[13]
  - Compliance required May 23, 2007.[14]
- The National Health Plan Identifier
  - Under development[15]
- The National Individual Identifier
  - Congressional hold on development[16]

---

11. The Employer Identification Number (EIN), issued by the Internal Revenue Service (IRS), was selected as the identifier for employers.

12. Small health plans had an additional year to comply, on August 1, 2005.

13. The National Provider Identifier (NPI) is a unique identification number for covered health care providers. Covered health care providers and all health plans and health care clearinghouses must use NPIs in administrative and financial transactions adopted under HIPAA. The NPI is a 10-position, intelligence-free numeric identifier (10-digit number), meaning that NPI numbers do not carry other information about health care providers, such as states in which they live or their medical specialties. NPI must be used in lieu of legacy provider identifiers in the HIPAA standard transactions. Covered providers also must share their NPI with other providers, health plans, clearinghouses, and any entity that may need it for billing purposes.

14. Small health plans had an additional year to comply, on May 23, 2008.

15. Please see the discussion in Chapter 2 about administrative simplification provisions of the Patient Protection and Affordable Care Act, enacted on March 23, 2010, for the new statutory effective date deadline of October 1, 2012, for the *unique health plan identifier.*

16. The National Individual Identifier is controversial. Congress has a long-standing hold on any regulatory action on this identifier. Prior to enactment of HIPAA, the

Identifiers are numeric electronic addresses for participants in health care electronic exchange. To learn more about identifiers, visit the Centers for Medicare & Medicaid Services (CMS) web site at www.cms.hhs.gov.

CHANGE IN FOCUS: ADMINISTRATIVE TO CLINICAL PROCESSES

In the early part of the first decade of the 21st century, the federal government initiated a fundamental shift in how it implemented health care policy, especially as it related to adoption of electronic processes. Previously, the federal government's focus was on administrative processes, using the authority of HIPAA Administrative Simplification. Although the federal government continued with its efforts to implement Administrative Simplification standards under the Administrative Procedures Act, the process was slow. The federal government also began implementing electronic *clinical* standards using a different approach.

In December 2002, the Bush Administration began implementing the E-Gov initiative, following enactment of HR 2458, the E-Government Act of 2002.[17] In July 2003, then HHS Secretary Tommy Thompson announced two initiatives designed for "building a national electronic healthcare system that will allow patients and their doctors to assess their complete medical records anytime and anywhere they are needed ..."[18]

> First, the Secretary announced that the Department has signed an agreement with the College of American Pathologists (CAP) to license the College's standardized medical vocabulary system and make it available without charge throughout the U.S. This action opens the door to establishing a common medical language as a key element in building a unified electronic medical records system in the U.S.
>
> Secondly, the Secretary announced that HHS has commissioned the Institute of Medicine to design a standardized model of an electronic health record. The health care standards development organization known as HL7 has been asked to evaluate the model once it has been designed. HHS will share the standardized model record at no cost with all components of the U.S. health care system. The Department expects to have a model record ready in 2004.
>
> Today's announcements are part of the ongoing HHS effort to develop the National Health Information Infrastructure by encouraging and facilitating the

---

(continued)

de facto individual identifier had been the Social Security number—which is the source of controversy about requiring it as a standard. Since enactment of HIPAA, a number of states have restricted the use of the Social Security number as an identifier in matters other than Social Security, and large health plans have developed unique individual identifiers for their members as a workaround.

17. Visit the National Archives site for more information on this Act at www.archives.gov/about/laws/egov-act-section-207.html.

18. Department of Health and Human Services, "HHS Launches New Efforts to Promote Paperless Healthcare System," news release, Tuesday, July 1, 2003, which is available at: www.hhs.gov/news/press/2003pres/20030701.html.

widespread use of modern information technology to improve the nation's health care system.

Then, in May 2004, Secretary Thompson announced the appointment of David Brailer, MD, PhD, as the first National Health Information Technology Coordinator to coordinate and accelerate US "health information technology efforts."[19] David Brailer wrote a foreword to this edition of *HIPAA Plain and Simple*.

In July 2004, Secretary Thompson initiated "a 10-year plan [known as the Decade of Health Information Technology (HIT), 2004–2014] to build a national electronic health information infrastructure in the United States" and outlined "four major collaborative goals" and "12 strategies for advancing and focusing future efforts."[20] We have discussed in detail these efforts in two of our books, and will not elaborate further here.[21]

In August 2006, the federal government celebrated the 10th anniversary of enactment of HIPAA Administrative Simplification. The question then was: if HIPAA Administrative Simplification could not be accomplished within 10 years, how likely would it be that it could achieve the objectives relating to the Decade of HIT, ending in 2014?

While the federal government was emphasizing clinical initiatives, the standards groups and health care stakeholders were busy at work trying to solve a number of problems that impeded the smooth working of electronic transactions from a business perspective. We discuss these issues in the next chapter.

On August 22, 2008, HHS published two Notices of Proposed Rulemaking (NPRMs): one related to a change in version of the transaction standards, and the other related to a change in code set from ICD-9 to ICD-10. Four days before the end of its term, the Bush Administration published the final rules related to these changes in the *Federal Register*. We discuss both the NPRMs and the final rules in the next chapter.

THE HITECH ACT

President Obama signed into law the American Recovery and Reinvestment Act of 2009 (ARRA) on February 17, 2009. Included in the so-called "stimulus bill" was the Health Information Technology for Economic and Clinical

19. Department of Health and Human Services, "Secretary Thompson, Seeking Fastest Possible Results, Names First Health Information Technology Coordinator," news release, Thursday, May 6, 2004, which is available at www.hhs.gov/news/press/2004pres/20040506.html.

20. Department of Health and Human Services, "The Decade of Health Information Technology: Delivering Consumer-Centric and Information-Rich Healthcare," fact sheet, Wednesday, July 21, 2004. Available at www.hhs.gov/news.

21. See Hartley CP, Jones ED. *EHR Implementation: A Step-by-Step Guide for the Medical Practice*. Chicago, IL: AMA Press, 2005; and Hartley CP, Jones ED, ENs D, and Whitt D. *Technical and Financial Guide to EHR Implementation*. Chicago, IL: American Medical Association, 2007(R).

Health Act (HITECH Act). The HITECH Act comprises Title XIII (Health Information Technology of Division A of ARRA (pp. 226–278) and Title IV (Medicare and Medicaid Health Information Technology; Miscellaneous Medicare Provisions) of Division B of ARRA (pp. 467–496).[22]

The HITECH Act provisions of ARRA in Title XIII include important changes in Privacy (Subtitle D), two of which are discussed here: Application of Security Provisions and Penalties to Business Associates of Covered Entities (Section 13401 on page 260 of ARRA) and Notification in the Case of Breach (Section 13402 on pages 260–263). We close our discussion of the HITECH Act with an outline of the increased civil penalties for noncompliance with the provisions of HIPAA and *in effect* privacy and security provisions of the HITECH Act, and enforcement provisions relating to breach notification that commenced on February 22, 2010, for breaches that are discovered on or after that date.

Security Rule and Business Associates

Because of the importance of this new HITECH Act requirement that business associates of covered entities had to comply with the HIPAA Security Rule by February 17, 2010, we reproduce below the definition of business associate.[23] You will note that the definition focuses on the handling of individually identifiable health information and covers a number of functions that a practice may contract outside of its workforce.

Definition of a Business Associate

(1) Except as provided in paragraph (2) of this definition, business associate means, with respect to a covered entity, a person who:

  (i) On behalf of such covered entity or of an organized health care arrangement (as defined in Sec. 164.501 of this subchapter, Administrative Data Standards and Related Requirements) in which the covered entity participates, but other than in the capacity of a member of the workforce of such covered entity or arrangement, performs, or assists in the performance of:

    (A) A function or activity involving the use or disclosure of individually identifiable health information, including claims processing or administration, data analysis, processing or administration, utilization review, quality assurance, billing, benefit management, practice management, and repricing; or

    (B) Any other function or activity regulated by this subchapter; or

22. ARRA, as signed by President Obama, is available at: www.gpo.gov:80/fdsys/pkg/PLAW-111publ5/pdf/PLAW-111publ5.pdf.

23. 45 CFR 160.103. Available at: http://edocket.access.gpo.gov/cfr_2004/octqtr/pdf/45cfr160.103.pdf. CFR is Code of Federal Regulations.

(ii) Provides, other than in the capacity of a member of the workforce of such covered entity, legal, actuarial, accounting, consulting, data aggregation (as defined in Sec. 164.501 of this subchapter), management, administrative, accreditation, or financial services to or for such covered entity, or to or for an organized health care arrangement in which the covered entity participates, where the provision of the service involves the disclosure of individually identifiable health information from such covered entity or arrangement, or from another business associate of such covered entity or arrangement, to the person.

(2) A covered entity participating in an organized health care arrangement that performs a function or activity as described by paragraph (1)(i) of this definition for or on behalf of such organized health care arrangement, or that provides a service as described in paragraph (1)(ii) of this definition to or for such organized health care arrangement, does not, simply through the performance of such function or activity or the provision of such service, become a business associate of other covered entities participating in such organized health care arrangement.

(3) A covered entity may be a business associate of another covered entity.

By no later than February 17, 2010, business associates were required statutorily to implement HIPAA Administrative Simplification Security Rule administrative, physical, and technical safeguards, based on having conducted a risk analysis; developed and implemented related policies, procedures, actions, and assessment; and complied with written documentation and workforce training requirements. Compliance "shall apply to a business associate of a covered entity in the same manner that such sections apply to the covered entity. The additional requirements of this title that relate to security and that are made applicable with respect to covered entities shall also be applicable to such a business associate and shall be incorporated into the business associate agreement between the business associate and the covered entity."[24] The additional requirements include application of civil and criminal penalties in the same manner that a covered entity would be subject, notification provisions for a breach, and application of "guidance on the most effective and appropriate technical safeguards" as determined by the Secretary of HHS, amongst other requirements.

---

24. 13401 *HITECH Act* 146. The North Carolina Healthcare Information and Communications Alliance, Inc., (NCHICA) has prepared a sample Amended and Restated Business Associate Agreement, which captures additions to the business associate agreement that are required under the HITECH Act. Available at: www.nchica.org.

Please be advised that additional enabling regulations pertaining to business associates as a result of the HITECH Act are forthcoming and are discussed briefly at the end of this chapter.

Application of the Security Rule to business associates of covered entities is a significant compliance change. Previous to the change, if there were a breach involving a business associate of which the covered entity were aware, then the covered entity could just terminate the contract if the breach was not remedied. Responsibility and liability rested with the covered entity. Now, with the change in the HITECH Act privacy provisions, the business associate, as well as the covered entity, has responsibility and liability directly for a breach.

COSTS RELATED TO BREACH

We recommend that physician practices and their business associates read an April 2009 *Baseline Magazine* article by Corinne Bernstein entitled "The Cost of Data Breaches."[25] This article reports on a Ponemon Institute study of incidents and costs incurred at 43 organizations in 17 industry sectors. Here are several highlights from the article:

- "Lost business accounted for nearly 70 percent of a data breach in 2008.
- "[S]ectors suffering the highest customer losses were health care ... and financial services.
- "The biggest cause of breaches ... is insider negligence ... 88% of all cases in 2008.
- "The number of breaches involving third-party organizations continues to climb."

The article concludes with the following quotation:

> "Organizations are getting better at detecting breaches," says the institute's Larry Ponemon. "But to reduce the incidence of data breaches, they need to use better security technologies, such as encryption and identity access management, and they must provide more training to their employees."

A more recent article analyzing the 2009 Ponemon Institute's annual study indicates that "[t]he cost of a data breach increased last year [2009] to $204 per compromised customer record. ... In tallying the cost of a data breach, Ponemon Institute looks at several factors including: the cost of lost business because of an incident; legal fees; disclosure expenses related to customer contact and public response; consulting help; and remediation expenses such as technology and training."[26]

So, in addition to responsibility and liability, physician practices—and all other covered entities—and their business associates must safeguard

---

25. Available at: www.baselinemag.com/c/a/Security/The-Cost-of-Data-Breaches-380742/?kc=rss.

26. Messmer, Ellen. "Data breach costs top $200 per customer record," *NetworkWorld*, January 25, 2010. Available at: www.networkworld.com/news/2010/012510-data-breach-costs.html.

individually identifiable health information and train their workforce members to protect their businesses and avoid the costs of losing customers because of a breach. In short, as the aforementioned articles indicate, a data breach will cost affected organization big dollars, customer losses, and maybe the business as well, particularly when breaches are publicly disclosed.

The HITECH Act requires that discovered breaches affecting 500 or more individuals be immediately reported to the HHS Office for Civil Rights (OCR) and "the Secretary [of HHS] shall make available to the public on the Internet website of the Department of Health and Human Services a list that identifies each covered entity involved in a breach. ..."[27] As of July 21, 2010, 108 breaches that affected 4,087,580 individuals have been posted on the OCR web site at www.hhs.gov/ocr/privacy/hipaa/administrative/breachnotificationrule/postedbreaches.html. Eighteen of the 108 reported breaches or to just under 17% involved business associates of the reporting covered entities. Of the 101 breaches that have a specified type of breach (paper or electronic records), approximately 75% of the breaches involved electronic records in stationary, portable, or mobile electronic devices, and 25% involved paper records. Eighty-three percent of electronic breaches involved loss or theft of records, with the largest number of those cases involving loss or theft of portable electronic devices, particularly laptops. As we discuss below with respect to the August 24, 2009, *Guidance Specifying the Technologies and Methodologies that Render Protected Health Information Unusable, Unreadable, or Indecipherable to Unauthorized Individuals*, there are available technologies and methods for securing hard copy and/or electronic PHI, which will provide a safe harbor from breach notification requirements and avoid potential reputational, financial, and other costs associated with having to publicly report a breach due to loss, theft, or other misuse of PHI.

Breach Notification[28]

The HITECH Act provides a new definition of a breach,[29] as follows:

(1) Breach

(A) In General. The term 'breach' means the unauthorized acquisition, access, use, or disclosure of protected health information which compromises the security or privacy of such information, except where an unauthorized person to whom such information is disclosed would not reasonably have been able to retain such information.

27. 13402(e)(4) *HITECH Act* 262.

28. Additional information and updates on breach notification are available at www.hhs.gov/ocr/privacy/hipaa/administrative/breachnotificationrule/index.html.

29. 13400 *HITECH Act* 258.

(B) Exceptions. The term 'breach' does not include-

(i) Any unintentional acquisition, access, or use of protected health information by an employee or individual acting under the authority of a covered entity or business associate if-

(I) Such acquisition, access, or use was made in good faith and within the course and scope of the employment or other professional relationship of such employee or individual, respectively, with the covered entity or business associate; and

(II) Such information is not further acquired, accessed, used, or disclosed by any person; or

(ii) Any inadvertent disclosure from an individual who is otherwise authorized to access protected health information at a facility operated by a covered entity or business associate to another similarly situated individual at same facility; and

(iii) Any such information received as a result of such disclosure is not further acquired, accessed, used, or disclosed without authorization by any person.

A breach requires notification, which is triggered when there is an incident of "unauthorized acquisition, access, use, or disclosure of unsecured protected health information."[30] Notification must be accomplished "without unreasonable delay and in no case later than 60 calendar days after the discovery of a breach by the covered entity involved (or business associate involved in the case of a notification [to the covered entity following discovery of a breach]."[31]

HHS Secretary Kathleen Sebelius published the Interim Final Rule for Breach Notification for Unsecured Protected Health Information in the

---

30. See 13402 *HITECH Act* 260–263. We strongly recommend that your practice's security official know the provisions of this section thoroughly and that your workforce members are familiar with them through training. Of particular importance is the requirement in Section 13402 (b) on p. 260 that a business associate notify its covered entity of a breach of "unsecured protected health information."

31. 13402 *HITECH Act* 260. The notification provision requires covered entities to notify affected parties directly and individually in a timely manner and to use appropriate public media for cases involving more than 500 individuals. A business associate that discover a breach is required to provide the covered entity with "identification of each individual whose unsecured protected health information" is breached, so that the covered entity can notify each individual and comply with additional notification requirements, as applicable. These notification requirements were not defined under HIPAA Administrative Simplification. Increased penalties for a breach by a covered entity or business associate were effective with enactment of the HITECH Act, with enforcement begun on February 22, 2010, for breaches on or after that date.

Federal Register on August 24, 2009.[32] The effective date of the Interim Final Rule was September 23, 2009. Here is the Summary of the Interim Final Rule:

> The Department of Health and Human Services (HHS) is issuing this interim final rule with a request for comments to require notification of breaches of unsecured protected health information. Section 13402 of the Health Information Technology for Economic and Clinical Health (HITECH) Act, part of the American Recovery and Reinvestment Act of 2009 (ARRA) that was enacted on February 17, 2009, requires HHS to issue interim final regulations within 180 days to require covered entities under the Health Insurance Portability and Accountability Act of 1996 (HIPAA) and their business associates to provide notification in the case of breaches of unsecured protected health information. For purposes of determining what information is 'unsecured protected health information,' in this document HHS is also issuing an update to its guidance specifying the technologies and methodologies that render protected health information unusable, unreadable, or indecipherable to unauthorized individuals.

As opposed to the statutory definition of breach above, the Interim Final Rule had revised wording that is reproduced here:

> Breach means the acquisition, access, use, or disclosure of protected health information in a manner not permitted [under the Privacy Rule] which compromises the security or privacy of the protected health information.
>
> (1) (i) For purposes of this definition, *compromises the security or privacy of the protected health information* means poses a significant risk of financial, reputational, or other harm to the individual.
>
> (ii) A use or disclosure of protected health information that does not include the [18] identifiers [that make up protected health information] [ie, de-identified data] does not compromise the security or privacy of the protected health information.[33]
>
> (2) Breach excludes:
>
> (i) Any unintentional acquisition, access, or use of protected health information by a workforce member or person acting under the authority of a covered

---

32. Department of Health and Human Services, Office of the Secretary, "45 Parts 160 and 164: Breach Notification for Unsecured Protected Health Information; Interim Final Rule," *Federal Register*, v.74, n.162, August 24, 2009, pp. 42739–42770. On May 14, 2010, HHS submitted a Breach Notification Final Rule to the Office of Management and Budget (OMB) for review. Its Regulation Identifier Number (RIN) is 0991-AB56. On July 28, 2010, HHS "withdrew" this rule "for further consideration, given the Department's experience to-date in administering the regulations.... We [HHS] intend to publish a final rule in the Federal Register in the coming months." Update is available at: www.hhs.gov/ocr/privacy/hipaa/administrative/breachnotificationrule/finalruleupdate.html and we recommend that you visit the breach notification Web site periodically for any further updates on the final rule. The Interim Final Rule continues in effect.

33. Identifiers comprising protected health information and de-identification are discussed in Chapter 3 on privacy.

entity or a business associate, if such acquisition, access, or use was made in good faith and within the scope of authority and does not result in further use or disclosure in a manner not permitted under [the Privacy Rule].

(ii) Any inadvertent disclosure by a person who is authorized to access protected health information at a covered entity or business associate to another person authorized to access protected health information at the same covered entity or business associate, or organized health care arrangement in which the covered entity participates, and the information received as a result of such disclosure is not further used or disclosed in a manner not permitted under [the Privacy Rule].

(iii) A disclosure of protected health information where a covered entity or business associate has a good faith belief that an unauthorized person to whom the disclosure was made would not reasonably have been able to retain such information.[34]

The key difference in the definition is the italicized wording that appears in the regulatory definition of breach but is absent in the statutory definition. As the preamble to the Interim Final Rule indicates, a covered entity or business associate that discovers a breach will have to conduct a risk analysis to determine the potential of harm to the affected individuals.

We recommend that your practice periodically visit the HHS Office for Civil Rights (OCR) web site (www.hhs.gov/ocr/privacy/hipaa/understanding/coveredentities/breachnotificationifr.html) to be apprised of provisions that may change with respect to the Breach Notification Rule as compliance audits and complaint investigations proceed, and if the OCR has a fix on the extent of breach notification compliance, in comparison to failures to comply. Remember, enforcement of the Breach Notification Rule commenced on February 22, 2010, for breach violations that occurred on or after that date.

GUIDANCE ON SECURING PROTECTED HEALTH INFORMATION

As required by Section 13402 (h)(2) of the HITECH Act,[35] the Secretary of HHS issued on April 27, 2009, Guidance Specifying the Technologies and Methodologies That Render Protected Health Information Unusable, Unreadable, or Indecipherable to Unauthorized Individuals for Purposes of the Breach Notification Requirements under Section 13402 of Title XIII (Health Information Technology for Economic and Clinical Health Act) of the American Recovery and Reinvestment Act of 2009.[36] The guidance is

34. 74 *Federal Register* 42767–42768.

35. *HITECH Act* 263.

36. Department of Health and Human Services, Office of the Secretary, "45 CFR Parts 160 and 164: Guidance Specifying the Technologies and Methodologies That Render Protected Health Information Unusable, Unreadable, or Indecipherable to Unauthorized Individuals for Purposes of the Breach

related to HHS and FTC "breach notification" regulations pertaining to "unsecured protected health information."

Here is the updated guidance that appears in the August 24, 2009, Breach Notification Interim Final Rule:

(B) *Guidance Specifying the Technologies and Methodologies that Render Protected Health Information Unusable, Unreadable, or Indecipherable to Unauthorized Individuals*

Protected health information (PHI) is rendered unusable, unreadable, or indecipherable to unauthorized individuals if one or more of the following applies:

(a) Electronic PHI has been encrypted as specified in the HIPAA Security Rule by 'the use of an algorithmic process to transform data into a form in which there is a low probability of assigning meaning without use of a confidential process or key'[37] and such confidential process or key that might enable decryption has not been breached. To avoid a breach of the confidential process or key, these decryption tools should be stored on a device or at a location separate from the data they are used to encrypt or decrypt. The encryption processes identified below have been tested by the National Institute of Standards and Technology (NIST) and judged to meet this standard.
   (i) Valid encryption processes for data at rest are consistent with NIST Special Publication 800-111, *Guide to Storage Encryption Technologies for End User Devices.*[38]
   (ii) Valid encryption processes for data in motion are those which comply, as appropriate, with NIST Special Publications 800-52, *Guidelines for the Selection and Use of Transport Layer Security (TLS) Implementations;* 800-77, *Guide to IPsec VPNs;* or 800-113, Guide to SSL VPNs, or others which are Federal Information Processing Standards (FIPS) 140-2 validated.[39]

(b) The media on which the PHI is stored or recorded has been destroyed in one of the following ways:
   (i) Paper, film, or other hard copy media have been shredded or destroyed such that the PHI cannot be read or otherwise cannot be

---

(continued)

Notification Requirements under Section 13402 of Title XIII (Health Information Technology for Economic and Clinical Health Act) of the American Recovery and Reinvestment Act of 2009; Guidance and Request for Information," *Federal Register*, v.74, n.79, April 27, 2009, pp. 19006–19010. www.hhs.gov/ocr/privacy/hipaa/understanding/coveredentities/federalregisterbreachrfi.pdf. or at www.hipaa.com, but has been supplanted by the Guidance published in the Interim Final Rule pertaining to Breach Notification (74 *Federal Register* 427339–42770, with the *Guidance* on pp. 42742–42743.)

37. 45 CFR 164.304, definition of "encryption."

38. Available at: http://.csrc.nist.gov; NIST Roadmap plans include the development of security guidelines for enterprise-level storage devices, and such guidelines will be considered in updates to this guidance, when available.

39. Available at: http://.csrc.nist.gov.

reconstructed. Redaction is specifically excluded as a means of data destruction.

(ii) Electronic media have been cleared, purged, or destroyed consistent with NIST Special Publication 800-88, *Guidelines for Media Sanitization*,[40] such that the PHI cannot be retrieved.

We provide excerpts here from the aforementioned Guidance that is germane to securing ePHI through encryption.

> The term "unsecured protected health information" includes PHI [protected health information] in any form that is not secured through the use of a technology or methodology specified in this guidance. This guidance, however addresses methods for rendering PHI in paper or electronic form unusable, unreadable, or indecipherable to unauthorized individuals.
>
> Data comprising PHI can be vulnerable to a breach in any of the commonly recognized data states: "data in motion" (i.e., data that is moving through a network, including wireless transmission); "data at rest" (i.e., data that resides in databases, file systems, and other structured storage methods); "data in use" (i.e., data in the process of being created, retrieved, updated, or deleted); or "data disposed" (e.g., discarded paper records or recycled electronic media).
>
> Encryption is one method of rendering electronic PHI unusable, unreadable, or indecipherable to unauthorized persons. The successful use of encryption depends upon two main features: the strength of the encryption algorithm and the security of the decryption key or process. The specification of encryption methods in this guidance includes the condition that the processes or keys that might enable decryption have not been breached. . . .[41]

As we discuss in Chapter 4 on the Security Rule, and in particular with respect to the two Technical Safeguard's addressable encryption implementation specifications, a covered entity physician practice must rely on outcomes of its risk analysis to determine whether encryption is necessary. In that risk analysis, the covered entity should evaluate potential risks and costs of breach of unsecured ePHI that becomes accessible to unauthorized users outside of the covered entity, *whether data at rest or data in motion*, which would trigger the new "breach notification" provisions of the HITECH Act. If a covered entity does not encrypt ePHI, then it must document its decision and explain why this implementation specification does not apply. Even in the absence of exposure to an open network, a covered entity should consider in its risk analysis, the costs and benefits of encrypting ePHI at rest on its closed electronic information system.

With expected increased use of electronic transactions in health care, such as e-prescribing, and electronic communications via e-mail, say, between a physician practice and a patient, most covered entities will be using open systems and will need encryption tools. We recommend that you contact your electronic information system hardware and software

40. Available at: http://.csrc.nist.gov.

41. *74 Federal Register* 19008 (of the April 27, 2009, preamble).

vendors for advice on encryption, and that you also consult the National Institute for Standards and Technology (NIST) Special Publication 800-53, Revision 3: *Recommended Security Controls for Federal Information Systems and Organizations (Initial Public Draft)*, February 2009,[42] and NIST Special Publication 800-66, Revision 1, *An Introductory Resource Guide for Implementing the Health Insurance Portability and Accountability Act (HIPAA) Security Rule*, October 2008.[43] Please refer to Appendix C for additional resources on encryption requirements.

Enforcement

On July 27, 2009, Secretary of HHS Kathleen Sebelius delegated enforcement of the HIPAA Security Rule to the HHS Office for Civil Rights (OCR), which had HIPAA Privacy Rule enforcement authority since the compliance date of the HIPAA Privacy Rule, April 14, 2003.[44] Then, on October 30, 2009, HHS published in the *Federal Register* its Interim Final Rule that strengthens HIPAA enforcement under HITECH Act civil financial penalty revisions enacted as part of the HITECH Act on February 17, 2009.[45] These HITECH Act revisions "significantly increase the penalty amounts the Secretary may impose for violations of the HIPAA rules and encourage prompt corrective action," according to the HHS press release.[46] The Interim Final Rule took effect on November 30, 2009, and OCR began to enforce the breach notification rule for notification violations of breaches that were discovered on or after February 22, 2010. Unified enforcement of the HIPAA Privacy, Security, and Breach Notification Rules and higher civil penalties increase the probability and severity of consequences for HIPAA noncompliance with those Rules.

Before enactment of the HITECH Act, civil penalties for HIPAA violations were $100 for each violation or $25,000 for all violations of the same provision in a calendar year.[47] Under the HITECH Act, penalties were

---

42. Available at: http://csrc.nist.gov/publications/drafts/800-53/800-53-rev3-markup-02-05-2009.pdf.

43. Available at: http://csrc.nist.gov/publications/nistpubs/800-66-Rev1/SP-800-66-Revision1.pdf or at www.hipaa.com.

44. Department of Health and Human Services, Office of the Secretary, "Office for Civil Rights; Delegation of Authority," *Federal Register*, v.74, n.148, August 4, 2009, p. 38630. Available at: www.hhs.gov/ocr/privacy/hipaa/administrative/securityrule/srdelegation.pdf.

45. Department of Health and Human Services, Office of the Secretary, "45 CFR Part 160—HIPAA Administrative Simplification: Enforcement; Interim Final Rule," *Federal Register*, v.74, n.209, October 30, 2009, pp. 56123–56131. Available at: www.hhs.gov;ocr/privacy/hipaa/administrative/enforcementrule/enfifr.pdf.

46. "HHS Strengthens HIPAA Enforcement," press release, October 30, 2009, which is available online at www.hhs.gov/news/press/2009pres/10/20091030a.html.

47. 74 *Federal Register* 56131.

markedly raised and have been divided into four tiers, with a maximum penalty of $1.5 million for all violations of an identical provision in a calendar year. That is a 60-fold increase over the previous maximum!

The tiered financial penalties are:

- $100–$50,000 if the covered entity **did not know** and, by exercising reasonable diligence, would not have known, that it violated such provision.
- $1,000–$50,000 if the violation was due to **reasonable cause** and not to willful neglect.
- $10,000–$50,000 if the violation was due to **willful neglect** and was corrected as required.[48]
- $50,000 or more if the violation was due to **willful neglect** and was **not corrected** as required.

According to OCR Director, Georgina Verdugo, "The Department's implementation of these HITECH Act enforcement provisions will strengthen the HIPAA protections and rights related to an individual's health information. ... This strengthened penalty scheme will encourage health care providers, health plans and other health care entities required to comply with HIPAA to ensure that their compliance programs are effectively designed to prevent, detect and quickly correct violations of the HIPAA rules."[49]

We recommend that readers periodically visit the OCR enforcement Web site, www.hhs.gov/ocr/privacy/hipaa/enforcement/index.html, for additional information and updates.

GETTING STARTED

As you begin to examine the detail of the HIPAA Administrative Simplification Transaction Standards and Code Sets and the Privacy and Security Rules in the following chapters, we would like you to always keep in mind the three fundamental properties[50] of privacy and security of PHI in oral, hard copy, or electronic form:

- *Confidentiality* is the property that data or information is not made available or disclosed to unauthorized persons or processes.
- *Integrity* is the property that data or information has not been altered or destroyed in an unauthorized manner.

48. "For a violation in which it is established that the violation was due to willful neglect and was corrected during the 30-day period beginning on the first date the covered entity liable for the penalty knew, or by exercising reasonable diligence, would have known that the violation occurred." 74 *Federal Register* 56131.

49. "HHS Strengthens HIPAA Enforcement." Press Release. October 30, 2009. Available at: www.hhs.gov/news/press/2009 pres/10/20091030a.html.

50. These definitions are from 45 CFR 164.304.

- *Availability* is the property that data or information is accessible and usable upon demand by an authorized person.

We also would like you to keep in mind that in the years ahead, there will be considerable regulatory activity related to enabling administrative simplification provisions of the HITECH Act, Patient Protection and Affordable Care Act (discussed at the end of Chapter 2), and perhaps other federal legislative initiatives. For example, as mentioned earlier in this chapter in footnote 32, HHS withdrew, on July 28, 2010, its final rule: HIPAA Administrative Simplification; Notification in the Case of Breach (Regulation Identifier Number (RIN) 0991-AB56) "for further consideration, given the Department's experience to date in administering the regulations.... We [HHS] intend to publish a final rule in the Federal Register in the coming months."[51] While the final rule continues in effect, we recommend that you visit the breach notification Web site periodically in coming months for further updates on the final rule. You also should be alert to any changes in the final rule regarding the encryption of and destruction methods of electronic and hard copy media for securing PHI that are specified in the *Guidance Specifying the Technologies and Methodologies that Render Protected Health Information Unusable, Unreadable, or Indecipherable to Unauthorized Individuals* (see 74 *Federal Register* 42742–42743).

On July 14, 2010, HHS published in the Federal Register the Notice of Proposed Rulemaking (NPRM): Modifications to the HIPAA Privacy, Security, and Enforcement Rules Under the Health Information Technology for Economic and Clinical Health Act.[52] According to the Summary of the NPRM: "[HHS] is issuing this [NPRM] to modify the standards for Privacy of Individually Identifiable Health Information (Privacy Rule), the Security Standards for the Protection of Electronic Protected Health Information (Security Rule), and the rules pertaining to Compliance and Investigations, Imposition of Civil Money Penalties, and Procedures for Hearings (Enforcement Rule) issued under [HIPAA]. The purpose of these modifications is to implement recent statutory amendments under the [HITECH Act], to strengthen the privacy and security protection of health information, and to improve the workability and effectiveness of these

---

51. Update is available at: www.hhs.gov/ocr/privacy/hipaa/administrative/breachnotificationrule/finalruleupdate.html. Also see, "Rethinking breach notices: HHS withdraws final rule for more consideration." *Modern Healthcare*, August 2, 2010:pp. 8–9.

52. Department of Health and Human Services, Office of the Secretary, "45 CFR Parts 160 and 164: Modifications to the HIPAA Privacy, Security, and Enforcement Rules Under the Health Information Technology for Economic and Clinical Health Act; Notice of proposed rulemaking," Federal Register, v.75, n.134, July 14, 2010, pp. 40867–40924. This document is available online at: http://edocket.access.gpo.gov/2010/pdf/2010-16718.pdf.

HIPAA Rules."[53] Comments on the NPRM can be submitted to HHS on or before September 13, 2010. It is likely that the Interim Final or Final Rule will be published in late 2010 or early 2011, with compliance likely beginning in mid-2011.

In addition, practices should prepare and expect to be busy with clinical initiatives relating to the HITECH Act, such as the financial incentives for adoption and meaningful use of certified electronic health record (EHR) technology.[54] Both the meaningful use criteria and the EHR certification programs are works in progress.

Stage 1 covers 2011–2012. For stage 1, the meaningful use objectives is, "Protect electronic health information created or maintained by the certified EHR technology through the implementation of appropriate technical capabilities," and the meaningful use measure is, "Conduct or review a security risk analysis per 45 CFR 164.308(a)(1) [discussed in Chapter 4] and implement security updates as necessary and correct identified security

---

53. On July 28, 2010, HHS published two final rules in the Federal Register pertaining to the HITECH Act EHR Incentive Programs and EHR Certification Standards and Criteria: Department of Health and Human Services, Centers for Medicare & Medicaid Services (CMS), "42 CFR Parts 412, 413, 422, and 495; Medicare and Medicaid Programs; Electronic Health Record Incentive Program; Final rule," Federal Register, v.75, n.144, July 28, 2010, pp. 44313–44588, which is available at: http://edocket.access.gpo.gov/2010/pdf/2010-17207.pdf; and Department of Health and Human Services, Office of the Secretary (on behalf of the Office of the National Coordinator for Health Information Technology (ONC), "45 CFR Part 170; Health Information Technology; initial Set of Standards, Implementation Specifications, and Certification Criteria for Electronic Health Record Technology; Final rule," Federal Register, v.75, n.144, July 28, 2010, pp. 44589–44654, which is available at: http://edocket.access.gpo.gov/2010/pdf/2010-17210.pdf. For further information and updates, we recommend that you visit the new Centers for Medicare & Medicaid Services (CMS) Official web site for the Medicare and Medicaid EHR Incentive Programs, which CMS launched on June 21, 2010, available at www.cms.gov/EHRIncentivePrograms/.

54. On July 28, 2010, HHS published two final rules in the Federal Register pertaining to the HITECH Act EHR Incentive Programs and EHR Certification Standards and Criteria: Department of Health and Human Services, Centers for Medicare & Medicaid Services (CMS), "42 CFR Parts 412, 413, 422, and 495; Medicare and Medicaid Programs; Electronic Health Record Incentive Program; Final rule," Federal Register, v.75, n.144, July 28, 2010, pp. 44313–44588, which is available at: http://edocket.access.gpo.gov/2010/pdf/2010-17207.pdf; and Department of Health and Human Services, Office of the Secretary (on behalf of the Office of the National Coordinator for Health Information Technology (ONC), "45 CFR Part 170; Health Information Technology; initial Set of Standards, Implementation Specifications, and Certification Criteria for Electronic Health Record Technology; Final rule," Federal Register, v.75, n.144, July 28, 2010, pp. 44589–44654, which is available at: http://edocket.access.gpo.gov/2010/pdf/2010-17210.pdf.

deficiencies as part of its risk management process."[55] In addition to conducting a risk assessment, there are eight security-related criteria within this objective-measure category that mirror provisions in the HIPAA Security Rule and for which eligible professionals (EPs) must attest compliance as part of the qualification process for receiving incentive payments for adoption of certified EHR technology.[56] We recommend that practices pay particular attention to these criteria as part of their overall compliance with the HIPAA Security Rule.

55. 75 Federal Register 44617.

56. See 45 CFR 170.302(o)-(v) and discussion related to those security certification criteria at 75 Federal Register 44652 and 44616–44623, respectively.

chapter 2

Transactions and Code Sets

This chapter describes the HIPAA transaction standards and code sets that went into effect for covered entities on October 16, 2003, and that are in effect today. We also outline the change in transaction version from 4010 to 5010 that requires compliance on January 1, 2012, and the conversion from ICD-9 to ICD-10 for diagnostic codes for all covered entities and for procedure codes for inpatient encounters. It is imperative that physician practices prepare ***now*** for implementation of these changes by developing an implementation strategy with their software vendors and health care clearinghouses for testing their standard electronic transactions and ICD-10 diagnostic codes with trading partners. Physician practices will continue to use CPT-4 and HCPCS codes for procedures. We close this chapter with an examination of statutory administrative simplification transaction and code set rule enhancements and additions in the Patient Protection and Affordable Care Act, enacted on March 23, 2010.

What You Will Learn in This Chapter

In this chapter you will learn about the Version 5010 transaction standards that require compliance by January 1, 2012. You also will learn that there are two broad categories of external code sets used in the standard transactions: medical and nonmedical. You will see a brief description of each. Many of these code sets are used in more than one of the ASC X12N standard transactions. You are not expected to memorize these external code sets, but it is important to know what they are, how they are defined and used, and where to find them. In Table 2.3, you will see a cross-tabulation of code sets by transaction standard for the 5010 version that requires compliance on January 1, 2012. ICD-10-CM external codes are included, but they do not require compliance by physician practices and other covered entities until October 1, 2013. You also will see the internal and external training timing requirements for achieving compliance with the Version 5010 transaction standards and the ICD-10 code set modification. Unlike the earlier compliance for the currently used transaction standards and code sets, the Department of Health and Human Services (HHS) has indicated that there will be no tolerance for transaction standards and ICD-10-CM noncompliance after the compliance dates of January 1, 2012, and October 1, 2013, respectively.

Key Terms

Code set	Data element
Code set maintaining organization	Data set
Compliance date	Descriptor
Data content	

HIPAA Administrative Simplification was enacted in August 1996. In the years that followed, the federal government promulgated transaction and code sets, as well as privacy, security, identifier, claim attachment, and enforcement standards, which we briefly discussed in Chapter 1. In this chapter, we examine in detail transaction standards and code sets and how they apply to the physician practice.

We have discussed the 4010/4010A transaction and code set standards in our earlier books, including the first edition of *HIPAA Plain and Simple: A Compliance Guide for Health Care Professionals,*[1] and *HIPAA Transactions: A Nontechnical Business Guide for Health Care.*[2] In this book, we outline the 4010/4010A transaction and code set standards, but focus more on the 5010 transaction and code set standards version that will require compliance on January 1, 2012, and the ICD-10-CM standard that will require compliance on October 1, 2013.

TRANSACTION STANDARDS

The overarching message with regard to transaction standards is that if a covered entity is sending or receiving *administrative* electronic transactions that relate to the claims process, it must use a HIPAA standard format.

What this means to health plans is:

- When requested by a covered entity, health plans must send and receive standard transactions.
- Health plans may not delay or reject any standard transaction solely because it is standard.
- Health plans may not reject standard transactions that contain situational data elements not used by the health plan.
- Health plans may use clearinghouses as business associates to accept standard transactions from other covered entities.

What this means to a physician practice is:

- If your practice conducts business using an electronic transaction, you must use the applicable standard transactions.[3]

1. Hartley, CP, Jones, ED. Chicago, IL: American Medical Association Press, 2004.
2. Jones, ED, Hartley, CP. Chicago, IL: American Medical Association Press, 2004.
3. "Under HIPAA, if a covered entity conducts one of the adopted transactions electronically, they must use the adopted standard. This means that they must

The final transaction and code set standard required compliance on October 16, 2003.[4] In understanding the HHS requirement for Version 5010 compliance on January 1, 2012, and ICD-10-CM compliance on October 1, 2013, it is important to look at what happened prior to and after the 2003 compliance date. In July 2003, the Centers for Medicare & Medicaid Services (CMS) determined that covered entities likely would not be compliant by the October 16, 2003, date.[5] On August 4, 2005, CMS announced that it "[would]not process incoming non-HIPAA-compliant electronic Medicare claims" after October 1, 2005. In its announcement, it reported: "As of June 2005 only about 0.5% of Medicare fee-for-service providers submitted non-HIPAA-compliant electronic claims. The highest rate of non-compliance as of May [2005] was from clinical laboratories, 1.72%. Only 1.45% of claims from hospitals were non-compliant and 0.45% from physicians. The high percentage among all provider types shows that everyone can become compliant. The law required all payers to conduct HIPAA-compliant transactions no later than October 16, 2003. However, only about 31% of Medicare claims were compliant at that time. Other payers had even lower numbers of compliant claims."[6] As you will see in the discussion that follows relating to Version 5010 and ICD-10-CM, HHS believes that there is—and has been since 2003—sufficient time for covered entities to increase the use of the electronic transaction standards and code sets and to achieve compliance.

(continued)

adhere to the content and format requirements of each standard." See *Overview: Transaction and Code Sets Standards* at the Centers for Medicare & Medicaid Services (CMS) web site: www.cms.hhs.gov/TransactionCodeSetsStands/.

4. The final rule was published in the *Federal Register* on August 17, 2000, and is cited in the references to Table 1.1 in Chapter 1. The history of the enabling regulations for the transaction and code set standards is covered in our books cited earlier in this chapter. There was a modification to the final rule that was published on February 20, 2003, and that is the document used for the discussion that follows. See Department of Health and Human Services, Office of the Secretary, "45 Part 162—Health Insurance Reform: Modifications to the Electronic Data Transaction Standards and Code Sets; Final Rule," *Federal Register*, v.68, n.34, February 20, 2003, pp. 8381-8399. Hereinafter, references to this document are in the format 68 *Federal Register* <page(s)>.

5. Jones, ED, and Hartley, CP. Appendix. In: *HIPAA Transactions: A Nontechnical Business Guide for Health Care*. Chicago, IL: American Medical Association Press; 2004: pp108-110.

6. See "2005.08.04: CMS Ending Contingency for Non-HIPAA-Compliant Medicare Claims," CMS Press Release, August 4, 2005, which is available at: www.cms.gov/apps/media/press/release.asp?Counter=1528&intNumPerPage=1000&checkDate=&checkKey=&srchType=1&numDays=0&srchOpt=0&srchData=&keywordType=All&chkNewsType=1%2C+2%2C+3%2C+4%2C+5&intPage=&showAll=1&pYear=1&year=2005&desc=false&cboOrder=date.

Need for Transaction and Code Set Modifications

On September 26, 2007, the National Committee on Vital and Health Statistics (NCVHS) made the following recommendations to then HHS Secretary Michael Leavitt: "The Secretary should **expedite** the development and issuance of a Notice of Proposed Rule Making (NPRM) to adopt the ASC X12N Version 5010 suite of transactions."[7] The NPRM was published in the *Federal Register* on August 22, 2008,[8] allowing 60 days for public comment, and the final rule was published in the *Federal Register* on January 16, 2009.[9] You will note in the next section that the proposed and final rules for ICD-10-CM were contiguous to the proposed and final Version 5010 rules, respectively, because the use of ICD-10-CM requires Version 5010. Below, we discuss both the proposed and final ICD-10 rulings.

The final Version 5010 rule required all covered entities to use Version 5010 standards:

> Except as otherwise provided in this part, if a covered entity conducts, with another covered entity that is required to comply with a transaction standard adopted under this part (or within the same covered entity), using electronic media, a transaction for which the Secretary has adopted a standard under this part, the covered entity must conduct the transaction as a standard transaction.[10]

For physician practices, these six typical electronic transaction standards are covered:

- Health Care Claim: Professional (837)[11]
- Health Care Eligibility Benefit Inquiry and Response (270/271)[12]

---

7. Letter from Simon P. Cohn, MD, MPH, Chair, NCVHS, to Michael O. Leavitt, Secretary, US Department of Health and Human Services, "Revisions to HIPAA Transactions Standards Urgently Needed," September 26, 2007. Available at: www.ncvhs.hhs.gov/070926lt.pdf.
8. Department of Health and Human Services, Office of the Secretary, "45 CFR Part 162: Health Insurance Reform; Modifications to the Health Insurance Portability and Accountability Act (HIPAA) Electronic Transaction Standards; Proposed Rule," *Federal Register*, v.73, n.164, August 22, 2008, pp. 49741–49793. Hereinafter, references to this document are in the format 73 *Federal Register* <page(s)>.
9. Department of Health and Human Services, Office of the Secretary, "45 CFR Part 162: Health Insurance Reform; Modifications to the Health Insurance Portability and Accountability Act (HIPAA); Final Rule," *Federal Register*, v.74, n.11, January 16, 2009, pp. 3295–3328. Hereinafter, references to this document are in the format 74 *Federal Register* <page(s)>.
10. 74 Federal Register 3325 and 45 CFR 162.923.
11. Accredited Standards Committee X12, Insurance Subcommittee, ASC X12N. *Health Care Claim: Professional (837)*. ASC Standards for Electronic Data Interchange Technical Report Type 3 (ASC X12N/005010X222), May 2006. Washington Publishing Company (www.wpc-edi.com).
12. Accredited Standards Committee X12, Insurance Subcommittee, ASC X12N. *Health Care Eligibility Benefit Inquiry and Response (270/271)*. ASC Standards for Electronic Data Interchange Technical Report Type 3 (ASC X12N/005010X279), April 2008. Washington Publishing Company (www.wpc-edi.com).

- Health Care Services Review—Request for Review and Response (278)[13]
- Health Care Claim Status Request and Response (276/277)[14]
- Health Care Claim Payment/Advice (835)[15]
- Coordination of Benefits Information[16].

The NPRM explained why the transaction standards that were in place since October 2003 were being modified:

> In addition to technical issues and business developments necessitating consideration of the new versions of the standards, there remain a number of unresolved issues that had been identified by the industry early in the implementation period for the first set of standards, and those issues were never addressed through regulation. . . .[17]

The focus in the following discussion is on the effect of those concerns on two modified standards because they have implications for policies and procedures in your practice that, over the next five years, may substantially enhance cash flow and reduce cost.[18] They are:

- Health Care Claim Payment/Advice (835)
- Health Care Claim Status Request and Response (276/277).

---

13. Accredited Standards Committee X12, Insurance Subcommittee, ASC X12N. *Health Care Services Review—Request for Review and Response (278).* ASC Standards for Electronic Data Interchange Technical Report Type 3 (ASC X12N/005010X217), May 2006. Washington Publishing Company (www.wpc-edi.com). This standard covers three types of transactions: "(a) A request from a health care provider to a health plan for the review of health care to obtain an authorization for the health care. (b) A request from a health care provider to a health plan to obtain authorization for referring an individual to another health care provider. (c) A response from a health plan to a health care provider to a request described in paragraph (a) or (b) of this section." 73 *Federal Register* 49791.

14. Accredited Standards Committee X12, Insurance Subcommittee, ASC X12N. *Health Care Claim Status Request and Response (276/277).* ASC Standards for Electronic Data Interchange Technical Report Type 3 (ASC X12N/005010X212), August 2006. Washington Publishing Company (www.wpc-edi.com).

15. Accredited Standards Committee X12, Insurance Subcommittee, ASC X12N. *Health Care Claim Payment/Advice (835).* ASC Standards for Electronic Data Interchange Technical Report Type 3 (ASC X12N/005010X221), April 2006. Washington Publishing Company (www.wpc-edi.com).

16. Accredited Standards Committee X12, Insurance Subcommittee, ASC X12N. *Health Care Claim: Professional (837).* ASC Standards for Electronic Data Interchange Technical Report Type 3 (ASC X12N/005010X222), May 2006. Washington Publishing Company (www.wpc-edi.com). Note that the ASC X12 transaction standard for the claim and for coordination of benefits is the same 837.

17. 73 *Federal Register* 49743.

18. In the first edition of HIPAA Plain & Simple: *A Compliance Guide for Health Care Professionals*, we introduced the concepts of raising the bridge and lowering the river. "*Raising the bridge* means generating more revenue per unit of service. *Lowering the river* means lowering costs per unit of service. Either, controlling for the other, will increase net revenue. Both will increase it even more." See Hartley CP, Jones ED. Chicago, IL: AMA Press, 2004, pp. 193–194.

Think about the effect on your practice of receiving your remittances and payments more quickly in electronic formats and having them automatically posted to your practice management system without human intervention. Also, think about making automated claim status inquiries without human intervention based on rules embedded in your software, thus eliminating the need for your workforce to spend time on the telephone with health plans.[19] The regulatory impact analysis that is part of the Version 5010 NPRM indicates that both health care providers and health plans receive a net gain in implementing electronic remittance and payments processing and claims status standards capabilities.[20]

What does the NPRM suggest as specific improvements underlying the modifications of the remittance and payments processing and claims status standards capabilities? Remember, unlike mandated policies and procedures required by other Rules,—eg, the Security Rule discussed in Chapter 4—your practice has a choice to jettison paper transactions and adopt 5010-transaction-based standard policies and procedures in how it processes remittances and payments from and how it makes claim status inquiries to health plan payers, based on business decisions. Your practice's software vendor(s) will play a key role in helping your practice address these policy and procedure business issues. Be sure to ask your software vendor(s) how your practice can prepare the information that will be needed to address these issues. Consider any expenditure of preparation time or money as an investment in your practice's business future, especially if your practice has waited until now to adopt electronic transactions.

Health Care Claim Payment/Advice (835)[21]

According to the NPRM, "[m]any of the enhancements in Version 5010 involve the Front Matter section of the Technical Report Type 3, which contains expanded instructions for accurately processing a compliant 835 transaction. Version 5010 provides refined terminology for using a standard, and enhances the data content to promote clarity." The NPRM highlights the following potential benefits of the refinements:

- More accurate use of the standard.
- Reduction of manual intervention.
- Motivation to vendors and billing services to provide more cost-effective solutions for electronic remittance advice transactions.

---

19. Does your practice know how much time and cost of workforce resources that it allocates to handling remittance, payment, and claims status issues with health plans?

20. 73 *Federal Register* 49757-49768, especially 49767-49768. The conclusion was confirmed in the final Version 5010 rule. See 74 *Federal Register* 3316-3317.

21. The NPRM discussion of this transaction standard is at 73 *Federal Register* 49748.

The NPRM goes on to highlight other changes:

- Tightened business rules and fewer code value options in Version 5010:
  - The current version "lacks standard definitions and procedures for translating remittance information and payments from various health plans to a provider, which makes automatic remittance posting difficult."
- New instructions for handling certain business situations in Version 5010:
  - "Version 5010 instructs providers on how to negate a payment that may be incorrect and post a correction."
- Flexibility to test the Version 5010 835 transaction with the existing Version 4010/4010A claim transaction:
  - This compatibility facilitates testing of the modified remittance standard with existing claims prior to the compliance date of January 1, 2012, for Version 5010, as "there may be a transition period with claims for services rendered before the compliance date that will be in the older version of the standard because data elements required in Version 5010 might not have been captured at the time services were rendered."
- Inclusion of a new Medical Policy segment in Version 5010:
  - This segment "provides more up-to-date information on payer policies and helps in detail management, appeals, and reduces telephone and written inquiries to payers."
  - This segment also "helps providers locate related published medical policies that are used to determine benefits by virtue of the addition of a segment for a payer's [Universal Resource Locator] URL for easy access to a plan's medical policies."
- Elimination of Not Advised codes in Version 5010:
  - In Version 4010/4010A, there was confusion in a payment context on the use of the code "debit," which was marked "Not Advised." In Version 5010, it is treated "as situational, with instructions on how and when to use the code."
- Clarification for use of claim status indicator codes in the Version 5010 835 transaction standard:
  - In Version 4010/4010A, there are "status codes that indicate a primary, secondary, or tertiary claim, but no instruction for the use of these codes," which "creates confusion when a claim is partially processed, or when a claim is processed but there is no payment."[22]

In general, these changes provide a practice more convenient access to health plan information that will facilitate submission of claims, thereby expediting remittance processing and payment. The final Version 5010 Rule concurred with the NPRM claims, noting that "[c]orrect implementation of

---

22. This and preceding quotations in this section on the 835 standard transactions are from 73 *Federal Register* 49748.

the X12 835 will reduce phone calls to health plans, reduce appeals due to incomplete information, eliminate unnecessary customer support, and reduce the cost of sending and processing paper remittance advices."[23] Finally, the NPRM estimates that costs savings for claim and remittance processing with the modification to standards for the claim (837) and remittance (835) components will amount to $0.55 per claim for providers and $0.18 for health plans, for a total of $0.73 per claim."[24]

Health Care Claim Status Request and Response (276/277)[25]

Unlike the 835 remittance advice standard transaction, which is estimated to be currently accepted by about 60% of all covered entities, the 276/277 claims status request and response is estimated to be currently accepted by only about 10% of all covered entities.[26] Version 5010 addresses the following issues in order to increase the percentage of acceptance:

- Identification of prescription numbers to determine which "prescription numbers are paid or not paid at the claim level" of the transaction.
  - "The ability to identify a prescription by the prescription number is important for pharmacy providers when identifying claims data in their systems."
- Elimination of some sensitive personal information that is extraneous to the purpose of checking claim status and that raises privacy and minimum necessary data issues under the HIPAA Privacy Rule, which is discussed in Chapter 3.
  - For example, the existing standard "requires the subscriber's date of birth and insurance policy number, which often is a Social Security number," which "is not needed to identify the subscriber because the policy number recorded for the patient already uniquely identifies the subscriber."
- Clarification of *situational data element* rules in Version 5010 in order to "reduce reliance on *companion guides*[27] and ensure consistency in the use of Implementation Guides," and to "reduce multiple interpretations."

---

23. 74 *Federal Register* 3298.

24. 73 *Federal Register* 49765.

25. The NPRM discussion of the 276/277 transaction standard is at 73 *Federal Register* 49750.

26. 73 *Federal Register* 49763.

27. "These deficiencies in the current implementation specifications have caused much of the industry to rely on 'companion guides' created by health plans to address areas of Version 4010/4010A that are not specific enough or require work-around solutions to address business needs. These companion guides are unique, plan-specific implementation instructions for the situational use of certain fields and/or data elements that are needed to support current business operations." 73 *Federal Register* 49746.

  - Physician practice reliance on identifying different interpretations of situational fields and data elements for properly submitting claims to their patients' multiple health plans is time consuming and costly. "For example, Version 5010 clarifies the relationships between dependents and subscribers, and makes a clear distinction between the term 'covered status' (whether the particular service is covered under the benefit package) and 'covered beneficiary' (the individual who is eligible for services)."

- Implementation of consistent rules across all standards "regarding the requirement to include both patient and subscriber information in the transaction."
  - If the dependent patient can be uniquely identified with an "individual identification number," then the subscriber identification is not necessary in the transaction: "to include the subscriber information with the dependent member information for a uniquely identifiable dependent is an administrative burden for the provider."

Version 5010 Health Care Claim Payment/Advice (835) and Health Care Claim Status Request and Response (276/277) have been the focus in this discussion of transaction standards for implementation by the physician practice because improvements in the implementation specifications have the promise to reduce time and cost regarding the receipt of payment from health plans for services rendered. In 2005, the Medical Group Management Association (MGMA) indicated that "it takes 45 days for a doctor to get an average payment."[28] With patient co-insurance at the front end of an encounter and health plan processing of a claim and a final payment from the patient, if any, after the delivery of service, it may actually take considerably longer for an account receivable to be reconciled and for a claim to be paid in full and closed.[29] Improvements to the Version 5010 Health Care Claim Payment/Advice (835) and Health Care Claim Status Request and Response (276/277) transaction standards have the potential to markedly speed up payment, which could favorably affect practice cash flow and claim and remittance processing costs.

Finally, for your reference online, CMS has made available comparisons of Version 4010/4010A with Version 5010, element by element.[30] The site for

---

28. Lieber R. "Asking Your Doc for Discounts: New Health Plans Mean It's Not As Farfetched As It Sounds," *The Wall Street Journal,* October 29–30, 2005, p. B1.
29. Effective February 18, 2010, as enacted in the HITECH Act, which is discussed in Chapter 1, a patient, who pays "out of pocket in full" for an encounter at time of service can request that his or her protected health information (related to the claim for that encounter) not be sent to a health plan if the disclosure is for "purposes of carrying out payment or health care operations (and is not for purposes of carrying out treatment)", and a health care provider *must* comply. (42 USC 17935) It is unclear what the incidence of this statutory requirement will be on patients paying out of pocket in full at time of service.
30. 73 *Federal Register* 49746.

Health Care Claim Payment/Advice (835), from which page one is illustrated as Figure 2.1, is available at www.cms.hhs.gov/ElectronicBillingEDITrans/Downloads/Remittance4010A1to5010.pdf. The site for Health Care Claim Status Request and Response (276/277) is available at www.cms.hhs.gov/ElectronicBillingEDITrans/Downloads/ClaimStatus4010A1to5010.pdf (see Figure 2.2). Also, visit the CMS web page, *Electronic Billing & EDI Transactions: 5010-D.0*, at www.cms.hhs.gov/ElectronicBillingEDITrans/18_5010D0.asp, for 4010/4010A to 5010 comparisons of the Health Care Claim: Professional (837) and Health Care Eligibility Benefit Inquiry and Response (270/271) and access to other information links inside and outside of CMS related to the Version 5010 transaction standards.

HIPAA TRANSACTION STANDARDS: FINAL RULE

On January 16, 2009, less than 5 months after publication of the NPRM—a very short period of time if calculated in "HIPAA-time"—the office of the Secretary of HHS published in the *Federal Register* final rules pertaining to Version 5010 and ICD-10. In part, the timing was due to the upcoming change from the Bush Administration to the Obama Administration. The Version 5010 final rule is discussed below and the ICD-10 rule in the next section. Please note that the discussion pertaining to the Version 5010/D.0 and ICD-10 NPRMs, except where noted, is unaffected by changes in the final rules.

The Version 5010 final rule adopted Accredited Standards Committee (ASC) X12 Version 5010 and National Council for Prescription Drug Programs (NCPDP) Versions D.0, 3.0, and 5.1 standards for electronic transactions, as shown in Table 2.1 (reproduced here from Table 1 in the final rule).[31]

Most of the transaction standards reflect updates. The Medicaid subrogation standard is newly adopted, and two standards are adopted for retail pharmacy supplies and professional services. Excluding the Medicaid pharmacy subrogation standard, Table 2.2 compares current transaction standard versions with modified or new transaction standard versions that will require compliance by covered entities beginning January 1, 2012.

Effective Dates of Final Rule

There were two effective dates for the final transaction rule. For all standards except the Medicaid Pharmacy Subrogation Transaction, the effective date was March 17, 2009. For the Medicaid Pharmacy Subrogation Transaction standard, the effective date was January 1, 2010. "[T]he effective date is the date that the policies set forth in this final rule take effect, and new policies are considered to be officially adopted."[32]

31. 74 *Federal Register* 3296-3297.

32. 74 *Federal Register* 3302.

FIGURE 2.1

Comparison Site for Health Care Claim Payment/Advice (835)

4010A1

Element Identifier	Description	ID	Min. Max.	Usage Reg.	Loop	Loop Repeat	Values
	835 4010A1						
ISA	**INTERCHANGE CONTROL HEADER**		1	R		1	
ISA01	Authorization Information Qualifier	ID	2--2	R			00,03
ISA02	Authorization Information	AN	10--10	R			
ISA03	Security Information Qualifier	ID	2--2	R			00,01
ISA04	Security Information	AN	10--10	R			
ISA05	Interchange ID Qualifier	ID	2--2	R			01,14,20,27, 28, 29, 30, 33, ZZ
ISA06	Interchange Sender ID	AN	15--15	R			
ISA07	Interchange ID Qualifier	ID	2--2	R			01,14,20,27, 28, 29, 30, 33, ZZ
ISA08	Interchange Receiver ID	AN	15--15	R			
ISA09	Interchange Date	DT	6--6	R			YYMMDD
ISA10	Interchange Time	TM	4--4	R			HHMM
ISA11	Interchange Control Standards ID	ID	1--1	R			U
ISA12	Interchange Control Version Number	ID	5--5	R			00401
ISA13	Interchange Control Number	N0	9--9	R			=IEA02
ISA14	Acknowledgement Requested	ID	1--1	R			0
ISA15	Usage Indicator	ID	1--1	R			P,T
ISA16	Component Element Separator		1--1	R			
GS	**Functional Group Header**		1	R	----------	1	
GS01	Functional Identifier Code	ID	2--2	R			HP
GS02	Application Sender's Code	AN	2--15	R			
GS03	Application Receiver's Code	AN	2--15	R			
GS04	Date	DT	8--8	R			CCYYMMDD
GS05	Time	TM	4--8	R			HHMM
GS06	Group Control Number	N0	1--9	R			=GE02
GS07	Responsible Agency Code	ID	1--2	R			X
GS08 GS08	Version/Release/Industry Id code Version/Release/Industry Id Code	AN	1--12	R			004010X091 004010X091A1

5010

Element Identifier	Description	ID	Min. Max.	Usage Reg.	Loop	Loop Repeat	Values
	835 5010						
ISA	**INTERCHANGE CONTROL HEADER**		1	R		1	
ISA01	Authorization Information Qualifier	ID	2--2	R			00,03
ISA02	Authorization Information	AN	10--10	R			
ISA03	Security Information Qualifier	ID	2--2	R			00,01
ISA04	Security Information	AN	10--10	R			
ISA05	Interchange ID Qualifier	ID	2--2	R			01,14,20,27, 28, 29, 30, 33, ZZ
ISA06	Interchange Sender ID	AN	15--15	R			
ISA07	Interchange ID Qualifier	ID	2--2	R			01,14,20,27, 28, 29, 30, 33, ZZ
ISA08	Interchange Receiver ID	AN	15--15	R			
ISA09	Interchange Date	DT	6--6	R			YYMMDD
ISA10	Interchange Time	TM	4--4	R			HHMM
ISA11	Interchange Control Standards ID	ID	1--1	R			U
ISA12	Interchange Control Version Number	ID	5--5	R			00401
ISA13	Interchange Control Number	N0	9--9	R			=IEA02
ISA14	Acknowledgement Requested	ID	1--1	R			0
ISA15	Usage Indicator	ID	1--1	R			P,T
ISA16	Component Element Separator		1--1	R			
GS	**Functional Group Header**		1	R	----------	1	
GS01	Functional Identifier Code	ID	2--2	R			HP
GS02	Application Sender's Code	AN	2--15	R			
GS03	Application Receiver's Code	AN	2--15	R			
GS04	Date	DT	8--8	R			CCYYMMDD
GS05	Time	TM	4--8	R			HHMM
GS06	Group Control Number	N0	1--9	R			=GE02
GS07	Responsible Agency Code	ID	1--2	R			X
GS08	Version Identifier Code	AN	1--12	R			005010X221

FIGURE 2.2

Comparison Site for Health Care Claim Status Request and Response (276/277)

4010A1

Element Identifier	Description	ID	Min. Max.	Usage Reg.	Loop	Loop Repeat	Values
276 4010A1							
ISA	INTERCHANGE CONTROL HEADER		1	R		1	
ISA01	Authorization Information Qualifier	ID	2-2	R			00, 03
ISA02	Authorization Information	AN	10-10	R			
ISA03	Security Information Qualifier	ID	2-2	R			00, 01
ISA04	Security Information	AN	10-10	R			
ISA05	Interchange ID Qualifier	ID	2-2	R			01, 14, 20, 27, 28, 29, 30, 33, ZZ
ISA06	Interchange Sender ID	AN	15-15	R			
ISA07	Interchange ID Qualifier	ID	2-2	R			01, 14, 20, 27, 28, 29, 30, 33, ZZ
ISA08	Interchange Receiver ID	AN	15-15	R			
ISA09	Interchange Date	DT	6-6	R			YYMMDD
ISA10	Interchange Time	TM	4-4	R			HHMM
ISA11	Interchange Control Standards ID	ID	1-1	R			U
ISA12	Interchange Control Version Number	ID	5-5	R			00401
ISA13	Interchange Control Number	N0	9-9	R			
ISA14	Acknowledgement Requested	ID	1-1	R			0, 1
ISA15	Usage Indicator	ID	1-1	R			P, T
ISA16	Component Element Separator	AN	1-1	R			
GS	FUNCTIONAL GROUP HEADER		1	R		>1	
GS01	Functional Identifier Code	ID	2-2	R			HR
GS02	Application Sender Code	AN	2-15	R			
GS03	Application Receiver Code	AN	2-15	R			
GS04	Date	DT	8-8	R			CCYYMMDD
GS05	Time	TM	4-8	R			HHMMSSDD
GS06	Group Control Number	N0	1-9	R			
GS07	Responsible Agency Code	ID	1-2	R			X
GS08	Version Identifier Code	AN	1-12	R			004010X093

5010

Element Identifier	Description	ID	Min. Max.	Usage Reg.	Loop	Loop Repeat	Values
276 5010							
ISA	INTERCHANGE CONTROL HEADER		1	R		1	
ISA01	Authorization Information Qualifier	ID	2-2	R			00, 03
ISA02	Authorization Information	AN	10-10	R			
ISA03	Security Information Qualifier	ID	2-2	R			00, 01
ISA04	Security Information	AN	10-10	R			
ISA05	Interchange ID Qualifier	ID	2-2	R			01, 14, 20, 27, 28, 29, 30, 33, ZZ
ISA06	Interchange Sender ID	AN	15-15	R			
ISA07	Interchange ID Qualifier	ID	2-2	R			01, 14, 20, 27, 28, 29, 30, 33, ZZ
ISA08	Interchange Receiver ID	AN	15-15	R			
ISA09	Interchange Date	DT	6-6	R			YYMMDD
ISA10	Interchange Time	TM	4-4	R			HHMM
ISA11	Repetition Seperator	AN	1-1	R			
ISA12	Interchange Control Version Number	ID	5-5	R			00501
ISA13	Interchange Control Number	N0	9-9	R			
ISA14	Acknowledgement Requested	ID	1-1	R			0, 1
ISA15	Usage Indicator	ID	1-1	R			P, T
ISA16	Component Element Separator	AN	1-1	R			
GS	FUNCTIONAL GROUP HEADER		1	R		>1	
GS01	Functional Identifier Code	ID	2-2	R			HR
GS02	Application Sender Code	AN	2-15	R			
GS03	Application Receiver Code	AN	2-15	R			
GS04	Date	DT	8-8	R			CCYYMMDD
GS05	Time	TM	4-8	R			HHMMSSDD
GS06	Group Control Number	N0	1-9	R			
GS07	Responsible Agency Code	ID	1-2	R			X
GS08	Version Identifier Code	AN	1-12	R			005010X212

TABLE 2.1

HIPAA Standards and Transactions

Standard	Transaction
ASC X12 837D	Health care claims—Dental
ASC X12 837P	Health care claims—Professional
ASC X12 837I	Health care claims—Institutional
NCPDP D.0	Health care claims—Retail pharmacy drug
ASC X12 837P and NCPDP D.0	Health care claims—Retail pharmacy supplies and professional services
NCPDP D.0	Coordination of benefits—Retail pharmacy drug
ASC X12 837D	Coordination of benefits—Dental
ASC X12 837P	Coordination of benefits—Professional
ASC X12 837I	Coordination of benefits—Institutional
ASC X12 270/271	Eligibility for a health plan (request and response)—Dental, professional, and institutional
NCPDP D.0	Eligibility for a health plan (request and response)—Retail pharmacy drugs
ASC X12 276/277	Health care claim status (request and response)
ASC X12 834	Enrollment and disenrollment in a health plan
ASC X12 835	Health care payment and remittance advice
ASC X12 820	Health plan premium payment
ASC X12 278	Referral certification and authorization (request and response)—Dental, professional, and institutional
NCPDP D.0	Referral certification and authorization (request and response)—Retail pharmacy drugs
NCPDP 5.1 and NCPDP D.0	Retail pharmacy drug claims (telecommunication and batch standards)
NCPDP 3.0	Medicaid pharmacy subrogation (batch standard)

TABLE 2.2

Comparison of Current and Modified or New Standard Transaction Versions

Standard	Transaction	Through Dec 31, 2011	From Jan 1, 2012
Health Care Claims or Equivalent Encounter Information Transaction	Retail pharmacy drug claims	NCPDP Telecommunication Standard Implementation Guide, Version 5, Release 1 (Version 5.1), Sept. 1999, and equivalent NCPDP Batch Implementation Guide, Version 1, Release 1 (Version 1.1), Jan. 2000, in support of Telecommunication Standard Implementation Guide, Version 5.1, for the NCPDP Data Record in the Detail Data Record	Telecommunication Standard Implementation Guide Version D, Release 0 (Version D.0), Aug. 2007 and equivalent Batch Standard Implementation Guide, Version 1, Release 2 (Version 1.2), NCPDP
	Dental health care claims	Accredited Standards Committee (ASC) X12N 837-Healthcare Claim: Dental, Version 4010, May 2000, WPC, 004010X097, and Addenda to Healthcare Claim: Dental, Version 4010, Oct. 2002, WPC, 004010X097A1	ASC X12 Standards for Electronic Data Interchange Technical Report Type 3-Health Care Claim: Dental (837), May 2006, WPC, 005010X224, and Type 1 Errata to Health Care Claim: Dental (837), ASC X12 Standards for Electronic Data Interchange Technical Report Type 3, Oct. 2007, WPC, 005010X224A1
	Professional health care claims	ASC X12N 837-Healthcare Claim: Professional, Volumes 1 and 2, Version 4010, May 2000, WPC, 004010X098, and Addenda to Healthcare Claim: Professional, Volumes 1 and 2, Version 4010, Oct. 2002, WPC, 004010X098A1	ASC X12 Standards for Electronic Data Interchange Technical Report Type 3-Health Care Claim: Professional (837), May 2006, WPC, 005010X222
	Institutional health care claims	ASC X12N 837-Healthcare Claim: Institutional, Volumes 1 and 2, Version 4010, May 2000, WPC, 004010X096, and Addenda to Healthcare	ASC X12 Standards for Electronic Data Interchange Technical Report Type 3-Health Care Claim: Institutional (837),

TABLE 2.2 (continued)

Comparison of Current and Modified or New Standard Transaction Versions

Standard	Transaction	Through Dec 31, 2011	From Jan 1, 2012
		Claim: Institutional, Volumes 1 and 2, Version 4010, Oct. 2002, WPC, 004010X096A1	May 2006, WPC, 005010X223, and Type 1 Errata to Health Care Claim: Institutional (837), ASC X12 Standards for Electronic Data Interchange Technical Report Type 3, Oct. 2007, WPC, 005010X223A1
	Retail pharmacy supplies and professional services claims		Telecommunication Standard Implementation Guide Version D, Release 0 (Version D.0), Aug. 2007, and equivalent Batch Standard Implementation Guide, Version 1, Release 2 (Version 1.2), NCPDP; and ASC X12 Standards for Electronic Data Interchange Technical Report Type 3-Health Care Claim: Professional (837), May 2006, WPC, 005010X222
Eligibility for a Health Plan	Retail pharmacy drugs	NCPDP Telecommunication Standard Implementation Guide, Version 5, Release 1 (Version 5.1), Sept. 1999, and equivalent NCPDP Batch Implementation Guide, Version 1, Release 1 (Version 1.1), Jan. 2000, in support of Telecommunication Standard Implementation Guide, Version 5.1, for the NCPDP Data Record in the Detail Data Record	Telecommunication Standard Implementation Guide Version D, Release 0 (Version D.0), Aug. 2007, and equivalent Batch Standard Implementation Guide, Version 1, Release 2 (Version 1.2), NCPDP

(continued)

TABLE 2.2 (continued)

Comparison of Current and Modified or New Standard Transaction Versions

Standard	Transaction	Through Dec 31, 2011	From Jan 1, 2012
	Dental, professional, and institutional health care eligibility benefit inquiry and response	ASC X12N 270/271-Healthcare Eligibility Benefit Inquiry and Response, Version 4010, May 2000, WPC, 004010X092, and Addenda to Healthcare Eligibility Benefit Inquiry and Response, Version 4010, Oct. 2002, WPC, 004010X092A1	ASC X12 Standards for Electronic Data Interchange Technical Report Type 3-Health Care Eligibility Benefit Inquiry and Response (270/271), April 2008, WPC, 005010X279
Referral Certification and Authorization	Retail pharmacy drugs	NCPDP Telecommunication Standard Implementation Guide, Version 5, Release 1 (Version 5.1), Sept. 1999, and equivalent NCPDP Batch Implementation Guide, Version 1, Release 1 (Version 1.1), Jan. 2000, in support of Telecommunication Standard Implementation Guide, Version 5.1, for the NCPDP Data Record in the Detail Data Record	Telecommunication Standard Implementation Guide Version D, Release 0 (Version D.0), Aug. 2007, and equivalent Batch Standard Implementation Guide, Version 1, Release 2 (Version 1.2), NCPDP
	Dental, professional, and institutional request for review and response	ASC X12N 278-Healthcare Services Review: Request for Review and Response, Version 4010, May 2000, WPC, 004010X094, and Addenda to Healthcare Services Review: Request for Review and Response, Version 4010, Oct. 2002, WPC, 004010X094A1	ASC X12 Standards for Electronic Data Interchange Technical Report Type 3-Health Care Services Review-Request for Review and Response (278), May 2006, WPC, 005010X217, and Type 1 Errata to Health Care Services Review-Request for Review and Response (278), ASC X12 Standards for Electronic Data Interchange Technical Report Type 3, April 2008, WPC, 005010X217E1

TABLE 2.2 (continued)

Comparison of Current and Modified or New Standard Transaction Versions

Standard	Transaction	Through Dec 31, 2011	From Jan 1, 2012
Health Care Claim Status	Dental, professional, institutional, and pharmacy	ASC X12N 276/277-Healthcare Claim Status Request and Response, Version 4010, May 2000, WPC, 004010X093, and Addenda to Healthcare Claim Status Request and Response, Version 4010, Oct. 2002, WPC, 004010X093A1	ASC X12 Standards for Electronic Data Interchange Technical Report Type 3-Health Care Claim Status Request and Response (276/277), Aug. 2006, WPC, 005010X212, and Type 1 Errata to Health Care Claim Status Request and Response (276/277), ASC X12 Standards for Electronic Data Interchange Technical Report Type 3, April 2008, WPC, 005010X212E1
Enrollment and Disenrollment in a Health Plan		ASC X12N 834-Benefit Enrollment and Maintenance, Version 4010, May 2000, WPC, 004010X095, and Addenda to Benefit Enrollment and Maintenance, Version 4010, Oct. 2002, WPC, 004010X095A1	ASC X12 Standards for Electronic Data Interchange Technical Report Type 3-Benefit Enrollment and Maintenance (834), Aug. 2006, WPC, 005010X220
Health Care Payment and Remittance Advice	Dental, professional, institutional, and pharmacy	ASC X12N 835-Healthcare Claim Payment/Advice, Version 4010, May 2000, WPC, 004010X091, and Addenda to Healthcare Claim Payment/Advice, Version 4010, Oct. 2002, WPC, 004010X091A1	ASC X12 Standards for Electronic Data Interchange Technical Report Type 3-Health Care Claim Payment/ Advice (835), April 2006, WPC, 005010X221
Health Plan Premium Payments		ASC X12N 820-Payroll Deducted and Other Group Premium Payment for Insurance Products, Version 4010, May 2000, WPC, 004010X061, and Addenda to Payroll Deducted and Other Group Premium Payment for Insurance Products, Version 4010, Oct. 2002, WPC, 004010X061A1	ASC X12 Standards for Electronic Data Interchange Technical Report Type 3-Payroll Deducted and Other Group Premium Payment for Insurance Products (820), Feb. 2007, WPC, 005010X218

(continued)

TABLE 2.2 (continued)

Comparison of Current and Modified or New Standard Transaction Versions

Standard	Transaction	Through Dec 31, 2011	From Jan 1, 2012
Coordination of Benefits Information	Retail pharmacy drug claims	NCPDP Telecommunication Standard Implementation Guide, Version 5, Release 1 (Version 5.1), Sept. 1999, and equivalent NCPDP Batch Implementation Guide, Version 1, Release 1 (Version 1.1), Jan. 2000, in support of Telecommunication Standard Implementation Guide, Version 5.1, for the NCPDP Data Record in the Detail Data Record	Telecommunication Standard Implementation Guide Version D, Release 0 (Version D.0), Aug. 2007 and equivalent Batch Standard Implementation Guide, Version 1, Release 2 (Version 1.2), NCPDP
	Dental health care claims	Accredited Standards Committee (ASC) X12N 837-Healthcare Claim: Dental, Version 4010, May 2000, WPC, 004010X097, and Addenda to Healthcare Claim: Dental, Version 4010, Oct. 2002, WPC, 004010X097A1	ASC X12 Standards for Electronic Data Interchange Technical Report Type 3-Health Care Claim: Dental (837), May 2006, WPC, 005010X224, and Type 1 Errata to Health Care Claim: Dental (837) ASC X12 Standards for Electronic Data Interchange Technical Report Type 3, Oct. 2007, WPC, 005010X224A1
	Professional health care claims	ASC X12N 837-Healthcare Claim: Professional, Volumes 1 and 2, Version 4010, May 2000, WPC, 004010X098, and Addenda to Healthcare Claim: Professional, Volumes 1 and 2, Version 4010, Oct. 2002, WPC, 004010X098A1	ASC X12 Standards for Electronic Data Interchange Technical Report Type 3-Health Care Claim: Professional (837), May 2006, WPC, 005010X222
	Institutional health care claims	ASC X12N 837-Healthcare Claim: Institutional, Volumes 1 and 2, Version 4010, May 2000, WPC, 004010X096, and Addenda to Healthcare Claim: Institutional, Volumes 1 and 2, Version 4010, Oct. 2002, WPC, 004010X096A1	ASC X12 Standards for Electronic Data Interchange Technical Report Type 3-Health Care Claim: Institutional (837), May 2006, WPC, 005010X223, and Type 1 Errata to

TABLE 2.2 (continued)

Comparison of Current and Modified or New Standard Transaction Versions

Standard	Transaction	Through Dec 31, 2011	From Jan 1, 2012
			Health Care Claim: Institutional (837), ASC X12 Standards for Electronic Data Interchange Technical Report Type 3, Oct. 2007, WPC, 005010X223A1

Compliance Dates for Final Rule

With one exception, all covered entities must comply with the standards in the final rule by January 1, 2012, less than two years from the date that this was written. The exception is that small health plans have an additional year, to January 1, 2013, to comply with the Medicaid Pharmacy Subrogation Standard. Note the following discussion in the preamble to the final rule:

> Covered entities are urged to begin preparations ***now***, to incorporate effective planning, collaboration and testing in their implementation strategies, and to identify and mitigate barriers long before the deadline. **While we have authorized contingency plans in the past,[33] we do not intend to do so in this case, as such an action would likely adversely impact ICD-10 implementation activities.** HIPAA gives us [HHS] authority to invoke civil money penalties against covered entities who do not comply with the standards, and we have been encouraged by industry to use our authority on a wider scale.[34] [Emphasis added]

As discussed in Chapter 1, the HITECH Act, enacted on February 17, 2009, increased civil financial penalties significantly for noncompliance, effective with enactment of the HITECH Act. Also, as discussed in Chapter 1, enforcement of those HITECH Act penalties was strengthened and enabled, effective November 30, 2009, through an Interim Final Rule published in the *Federal Register* on October 30, 2009. Accordingly, your practice should discuss with your software vendor(s) and other related business associates,[35] such as your health care clearinghouse, how the Version 5010 changes will affect your practice's policies and procedures and how

33. See the discussion earlier in this chapter about the contingency plan regarding the October 2003 transactions and code set compliance date.

34. 74 *Federal Register* 3303.

35. Be sure to update your business associate agreements to bolster the "satisfactory assurances" pertaining to security and privacy obligations required of business associates statutorily under the HITECH Act, which are discussed in Chapter 1.

testing of the transactions will occur with your trading partners (eg, health plans and other health care providers, if applicable).

Testing Requirements and Dates in Final Rule

Again, referring to the preamble of this final rule, HHS outlines *expectations* for covered entities to conduct two levels of testing of the standard transactions.[36] To facilitate testing from the effective date (March 17, 2009) until the compliance date (January 1, 2012) of the final rule, HHS permits, subject to trading partner agreement, "dual use of standards during that timeframe, so that either Version 4010/4010A1 or Version 5010, and either Version 5.1 or D.0, may be used."[37]

Two levels of testing are required under the final rule.

> **Level 1 Testing.** "The Level 1 testing period is the period during which covered entities perform all of their internal readiness activities in preparation for testing the new versions of the standards with their trading partners. When we refer to compliance with Level 1, we mean that a covered entity can demonstrably create and receive compliant transactions, resulting from the completion of all design/build activities and internal testing."[38]

You should have completed your practice's internal readiness activities (eg, gap analysis, design, development, internal testing) by now. If you haven't started, start now!

By the end of 2010, you should have completed internal testing for Versions 5010 and D.0. That means Achieve Level 1 compliance (covered entities have completed internal testing and can send and receive compliant transactions) for Versions 5010 and D.0.

> **Level 2 Testing.** "The Level 2 testing period is the period during which covered entities are preparing to reach full production readiness with all trading partners. When a covered entity is in compliance with Level 2, it has completed end-to-end testing with each of its trading partners, and is able to operate in production mode with the new versions of the standards by the end of that period. By 'production mode,' we mean that covered entities can successfully exchange (accept and/or send) standard transactions and, as appropriate, be able to process them successfully."[39]

- **January 1, 2011.** Begin Level 2 testing period activities (end-to-end testing with trading partners, achieve production mode exchange of appropriate standard transactions with trading partners).
- **January 1, 2012.** "[A]ll covered entities will have reached Level 2 compliance, and must be fully compliant in using Versions 5010 and D.0 exclusively."[40]

---

36. 74 *Federal Register* 3302-3303.
37. 74 *Federal Register* 3306.
38. 74 *Federal Register* 3302.
39. 74 *Federal Register* 3302-3303.
40. 74 *Federal Register* 3303.

AN OVERVIEW OF CODE SETS

"Each year, in the United States, health care insurers process over 5 billion claims for payment. For Medicare and other health insurance programs to ensure that these claims are processed in an orderly and consistent manner, standardized coding systems are essential."[41]

A *code set* is a body of information "used to encode data elements" that is created and maintained by a code set maintaining organization. A code set has predetermined values, which are distinguished from data that would be used to encode data elements based on values drawn, for example, from information about a person such as age.

An example of a code set that is easily recognized is a zip code. A zip code directory, created and maintained by the US Postal Service, is a code set from which you would select a predetermined value based on the location of a particular address. For example, if you knew an address in Charleston, South Carolina, you could go to the zip code directory, look up the street name, and find the zip code.[42] In contrast, age is a value based on personal knowledge that is self-reported or otherwise imparted to you. Both types of values are critical to implementation of standards and populating underlying data elements.

External code sets are integral to the establishment and use of standard transactions. You are not expected to know vast bodies of information that will facilitate an exchange of information in a transaction. You also are not expected to develop your own description of a place or an event because the other party to the transaction may not understand your description. Think what would happen if instead of using a zip code each person used his or her own location rule or description of an event. Usually, an outside body that is recognized as an authority and that has expertise in a particular area or ability to define a common system of rules that will be widely used, either by acceptance or mandate, constructs the rules and values, like zip code. Zip code shall have five numeric characters (numbers) and cover the United States, and zip +4 shall have five numeric characters, a hyphen, and four trailing numeric characters and cover the United States. We learn zip code values from a directory or computer file, write them in correspondence in addresses and return addresses, and everybody uses them. We learn values that define the numeric characteristic of age at an early age, based on a common understanding of implicit rules. Everybody uses zip codes and everybody defines the numeric characteristic of age in round numbers, say between 1 and 80, but we just get the values from different sources.

---

41. See *Healthcare Common Procedure Coding System (HCPCS)*-General Information, which is available at: www.cms.gov/MedHCPCSGENInfo/.

42. At the Web site, www.usps.com, you can click on "Find a Zip Code," enter the number and street address, city, and state, and receive a Zip+4 code in response. This is an example of accessing an external code set. You will learn in Chapter 3 that zip code is one of eighteen (18) protected health information (PHI) identifiers when used in conjunction with other PHI identifiers.

Explicit code sets such as zip code and implicit rules such as age are both subject to explicit rules on how they are used in HIPAA transaction standards.

Code Sets in the Physician's Office

If you work in a physician's practice, you may only use a small subset of procedure codes, with which you will become familiar over a period of time. Similarly, a back office coder in a physician's office or in a payer's office will develop a working knowledge of these code sets over time. It is important that within the physician's practice that the service rendered is translated into the appropriate procedure code and that procedure code is accurately reflected in the data set comprising the standard transaction for a claim.[43] Knowledge of the rules of how procedure codes are handled in electronic standard transactions (eg, the claim transaction) will enhance the likelihood that transaction standards are transmitted error free from the physician's practice. Doing so will speed up the response from the payer, minimize time in the practice correcting errors and resubmitting claims, or, for that matter, transactions such as an eligibility inquiry or claim status inquiry.

BUSINESS TIP

Knowledge of the rules of how procedure codes are handled in electronic standard transactions in the practice will enhance the likelihood that transaction standards are transmitted error free, will elicit quick response from the payer, and minimize time correcting errors and resubmitting claims.

Whether you are in a practice or in a health plan payment environment, you also will want to ensure that your software vendor is knowledgeable about the code sets and the rules by which they are used in the transaction standards. Remember, as the covered entity, the health care provider and health plan are responsible for compliant transactions, so the vendor's activities are your responsibility.[44]

---

43. With increasing deployment of electronic health record (EHR) systems and integration or interface with practice management systems in the coming decade, the appropriate procedure code(s) will be automatically determined by the entries in the EHR that characterize the rendering of services by the physician during the encounter.

44. Your practice's software vendor or clearinghouse, in a business associate role, may be subject to civil penalties for violations of standard transaction rules beginning February 17, 2010, when business associates, as required by the HITECH Act, are statutorily regulated directly by the federal government rather than indirectly by covered entities with respect to the HIPAA Security Rule and certain provisions of the HIPAA Privacy Rule, including Breach Notification. Such violations could be discovered during a security or privacy compliance audit or complaint investigation, conducted by the Department of Health and Human Services (HHS) Office for Civil Rights (OCR), and referred to the Centers for Medicare & Medicaid Services (CMS), which has responsibility for enforcing compliance with standard transactions and code sets rules.

CODE SET CATEGORIES

There are two categories of code sets:

- Medical data code sets that are *specified* in the Transactions and Code Sets Final Rule and in the implementation guides
- Nonmedical data code sets, which are *described* in the implementation guides

Each of these types of code sets is discussed here.

Medical Data Code Sets

Each of the standard transactions involves an exchange of information between a health care provider and a health plan, regarding the delivery of health care or the financing of health care or health care benefits. To make the exchange meaningful and understandable, each party to the exchange has to be able to interpret precisely what the other is conveying. With the complexity and variety of actions in the health care field, the common language is a set of four broad types of medical data code sets:

- Coding systems for diseases, impairments, or other health-related problems
- Causes of injury, disease, impairment, or other health-related problems
- Actions taken to prevent, diagnose, treat, or manage diseases, injuries, and impairments
- Any substances, equipment, supplies, or other item used to perform these actions.

The Secretary of HHS has adopted these specified code sets that encompass the four types of medical data code sets identified above.[45]

- *International Classification of Diseases*, 9th Edition, *Clinical Modification* (ICD-9-CM), Volumes 1 and 2, as updated and distributed by HHS for the following conditions:
  - Diseases
  - Injuries
  - Impairments
  - Other health-related problems and their manifestations
  - Causes of injury, disease, impairment, or other health-related problems.
- *International Classification of Diseases*, 9th Edition, *Clinical Modification* (ICD-9-CM), Volume 3, Procedures, as updated and distributed by HHS for procedures or actions taken for diseases, injuries, and impairments on *hospital* inpatients reported by hospitals, such as:
  - Prevention
  - Diagnosis

45. See Center for Medicare & Medicaid Services (CMS), *Transaction and Code Sets Standards*, which is available at: www.cms.hhs.gov/TransactionCodeSetsStands/.

- ☐ Treatment
- ☐ Management.

- National Drug Codes (NDC), as maintained and distributed by HHS for reporting by retail pharmacies on drugs and biologics.[46]
- Code on Dental Procedures and Nomenclature, as maintained and distributed by the American Dental Association (ADA) for dental services.[47]
- The combination of Healthcare Common Procedure Coding System (HCPCS), as maintained and distributed by HHS, and *Current Procedural Terminology* (CPT®) coding system, as maintained and distributed by the American Medical Association (AMA) for physician and other health care services, including, but not limited to:
  - ☐ Physician services
  - ☐ Physical and occupational therapy services
  - ☐ Radiologic procedures
  - ☐ Clinical laboratory tests
  - ☐ Other medical diagnostic procedures
  - ☐ Transportation services, including ambulance.
- HCPCS Level II,[48] as maintained and distributed by HHS, for all other substances, equipment, supplies, or other items used in health care services, with the exception of drugs and biologics, including, but not limited to:
  - ☐ Medical supplies
  - ☐ Orthodontic and prosthetic devices
  - ☐ Durable medical equipment.

An issue regarding use of NDC and HCPCS codes was resolved with publication of the modification to the final rule on February 20, 2003, namely, the adoption of the NDC standard for Retail Pharmacy transactions and no standard for non-Retail Pharmacy transactions.[49] In the final Transaction and Code Set Standard (TCS) Rule published on August 17, 2000, Retail Pharmacy and non-Retail Professional, Institutional, and Dental transactions had to use the NDC.[50] In the proposed modification published

---

46. See U.S. Food and Drug Administration (FDA), *National Drug Code Directory*, which is available at: www.fda.gov/Drugs/InformationOnDrugs/ucm142438.htm.
47. See American Dental Association (ADA), *Code on Dental Procedures and Nomenclature*, which is available at: www.ada.org/3827.aspx. "The version of the *Code* that is effective January 1, 2009 through December 31, 2010 is published by the ADA in the manual titled *CDT 2009/2010*."
48. See *Healthcare Common Procedure Coding System (HCPCS)* Level II Coding Procedures, Revision December 18, 2009, which is available at: www.cms.gov/MedHCPCSGenInfo/.
49. 68 *Federal Register* 8381–8399.
50. 65 *Federal Register* 50370.

on May 31, 2002, NDC would be the standard code only for Retail Pharmacy transactions, with no standard for non-Retail Pharmacy transactions. However, HHS also solicited comments from the public on whether using HCPCS for non-Retail Pharmacy transactions should be the standard in lieu of having no standard for those transactions.[51]

In its decision-making process, HHS considered a variety of comments from the public.[52] HHS noted that "the NDC and HCPCS remain two of the most prevalent and useful code sets for reporting drugs and biologics in non-Retail Pharmacy transactions," and that in the absence of a standard, "the selection of the code set to be used would likely be specified by health plans via trading partner agreements, as long as the Implementation Guides permitted that selection."[53] Implementation Guides permit the use of NDC or HCPSC in non-Retail Pharmacy transactions.

Another important factor in the decision-making process was fostering development of new code sets:

> Another significant advantage to repealing the adoption of the NDC for reporting drugs and biologics in non-retail pharmacy standard transactions and not adopting a replacement standard code set at this time is that the industry and HHS will have time to explore the development of a new drug coding system to meet current and future needs of this sector of the health care industry.[54]

Any new code set would have to be included in the Implementation Guides, which would involve, as a first step, proposing the code set and supporting its business case as part of the Designated Standard Maintenance Organization (DSMO) process.[55]

Another important issue with regard to code sets concerned the use of HCPCS Level 3 codes on a local basis. Health care delivery is essentially local, so over time codes evolved for alterations or modifications to procedures that had a local or regional character. Local or regional private payers or state payers such as Medicaid could accommodate these codes in a nonstandard, proprietary electronic environment in which both the health care provider and payer recognized the codes. However, with national standards, local codes should not be used. As a result, HIPAA Administrative Simplification transaction standards do not permit their use. If users can justify on business grounds the use of new national codes, they can apply to CMS for HCPCS and AMA for CPT® consideration of the new codes, which would then go through the DSMO process for validation of business

---

51. 67 *Federal Register* 38044–38050.

52. 68 *Federal Register* 8385–8387.

53. 68 *Federal Register* 8386.

54. 68 *Federal Register* 8387.

55. While it is beyond the scope of the discussion here, information on the DSMO process is available at 68 *Federal Register* 8382. Also, see *HIPAA-DSMO Transaction Change Request System*, which is available at: www.hipaa-dsmo.org/Main.asp.

need. We shall see later in this chapter how ICD-10 codes will supplant ICD-9 codes beginning on October 1, 2013.

Nonmedical Data Code Sets

To conduct any of the standard transactions, there are a variety of nonmedical data code sets that must accompany the exchange of medical information. For example, in identifying the location of a physical address, all standard transactions require the use of a zip code, which is a commonly known nonmedical data code set. A less well-known code set is a US Department of Defense (DOD) *pay grade*, known as DOD2, which is only used in the Health Care Eligibility Benefit Inquiry and Response (270/271) transaction standard.

HOW TO READ CODE SETS

Nonmedical and medical data code sets are listed in "Appendix A: External Code Sources," of each of the ASC X12N 5010 Implementation Guides.[56] Table 2.3 lists the external data code sets and shows their applicability for each of the ASC X12N transaction standards that an Implementation Guide represents.

"Appendix A: External Code Sources" in each of the Technical Reports Type 3 identifies each code set by a *code source number* and *code set name*, and categorizes each code set in four ways:

- Simple data element/code references
- Source
- Available from
- Abstract.[57]

We reproduced two examples from Appendix A of the ASC X12N Implementation Guide: *Health Care Services Review—Request for Review and Response (278)*, ASC X12N/005010X217, May 2006:[58]

---

56. These External Code Sets require compliance on January 1, 2012, when 5010 transactions standards must be used. A similar table for External Code Sets in use through December 31, 2011, can be found in Table 4.1 (pp. 65–67) of our book: Jones, ED and Hartley, CP. *HIPAA Transactions: A Nontechnical Business Guide for Health Care.* Chicago, IL: American Medical Association Press, 2004.

57. The abstract is the descriptor of a code set.

58. Accredited Standards Committee X12, Insurance Subcommittee, ASC X12N, as referenced in text. For more information, visit the Web site for Washington Publishing Company at www.wpc-edi.com.

TABLE 2.3

Version 5010 External Codes

External Set	212	217	218	220	221	222	223	224	279
4 ABA Routing Number			X		X				
5 Countries, Currencies and Funds		X	X	X	X	X	X	X	X
16 D-U-N-S Number			X						
22 States and Provinces		X	X	X	X	X	X	X	X
51 Zip Code		X	X	X	X	X	X	X	X
60 (DFI) Identification Code			X		X				
91 Canadian Financial Institution Branch and Institution Number			X		X				
94 International Organization for Standardization (Date and Time)				X					
102 Languages				X					
121 Health Industry Number					X				
130 Healthcare Common Procedural Coding System	X	X			X	X	X		X
131 International Classification of Diseases, 9th Revision, Clinical Modification (ICD-9-CM)		X		X		X	X	X	X
132 National Uniform Billing Committee (NUBC) Codes	X				X	X	X		
133 Current Procedural Terminology (CPT) Codes									X
135 American Dental Association	X	X			X			X	X
139 Claim Adjustment Reason Code					X	X	X	X	
206 Government Bill of Lading Office Code				X					X
229 Diagnosis Related Group Number		X			X		X		
230 Admission Source Code		X					X		
231 Admission Type Code		X					X		
235 Claim Frequency Type Code		X			X	X	X	X	
236 Uniform Billing Claim Form Bill Type		X					X		
237 Place of Service Codes for Professional Claims		X				X		X	X
239 Patient Status Code		X					X		
240 National Drug Code by Format	X	X			X	X	X		X
245 National Association of Insurance Commissioners (NAIC)					X	X	X	X	

(continued)

TABLE 2.3 (continued)

Version 5010 External Codes

External Set	212	217	218	220	221	222	223	224	279
284 Nature of Injury Code									x
307 National Council for Prescription Drug Programs Pharmacy Number				x	x				x
327 Society for Worldwide Interbank Financial Telecommunication (SWIFT)			x						
359 Treatment Codes							x		
407 Occupational Injury and Illness Classification Manual									x
411 Remittance Advice Remark Codes					x	x	x	x	
457 NISO Z39.53 Language Code List				x					
468 Ambulatory Payment Classification					x				
507 Health Care Claim Status Category Code	x								
508 Health Care Claim Status Code	x								
513 Home Infusion EDI Coalition (HIEC) Product/Service Code List	x	x			x	x	x		x
530 National Council for Prescription Drug Programs Reject/Payment Codes	x				x				
537 Centers for Medicare and Medicaid Services (CMS) National Provider Identifier	x	x		x	x	x	x	x	x
540 CMS PlanID	x	x	x	x	x	x	x	x	x
576 Workers Compensation Specific Procedure and Supply Codes	x				x	x	x	x	
582 CMS Durable Medical Equipment Regional Carrier (DMERC) Certificate of Medical Necessity (CMN) Forms						x			
656 Form Type Codes						x			
663 Logical Observation Identifier Names and Codes (LOINC)		x							
682 Health Care Provider Taxonomy		x				x	x	x	x

TABLE 2.3 (continued)

Version 5010 External Codes

External Set	212	217	218	220	221	222	223	224	279
716 Health Insurance Prospective Payment System (HIPPS) Rate Code for Skilled Nursing Facilities	X				X		X		
843 Advanced Billing Concepts (ABC) Codes	X	X			X	X	X		
844 Eligibility Category									X
859 Classification of Race or Ethnicity				X					
860 Race or Ethnicity Collection Code				X					
886 Health Care Service Review Decision Reason Codes		X							
896 International Classification of Diseases, 10th Revision, Procedure Coding System (ICD-10-PCS)				X			X		X
897 International Classification of Diseases, 10th Revision, Clinical Modification (ICD-10-CM)		X				X	X	X	X
932 Universal Postal Codes		X	X	X	X	X	X	X	X
DOD1 Military Rank and Health Care Service Region									X
DOD2 Paygrade									X

Legend

212: Health Care Claim Status Request and Response (276/277), WPC, August 2006.

217: Health Care Services Review--Request for Review and Response (278), WPC, May 2006.

218: Payroll Deducted and Other Group Premium Payment for Insurance Products (820), WPC, February 2007.

220: Benefit Enrollment and Maintenance (834), WPC, August 2006.

221: Health Care Claim Payment/Advice (835), WPC, April 2006.

222: Health Care Claim: Professional (837), WPC, May 2006.

223: Health Care Claim: Institutional (837), WPC, May 2006.

224: Health Care Claim: Dental (837), WPC, May 2006.

279: Health Care Eligibility Benefit Inquiry and Response (270/271), WPC, April 2008.

Source

Accredited Standards Committee (ASC) X12, Insurance Subcommittee, ASC X12N. "Appendix A: External Code Sources" of Documents Referenced in Legend. Washington Publishing Company (WPC), www.wpc-edi.com.

Code Source Number 51: Code Set Name: Zip Code

- *Simple Data Element/Code References*[59]
  - 116, 66/16, 309/PQ, 309/PR, 309/PS, 771/010
- *Source*
  - National Zip Code and Post Office Directory, Publication 65, The USPS Domestic Mail Manual
- *Available From*
  - US Postal Service, Washington, DC 20260; New Orders, Superintendent of Documents, P.O. Box 371954, Pittsburgh, PA 15250-7954
- *Abstract*

The zip code is a geographic identifier of areas within the United States and its territories for purposes of expediting mail distribution by the US Postal Service. It is five or nine numeric digits. The zip code structure divides the US into ten large groups of states. The left-most digit identifies one of these groups. The next two digits identify a smaller geographic area within the large group. The two rightmost digits identify a local delivery area. In the nine-digit zip code, the four digits that follow the hyphen further subdivide the delivery area. The two leftmost digits identify a sector, which may consist of several large buildings, blocks, or groups of streets. The rightmost digits divide the sector into segments such as a street, a block, a floor of a building, or a cluster of mailboxes.

The USPS Domestic Mail Manual includes information on the use of the new 11-digit zip code.

Code Source Number 897: Code Set Name: International Classification of Diseases, 10th Revision, Clinical Modification (ICD-10-CM)

- *Simple Data Element/Code References*
  - 235/DC, 1270/ABF, 1270/ABJ, 1270/ABK, 1270/ABN, 1270/ABU, 1270/ABV, 1270/ADD, 1270/APR, 1270/ASD, 1270/ATD.
- *Source*
  - *International Classification of Diseases*, 10th Revision, *Clinical Modification* (ICD-10-CM)
- *Available From*

  OCD/Classifications and Public Health Data Standards
  National Center for Health Statistics
  3311 Toledo Road
  Hyattsville, MD 20782
- *Abstract*

  The International Classification of Diseases, 10th Revision, *Clinical Modification* (ICD-10-CM), describes the classification of morbidity and

59. The category, Simple Data Element/Code References identifies where in the transaction the code set is used.

mortality information for statistical purposes and for the indexing of hospital records by diseases.

Zip code is used with each of the transaction standards, except *Health Care Claim Status and Response (276/277)* (ASC X12N/005010X212), when these standard transactions require compliance on January 1, 2012. ICD-10-CM is used with the following transactions:

- *Health Care Services Review—Request for Review and Response (278)*(ASC X12N/005010X217)
- *Health Care Claim: Professional (837)*(ASC X12N/005010X222)
- *Health Care Claim: Institutional (837)*(ASC X12N/005010X223)
- *Health Care Claim: Dental (837)* (ASC X12N/005010X224)
- *Health Care Eligibility Benefit Inquiry and Response (270/271)* (ASC X12N/005010X279).

Note that the ICD-10-CM code set for diagnosis coding requires compliance on October 1, 2013.[60]

When checking on any external code, it is important to examine in which standard transactions that it is used and where. The "where" is found in the *Simple Data Element/Code References* category, and the entries are the same across standard transactions in which a specified code set is used.

The best way to find these is to use in the current 4010 version the *Health Care Data Element Dictionary*, which is available for Internet download from Washington Publishing Company (WPC) in portable document format (pdf) for $175.[61]

ICD-10: Code Set Standards Modification

Introduction. The Notice of proposed rulemaking (NPRM) for ICD-10 was published in the *Federal Register* on August 22, 2008,[62] the same day that the NPRM for Version 5010 was published in the *Federal Register*. Then, on

60. Physicians will be required to use ICD-10-CM on and after October 1, 2013, to code diagnosis, but will not be required to use ICD-10-PCS procedure codes in a nonpatient (ambulatory) setting.

61. For more information, please visit Washington Publishing Company (WPC) at www.wpc-edi.com. This document also is available in book or CD versions. According to e-mail correspondence between Steve Bass of Washington Publishing Company and Ed Jones dated February 8, 2010, WPC plans to publish a 5010-data dictionary later in 2010.

62. Department of Health and Human Services, Office of the Secretary, "45 CFR Parts 160 and 162—HIPAA Administrative Simplification: Modification to Medical Data Code Set Standards to Adopt ICD-10-CM and ICD-10-PCS; Proposed Rule," *Federal Register*, v.73, n.164, August 22, 2008, pp. 49795–49832. Hereinafter, citations will be in the standard format 73 *Federal Register* <page(s)>.

January 16, 2009, the final ICD-10 rule was published,[63] again on the same day as the final rule for Version 5010. These two rules go together: ICD-10 cannot work with the existing 4010/4010A transaction standards, and 5010 needs to be in place before to accommodate a different ICD-10 data element character length. Below, we discuss both the proposed and final ICD-10 rulings.

The ICD-10 rule comprises two parts:

- International Classification of Diseases, Tenth Revision, Clinical Modification (ICD-10-CM) for diagnosis coding
- International Classification of Diseases, Tenth Revision, Procedure Coding System (ICD-10-PCS) for inpatient hospital procedure coding only.[64]

Only ICD-10-CM is germane to physician practice generated transactions. However, physicians that practice in hospitals, on staff or privileged, will have to have acquaintance with the structure of the ICD-10-PCS procedural codes.

International Classification of Diseases (ICD) is developed and maintained by the World Health Organization. The National Center for Health Statistics (NCHS), part of the Centers for Disease Control and Prevention (CDC), has responsibility for implementation of the ICD.

The currently used ICD-9-CM diagnosis codes, were "adopted as a HIPAA [code set] standard in 2000 for reporting diagnoses, injuries, impairments, and other health problems and their manifestations, and causes of injury, disease, impairment or other health problems in standard transactions."[65] ICD-9-CM diagnoses codes, of which there are approximately 13,000[66] are 3 to 5 digits in length.

The ICD-9-CM code set functionality "has been exhausted" and "is nearing the end of its useful life."[67] In addition to space limitations, there are three other key reasons to replace it[68]:

- Effects of Work-arounds on Structural Hierarchy
  - Some parts of the ICD-9-CM are full, so codes "must be assigned to other topically unrelated chapters," making the codes sometimes difficult to find.

63. Department of Health and Human Services, Office of the Secretary, "45 CFR Part 162—HIPAA Administrative Simplification: Modifications to Medical Data Code Set Standards to Adopt ICD-10-CM and ICD-10-PCS; Final Rule," *Federal Register*, v.74, n.11, January 16, 2009, pp. 3328–3362. Hereinafter, citations will be in the standard format 74 *Federal Register* <page(s)>.

64. Non-inpatient (ambulatory) providers will continue to use CPT-4 and HCPCS codes for coding procedures.

65. 73 *Federal Register* 49798.

66. 73 *Federal Register* 49799.

67. Ibid.

68. Ibid.

- Lack of Detail:
  - "[I]n an age of electronic health records, it does not make sense to use a coding system that lacks specificity and does not lend itself well to updates.... Emerging health care technologies, new and advanced terminologies, and the need for interoperability amid the increase in electronic health records (EHRs) and personal health records (PHRs) require a standard code set that is expandable and sufficiently detailed to accurately capture current and future health care information."
- Obsolescence
  - ICD-9-CM is no longer supported or maintained by the World Health Organization: "As we [United States] become a global community, it is vital that our health care data represent current medical conditions and technologies, and that they are compatible with the international version of ICD-10."

In contrast to the ICD-9-CM, "ICD-10-CM diagnosis codes are three (3) to seven (7) alphanumeric characters," and "the number of ICD-10-CM codes is approximately 68,000. The ICD-10-CM code set provides much more information and detail within the codes than ICD-9-CM, facilitating timely electronic processing of claims by reducing requests for additional information."[69] This last point is very important: in conjunction with Version 5010 transaction standards modifications, ICD-10-CM will facilitate better information exchange between health care stakeholders, thereby leading to more efficient processing of claims and payments. Looking to the future, the ICD-10 NPRM concludes that "ICD-10 code sets provide a standard coding convention that is flexible, providing unique codes for all substantially different procedures of health conditions and allowing new procedures and diagnoses to be easily incorporated as new codes for both existing and future clinical protocols."[70]

The ICD-10 NPRM provided a compliance date of October 1, 2011, for use of ICD-10-CM in physician practices and by other covered entities. During the public comment period, the Workgroup for Electronic Data Interchange (WEDI), in its advisory role to HHS under the HIPAA Administrative Simplification legislation and enabling regulations, submitted comments on the ICD-10 NPRM to HHS, indicating that the compliance date did not provide sufficient time for a successful implementation in the health care industry.[71] Instead, WEDI "recommends that a minimum of four years will be needed after completion of transaction upgrades and a total of six years after publication of the final rules for upgrades of transactions and medical code sets (October 1 after the anniversary of the sixth year).[72] That would make the compliance

69. 73 *Federal Register* 49801.

70. 73 *Federal Register* 49800.

71. Letter from Jim Whicker, Chairman, WEDI, to Centers for Medicare & Medicaid Services, October 20, 2008. See www.wedi.org.

72. Ibid.

date near or several years after the end of the "Decade of Health Information Technology" in 2014. By taking so long, the US health care industry would be unable to achieve in a timely manner the objectives of implementing electronic health records (EHRs)[73] and interoperability, which cannot be done without updating its code sets. As we shall see in the discussion below on the final ICD-10 rule, the compliance date is October 1, 2013, just prior to the completion of the Decade of HIT.

In 2005, Linda Kloss, CEO of Chicago-based American Health Information Management Association (AHIMA), made the following statement:

> The full benefits of an EHR can only be realized if we improve the quality of data that EHRs are designed to manage. The current classification coding system used in the US, ICD-9-CM is a 30-year-old system and can no longer accurately describe today's practice of medicine. Continuing to use this system jeopardizes the ability to effectively collect and use accurate, detailed healthcare data and information for the betterment of domestic and global healthcare. By failing to upgrade, we could find ourselves building an infrastructure that does not provide the information necessary to meet the healthcare demands of the 21st century.[74]

On November 5, 2003, the National Committee on Vital and Health Statistics (NCVHS) recommended in a letter to then Secretary of the HHS, Tommy Thompson, that ICD-10-CM be adopted as a HIPAA Administrative Simplification code set standard.[75] NCVHS made the following observation in its letter:

> Benefits are harder to quantify, but appear to outweigh the costs. They include facilitating improvements to the quality of care and patient safety, fewer rejected claims, improved information for disease management, and more accurate reimbursement rates for emerging technologies. These costs and benefits and related issues also have been substantially documented in testimony before the Subcommittee, as well as in a cost/benefit study by the RAND Corporation (RAND)[76] that was specially commissioned by NCVHS.

---

73. The HITECH Act discussed in Chapter 1 and final enabling regulations pertaining to Stage 1 "meaningful use" criteria and 2011–2014 "incentives" for EHR adoption that were published in the Federal Register on July 28, 2010 and referenced in that chapter, clearly emphasize federal urgency in moving forward with EHR adoption sooner rather than later. See 75 Federal Register 44313–44588 and 75 Federal Register 44589–44654, both published on July 28, 2010.

74. Linda Kloss, "The Promise of ICD-10-CM. *Health Management Technology*, July 2005, p.48. This article is available at www.healthmgttech.com.

75. This letter is available at www.ncvhs.hhs.gov/031105lt.htm.

76. The referenced RAND study is MC Libicki and IT Brahmakulam, *The Costs and Benefits of Moving to the ICD-10 Code Sets*. TR-132-DHS. Santa Monica, CA: RAND Corporation, March 2004. This report is available at: www.rand.org/pubs/technical_reports/2004/RAND_TR132.sum.pdf.

The ICD-10 NPRM highlights projected benefits,[77] summarized as:

- More accurate payments for new procedures
- Fewer rejected claims
- Fewer improper claims
- Better understanding of new procedures
- Improved disease management
- Better understanding of health conditions and health care outcomes.

For physician practices, the NPRM analysis estimates that the practices on average will experience costs of 0.04 percent of revenue/receipts, which "include a portion of the coding training costs and productivity losses in addition to costs directly allocated to physicians and practice expenses."[78]

The costs and benefits will have to be determined by each practice. However, it appears reasonable to assume that if ICD-9-CM is "exhausted" and that benefits would accrue to use of ICD-10-CM, in contrast to WEDI's recommendation of further delay to the future, that the federal government and the health care industry may wish to proceed with all deliberate speed in a concentrated effort to implement ICD-10-CM sooner rather than later! The October 1, 2013, compliance date is a step in the right direction.

ICD-10 Final Rule. The final rule adopts modifications to two code set standards in the Transactions and Code Sets final rule that required compliance by covered entities on or after October 16, 2003. The new final rule, published in the *Federal Register* on January 16, 2009, modifies standard medical data code sets for coding diagnoses (ICD-10-CM)[79] and inpatient hospital procedures (ICD-10-PCS).[80] Noninpatient (ambulatory) procedures continue to be coded under the existing and new final rules using Current Procedural Terminology, 4th Edition (CPT-4) and Healthcare Common Procedure Coding Systems (HCPCS). Table 2.4 compares code sets under existing and modified rules.

77. 73 *Federal Register* 49821.

78. 73 *Federal Register* 49820.

79. ICD-10-CM means International Classification of Diseases, 10th Revision, Clinical Modification for diagnosis coding, including the Official ICD-10-CM Guidelines for Coding and Reporting, as maintained and distributed by the U.S. Department of Health and Human Services (HHS).

80. ICD-10-PCS means International Classification of Diseases, 10th Revision, Procedure Coding System for inpatient hospital procedure coding, including the Official ICD-10-PCS Guidelines for Coding and Reporting, as maintained and distributed by HHS.

TABLE 2.4

Modification of Transaction and Code Set Rule Diagnosis and Procedure Codes

	Current Code Set Rule	Modified Code Set Rule
All Diagnoses	International Classification of Diseases, 9th Revision, Clinical Modification, Volumes 1 and 2, including the Official ICD-9-CM Guidelines for Coding and Reporting, known as ICD-9-CM Volumes 1 and 2.	ICD-10-CM
Inpatient Procedures	International Classification of Diseases, 9th Revision, Clinical Modification, Volume 3, including the Official ICD-9-CM Guidelines for Coding and Reporting, known as ICD-9-CM Volume 3.	ICD-10-PCS
Non-Inpatient (Ambulatory) Procedures	CPT-4 and HCPCS	CPT-4 and HCPCS

Effective Date. The effective date of the ICD-10 final rule was March 17, 2009. "The effective date is the date that the policies herein take effect, and new policies are considered to be officially adopted."[81]

Compliance Date. The compliance date for the modification of the diagnosis and procedure code rule from ICD-9 to ICD-10 is **October 1, 2013**. "The compliance date is the date on which entities are required to have implemented the policies adopted in this rule."[82]

October 1 was chosen to coincide with the effective date of the annual Medicare Inpatient Prospective Payment System. The ICD-10 compliance date is 21 months after the compliance date for the 5010 Rule. Based on health care industry input, "it appears that 24 months (2 years) is the minimum amount of time that the industry needs to achieve compliance with ICD-10 once Version 5010 has moved into external (Level 2) testing,"[83] which commences January 1, 2011 (33 months before the ICD-10 compliance date).

> HHS has concluded that it would be in the health care industry's best interests if **all entities** [emphasis added] were to comply with the ICD-10 code set standards at the same time to ensure the accuracy and timeliness of claims and transaction processing.... The availability and use of crosswalks, mappings and guidelines should assist entities in making the switchover from ICD-9 to ICD-10 code sets on October 1, 2013, without the need for the concurrent use of both code sets [ICD-9 and ICD-10] in claims processing, medical record and related systems with respect to claims for services provided on the same day.... HHS believes that different compliance dates

81. 74 *Federal Register* 3328.

82. Ibid.

83. 74 *Federal Register* 3334.

based on the size of a health plan would also be problematic since a provider has no way of knowing if a health plan qualifies as a small health plan or not.[84]

As is presently the case, coding before, on, or after the compliance date is based on the *date of discharge*.

Testing. "HHS has not established dates for Level 1 and Level 2 testing compliance for ICD-10 implementation. We encourage all industry segments to be ready to test their systems with ICD-10 as soon as it is feasible."[85] Recalling definitions of Level 1 and 2 testing from the 5010 final rule:

> *Level 1 Testing:* "The level 1 testing period is the period during which covered entities perform all of their internal readiness activities in preparation for testing the new versions of the standards with their trading partners. When we refer to compliance with Level 1, we mean that a covered entity can demonstrably create and receive compliant transactions, resulting from the completion of all design/build activities and internal testing."[86]
>
> *Level 2 Testing:* "The Level 2 testing period is the period during which covered entities are preparing to reach full production readiness with all trading partners. When a covered entity is in compliance with Level 2, it has completed end-to-end testing with each of its trading partners, and is able to operate in production mode with the new versions of the standards by the end of that period. By 'production mode,' we mean that covered entities can successfully exchange (accept and/or send) standard transactions and as appropriate, be able to process them successfully."[87]

Crosswalks. HHS acknowledges that crosswalks or mappings of data element code values between ICD-9 and ICD-10 "will be critical." HIPAA Administrative Simplification requires under Section 1174(b)(2)(B)(ii) of the Act that "if a code set is modified under this subsection, the modified code set shall include instructions on how data elements of health information that were encoded prior to the modification may be converted or translated so as to preserve the informational value of the data elements that existed before the modification ... and in a manner that minimizes the disruption and cost of complying with such modification."[88] Bi-directional crosswalks that can translate from the old code to the new or from the new to the old are referred to as *General Equivalency Mappings*.

The National Center for Health Statistics (NCHS) of the Centers for Disease Control and Prevention (CDC) is responsible in the United States for use of the International Statistical Classification of Diseases, Tenth Revision, Clinical Modification (ICD-10-CM), and has a Web site at www.cdc.gov/nchs/icd/icd10cm.htm#10update. As this is written in

84. 74 Federal Register 3335.

85. 74 *Federal Register* 3336.

86. 74 *Federal Register* 3302.

87. Ibid.

88. 74 *Federal Register* 3337.

late-July 2010, the ICD-10-CM site indicates that it is current as of the latest update, April 22, 2010. We reproduce here detail from the ICD-10 site:

> The ICD-10 is copyrighted by the World Health Organization (WHO), which owns and publishes the classification. WHO has authorized the development of an adaptation of ICD-10 for use in the United States for U.S. Government purposes. As agreed, all modifications to the ICD-10 must conform to WHO conventions for the ICD. ICD-10-CM was developed following a thorough evaluation by a Technical Advisory panel and extensive additional consultation with physician groups, clinical coders, and others to assure clinical accuracy and utility.

The entire draft of the Tabular List of ICD-10-CM, and the preliminary crosswalk between ICD-9-CM and ICD-10-CM were made available on the NCHS web site for public comment. The public comment period ran from December 1997 through February 1998. The American Hospital Association [AHA] and the American Health Information Management Association [AHIMA] conducted a field test for ICD-10-CM in the summer of 2003, with a subsequent report of their findings.[89] All comments and suggestions from the open comment period and the field test were reviewed, and additional modifications to ICD-10-CM were made based on these comments and suggestions. Additionally, new concepts have been added to ICD-10-CM based on the established update process for ICD-9-CM (the ICD-9-CM Coordination and Maintenance Committee) and the World Health Organization's ICD-10 (the Update and Revision Committee). This represents ICD-9-CM modifications from 2003–2009 and ICD-10 modifications from 2002–2008.

The clinical modification represents a significant improvement over ICD-9-CM and ICD-10. Specific improvements include: the addition of information relevant to ambulatory and managed care encounters; expanded injury codes; the creation of combination diagnosis/symptom codes to reduce the number of codes needed to fully describe a condition; the addition of sixth and seventh characters; incorporation of common 4th and 5th digit subclassifications; laterality; and greater specificity in code assignment. The new structure will allow further expansion than was possible with ICD-9-CM.

> **"2010 Update of ICD-10-CM**
>
> [The] files linked below are the 2010 update of the ICD-10-CM. Content changes to the Tabular and to the General Equivalence Mapping Files are described in separate files that are included along with the main files compressed in zip format....
>
> **Although this release of ICD-10-CM is now available for public viewing, the codes in ICD-10-CM are not currently valid for any purpose or use. The effective implementation date for ICD-10-CM (and ICD-10-PCS) is October 1, 2013. Updates to this version [2010] are anticipated prior to implementation of ICD-10-CM."** [Emphasis added]

---

89. AHA and AHIMA, *ICD-10-CM Field Testing Project: Report on Findings—Perceptions, Ideas and Recommendations from Coding Professionals Across the Nation*, September 23, 2003, which is available at: www.ahima.org/icd10/documents/FinalStudy_000.pdf.

The 2010 files that currently are available on the ICD-10-CM web site are the following:

- Preface
- Guidelines
- Index to Diseases and Injury
- Tabular List
- Index to External Causes of Injury
- Table of Drugs and Chemicals
- Table of Neoplasms
- General Equivalence Mapping Files
- Tabular Addenda
- Tabular Addenda Errata
- Index Addenda.

We recommend that you refer to the ICD-10-CM files periodically—and in particular the General Equivalence Mapping Files—to keep abreast of changes in ICD-10-CM before the implementation date of October 1, 2013, and to be familiar with the way ICD-10-CM differs in format and content with ICD-9-CM.

CMS also has a useful ICD-10 Provider Resources web page, www.cms.gov/ICD10/05a_ProviderResources.asp#TopOfPage, which provides guidance for practices preparing to implement ICD-10 and links to useful downloads.[90] For reference, we recommend that you download the April 2010 document, *General Equivalence Mappings: Frequently Asked Questions* at www.cms.gov/ICD10/Downloads/GEMs-CrosswalksBasicFAQ.pdf, and the April 2010 document, *General Equivalence Mappings: Top 10 Questions and Answers* at www.cms.gov/ICD10/Downloads/GEMs-CrosswalksTechnicalFAQ.pdf.

WHAT 5010 AND ICD-10-CM MEAN TO YOUR PRACTICE

The clock is ticking! Each final rule proposed that health care covered entities begin no later than the effective dates of March 17, 2009, to test activities, starting with a gap analysis. Accordingly, your practice should begin to think about how these changes will impact your practice, especially business-related policies and procedures. You will want help from your IT vendor as the 5010 and ICD-10 modifications will have significant impacts on your software related to standard transactions and how you identify diagnoses in your electronic health record systems.

The final 5010 and ICD-10 transaction and code set rule modifications will have a significant impact on your practice's *administrative* policies and procedures. Again, the time from today to each rule's

90. As this is written in late-July 2010, note that this site was last updated on June 22, 2010. We recommend that you check for ICD-10 updates on a regular basis.

compliance date(s) will go by quickly—as this is written, 5010 requires compliance in less than 2 years. Furthermore, the federal health information technology initiatives will compound your workload as your practice examines how your *clinical* workflows, policies, and procedures will change as you introduce more and more electronic tools and records for collecting, compiling, analyzing, and reporting data. If you haven't already, ask your software vendors **now** how they plan to handle 5010 and ICD-10-CM by the compliance dates, including required testing, and get answers and milestones of accomplishment with respect to achieving compliance, in writing, especially in any contract that you execute for software.

While your first concern needs to be the looming Version 5010/D.0 and ICD-10 compliance dates, you also must be aware of future additions and enhancements to administrative simplification standards outlined in the Patient Protection and Affordable Care Act, which we will discuss next.

IMPACT OF HEALTH INSURANCE REFORM ON ADMINISTRATIVE SIMPLIFICATION TRANSACTIONS

The Patient Protection and Affordable Care Act as H.R. 3590 was signed into law by President Obama on March 23, 2010, as Public Law 111-148. The follow-up Health Care and Education Reconciliation Act of 2010 was signed into law by President Obama on March 30, 2010, as Public Law 111-152.[91] Together, these two laws are commonly referred to as Health Insurance Reform.

Our focus in the closing section of this chapter is on 12 of the 906 pages of the Patient Protection and Affordable Care Act (H.R. 3590 as passed[92]) that relate to Administrative Simplification:

- Sections 1104 (Administrative simplification) and 1105 (Effective Date) in Subtitle B—Immediate Actions to Preserve and Expand Coverage of Title I—Quality, Affordable Health Care for All Americans, pp. 28-36.
- Section 10109 (Development of standards for financial and administrative transactions) in Subtitle A—Provisions Relating to Title I of Title X—Strengthening Quality, Affordable Health Care for All Americans, pp. 797-799.

The effective date of the administrative simplification provisions was the enactment date of March 23, 2010.

91. Public Law 111-152 (H.R. 4872) is available at: http://frwebgate.access.gpo.gov/cgi-bin/getdoc.cgi?dbname=111_cong_bills&docid=f:h4872enr.txt.pdf.

92. Public Law 111-148 (H.R. 3590) is available at: http://frwebgate.access.gpo.gov/cgi-bin/getdoc.cgi?dbname=111_cong_bills&docid=f:h3590enr.txt.pdf.

Section 1104. The provisions of this section modify existing and add new legal requirements relating to HIPAA Administrative Simplification. Section 1104(a) amends the Purpose of Administrative Simplification, as indicated by the bold texts: 'To improve efficiency and effectiveness of the health care system, by encouraging the development of a health information system through the establishment of **uniform** standards and requirements for the electronic transmission of certain health information **and to "reduce the clerical burden on patients, health care providers, and health plans**."' [93]

In short, based on the authors' years of experience with HIPAA, the amendments' focus is on moving toward minimization or elimination of variance in the application and use of standards, by requiring **uniform** standards; and, coinciding with that and further adoption of electronic business processes in lieu of paper-based transactions, minimizing or eliminating nonproductive workflows currently experienced by the health care workforce.

The substantive part of Section 1104 for accomplishing the amended purpose is in Section 1104(b), Operating Rules for Health Information Transactions.[94]

Operating Rules are defined as "the necessary business rules and guidelines for the electronic exchange of information that are not defined by a standard or its implementation specifications as adopted for purposes of this part."[95]

In addition to the existing HIPAA transaction standards, Section 1104(b) also specifies a new standard for *Electronic funds transfers* and lays out the requirements for financial and administrative transactions:

"(A) In General—The standards and associated operating rules adopted by the Secretary shall—

(i) to the extent feasible and appropriate, enable determinations of an individual's eligibility and financial responsibility for specific services prior to or at the point of care;

(ii) be comprehensive, requiring minimal augmentation by paper or other communications;

93. See H.R. 3590, p. 28.

94. See H.R. 3590, pp. 28-35.

95. See H.R.3590, p. 29. Also, visit the Council for Affordable Quality Healthcare (CAQH) web site at www.caqh.org for additional information on operating rules as they pertain to the Committee on Operating Rules for Informational Exchange (CORE): "Operating rules build on existing standards to make electronic transactions more predictable and consistent, regardless of the technology. Rights and responsibilities of all parties, security, transmission standards and formats, response time standards, liabilities, exception processing, error resolution and more must be clearly defined in order to facilitate successful interoperability. Beyond reducing cost and administrative hassles, operating rules foster trust among all participants." Available at: www.caqh.org/CORE_rules.php.

(iii) provide for timely acknowledgment, response, and status reporting that supports a transparent claims and denial management process (including adjudication and appeals); and

(iv) describe all data elements (including reason and remark codes) in unambiguous terms, require that such data elements be required or conditioned upon set values in other fields, and prohibit additional conditions (except where necessary to implement State or Federal law, or to protect against fraud and abuse)." [96]

Following the layout of requirements, Section 1104(b) outlines the procedures for the development of operating rules; review and recommendations from the National Committee on Vital and Health Statistics (NCVHS) to the Secretary of HHS for adoption; adoption, effective, and compliance date deadlines, which are outlined in Table 2.5; compliance with operating rules, including health plan certification and documentation requirements; provisions for review and modification of operating rules based on usage; and penalties for noncompliance. In addition, the Secretary of HHS is directed to issue final rules by certain dates, with discretion to use interim final rules, if necessary.

In addition to the foregoing, Section 1104(c) provides for promulgation of three new final rules[97]:

- Unique Health Plan Identifier, to "be effective not later than October 1, 2012, which "[t]he Secretary may do so on an interim final basis."
- Electronic Funds Transfer, to be adopted "not later than January 1, 2012, in a manner ensuring that such standard is effective not later than January 1, 2014," which may be "on an interim final basis."
- Health Claims Attachments[98] to "establish a transaction standard and a single set of associated operating rules... that is consistent with the X12 Version 5010 transaction standards," ... to be adopted "not later than January 1, 2014, in a manner ensuring that such standard is effective not later than January 1, 2016, which may be "on an interim final basis."

Section 10109. Section 10109. This section, in three subsections, outlines additional considerations relating to development of standards for financial and administrative transactions. Section 10109(a) requires the Secretary of HSS to solicit, "not later than January 1, 2012, and not less than every 3 years thereafter, input from [NCVHS, the Health Information Technology Policy Committee, the Health Information Technology Standards Committee, standard setting organizations, and healthcare

96. See H.R. 3590, p. 29.

97. See H.R. 3590, p. 35.

98. The Secretary of HHS issued a Notice of Proposed Rulemaking (NPRM) for a claim attachment on September 23, 2005. This NPRM was "withdrawn" on January 1, 2010 (see HHS, "Completed Actions, Number 182: Electronic Claims Attachments Standards," 75 Federal Register 21804. Available at: http://edocket.access.gpo.gov/2010/pdf/2010-8934.pdf).

TABLE 2.5

Adoption, Effective, and Compliance Dates for Operating Rules

Standard	Adoption Date*	Effective Date*	Health Plan Compliance Date***
Eligibility for a Health Plan	July 1, 2011	January 1, 2013	December 31, 2012***
Health Claim Status	July 1, 2011	January 1, 2013	December 31, 2012***
Electronic Funds Transfers	July 1, 2012	January 1, 2014	December 31, 2013
Health Care Payment and Remittance Advice	July 1, 2012	January 1, 2014	December 31, 2013
Health Claims or Equivalent Encounter Information	July 1, 2014	January 1, 2016	December 31, 2015
Enrollment and Disenrollment in a Health Plan	July 1, 2014	January 1, 2016	December 31, 2015
Health Plan Premium Payments	July 1, 2014	January 1, 2016	December 31, 2015
Referral Certification and Authorization	July 1, 2014	January 1, 2016	December 31, 2015

*Not later than

** Not later than. Requires written certification of compliance provided to Secretary of HHS.

*** The "December 31, 2012" dates for Eligibility for a Health Plan and Health Claim Status have the same endnote: Not later than. (h)(1)(A) on p. H.R.3590—31 specifies a date of "December 31, 2013," which conflicts with the effective dates for these standards and with (h)(5)(B) on p. H.R.3590—32: "Date of Compliance—A health plan shall comply with such requirements not later than the effective date of the applicable standard or operating rule." Hence, we use "December 31, 2012" in the table.

stakeholders] whether there could be greater **uniformity** in financial and administrative activities... and whether such activities should be considered financial and administrative transactions for which the adoption of standards and operating rules would improve the operation of the health care system and reduce administrative costs."[99]

For initial evaluation by January 1, 2012, of "activities and items" vis-à-vis "greater uniformity" and/or consideration as operating rules and transaction standards, Section 10109(b) outlines five areas:

- Application process for enrollment of health care providers by health plans.
- Health care transactions of automobile insurance.
- Financial audits required by health plans, federal and state agencies, and others determined by the Secretary of HHS.

99. See H.R. 3590, pp. 797-798.

- Greater transparency and consistency of methodologies and processes used to establish claim edits used by health plans.
- Health plan publication of timeliness of payment rules.

Finally, Section 10109(c) requires the Secretary of HHS to "task the ICD-9-CM Coordination and Maintenance Committee to convene a meeting, not later than January 1, 2011, to receive input from appropriate stakeholders (including health plans, health care providers, and clinicians) regarding the crosswalk between ICD-9 and ICD-10 that is posted on the website of the Centers for Medicare & Medicaid Services (CMS), and make recommendations about appropriate revisions to it.[100] Such revisions would be posted on the CMS web site, the revised crosswalk would be deemed a code set standard, and any subsequent revised crosswalks would be posted on the CMS web site prior to "implementation of such subsequent revision."

In this chapter we have reviewed administrative simplification transaction and code set standards and their modifications, which will go into effect on January 1, 2012 (Version 5010/D.0) and October 1, 2013 (ICD-10), and new operating rules and a new *electronic funds transfers* standard that is outlined in the Patient Protection and Affordable Care Act. It is important for your practice to carefully follow regulatory initiatives and developments related to these administrative simplification transactions and code sets in the coming years. To keep your practice informed, we recommend that you subscribe—at no cost—to the California HealthCare Foundation's excellent daily electronic newsletter, *iHealthBeat*, which is available at www.ihealthbeat.org. Your practice can also follow federal regulatory initiatives and developments that will affect your practice, at www.cms.hhs.gov, www.ama-assn.org/go/5010, and www.hipaa.com.

We also recommend that your practice develop a game plan and have periodic meetings with the workforce to discuss administrative and clinical aspects of moving more toward electronic business tools in your practice. As a first step, if you have not done so already, have your software vendor attend and outline its plan for enabling in your software 5010 transaction and ICD-10 code set standards. Plan to meet monthly to check progress, and make sure that key workforce members in your practice read and understand the final rules. We have discussed how to go about planning for these changes and assessing their affects in other chapters of this book, our other books mentioned earlier in this chapter, and in *EHR Implementation: A Step-by-Step Guide for the Medical Practice*[101] and *Technical and Financial Guide to EHR Implementation*.[102]

---

100. See H.R. 3590, pp. 798–799.

101. Hartley, CP, Jones, ED. Chicago, IL: American Medical Association, 2005.

102. Hartley, CP, Jones, ED, Ens, D, and Whitt, D. Chicago, IL: American Medical Association, 2007(R).

chapter 3

The Privacy Team

Respecting a patient's privacy and confidentiality has always been part of the culture of a physician's practice. Initially, the actions surrounding rules and enforcement activities around privacy practices seemed to be an affront to many workforce members. But you completed the tasks, consulted legal advice, built the Notice of Privacy Practices and implemented authorizations and consent forms, and built new habits.

Between 2003 and now, an expanded electronic environment has become commonplace, not just to individuals but also to health care providers.

- Electronic health record (EHR) systems are replacing paper charts, and there's reimbursement money now to support the transition.
- Regional health information organizations (RHIOs) provide a secure network for providers, payers, and patients to exchange electronic protected health information (ePHI).
- Social networking sites provide a means for individuals to exchange wellness updates, and if they wish, their own confidential health information. (Individuals are not covered entities.)
- Employers are supporting employees in wellness activities and in-house clinics.
- ePrescribing networks store individual's prescriptions and send automatic patient alerts to avoid interactions and allergies while reconciling medications the patient has picked up from the pharmacy.
- A SIM (Subscriber Identity Module) card that once stored telephone numbers in a mobile phone now integrates with other functions to sync stored information into servers and computers. Providers can access patient records from anywhere in the world, if service is available.

In an effort to stay current with, and forecast emerging technology while also creating incentives for physicians to adopt technology, regulations safeguarding PHI had to be updated as well.

What You Will Learn in This Chapter

This chapter, loaded with lists, charts, diagrams, and insider tips on how to manage patient privacy, gives you step-by-step instructions on current HIPAA Privacy Regulations, and a starburst to show you what's new. We've divided the updates for your privacy implementation into 10 steps.

Step 1: Build the foundation for privacy management.

Step 2: Learn when you are permitted to use and disclose protected health information (PHI) without authorization.

Step 3: Identify uses and disclosures of PHI that require authorizations. This includes guidelines on what you can share with family and friends, disaster relief agencies, and enforcement agencies.

Step 4: Identify personal identity authentication issues, such as verification of personal representatives, guidance on custody agreements, and guidance about how to deny a use or disclosure to someone you think may cause substantial harm to the patient.

Step 5: Update your HIPAA Privacy safeguards.

Step 6: Update new patient rights, including rights provided in the HITECH and Breach Notification Rules.

Step 7: Update business associate contracts in light of their new compliance status.

Step 8: Revise and protect marketing activities with rules that close loopholes in prior marketing activities.

Step 9: Train your staff on new issues, including details included in the Breach Notification Rule and provide refreshers for old privacy.

Step 10: Implement your updated plan, and safeguard your assets.

With each step, you'll find "What to Do" and "How to Do It" sections to use as a foundation for writing simple policies and procedures for a small to midsize physician practice. The procedures in this chapter can also be used in a long-term care facility, and some of them can be used in home health care. Real scenarios show you how the situation may look so that you can see why the policy or procedure is necessary.

Key Terms

In this chapter, we will introduce terms, many of which have been updated in the HITECH and Breach Notification Rules. Here, you will see a list of terms, and in the Glossary, you'll find definitions for each.

Designated record sets

Electronic Protected Health Information (ePHI)

Department of Health and Human Service (HHS)

Incidental use and disclosure

Office for Civil Rights (OCR)
Patient rights
Personal representative
Protected health information (PHI)
Treatment, payment, and health care operations
Use and disclosure

STEP 1: BUILD THE FOUNDATION FOR PRIVACY MANAGEMENT

HIPAA's Privacy Rule establishes the foundation upon which layers of electronic transactions can be built. Technology already exists whereby physicians can order a CBC panel, and within moments receive lab results, even if the blood is drawn at a hospital across town. To set the stage for your electronic exchange, begin by identifying a privacy official.

Step 1A: Identify a Privacy Official

As of April 14, 2003, your organization has been required to identify a privacy official who is responsible for developing and implementing your privacy policies and procedures. If your privacy official has taken another position elsewhere, you must name another person to manage this job.

The privacy official is also the contact person or office responsible for receiving complaints and providing individuals with further information about matters contained in the organization's Notice of Privacy Practices.

A privacy official must continually update knowledge of the Privacy Rule guidelines, updates, and new regulations and train the workforce on requirements. The privacy official also is responsible for training the workforce on those policies and procedures, including imposing sanctions on workforce members that breach an individual's privacy.

Privacy officials must have the support of the organization's leadership, and in many cases, the privacy official reports directly to the president, board of directors, or managing partner.

While the privacy official is responsible for privacy management, he or she may delegate responsibilities to others within the organization if they are trained and communicate promptly with the privacy official on these matters.

There are ten implementation specifications in the privacy management component of HIPAA's Privacy Rule. We'll discuss each one and provide guidance on how to complete each specification.

Personnel Designations (Privacy Official)

Standard	Code of Federal Regulations	Privacy Management
Personnel designations (privacy official)	45 CFR 164.530 (a)	Administrative requirements

What to Do:

Assign an individual to be your privacy official.

How to Do It:

1. The practice's management team creates a job description for the privacy official. A job description is included in Figure 3.1.

FIGURE 3.1

Privacy Official Job Description

The Privacy Official (Small practice)

The privacy official will report directly to the managing partner of the practice and will be responsible for the implementation and day-to-day administration and oversight of our HIPAA Privacy compliance program. The privacy officer is also responsible for coordinating HIPAA Privacy activities with HIPAA Security and Breach Notification activities.

Critical Functions

Our privacy official is responsible for the following activities:

- Maintain an inventory of how we use and disclose all protected health information (PHI).
- Work with legal counsel to ensure compliance documents are drafted, reviewed, and approved, including the Notice of Privacy Practices and relevant updates, Acknowledgement Forms, Authorizations, Consents, and other forms as required.
- Establish policies and procedures to ensure individual rights guaranteed by HIPAA and the Breach Notification Rule are set up, including a complaint process and sanctions.
- Develop a training program.
- Maintain an inventory of all business associate agreements. Working with legal counsel, draft an amended and/or new agreements that address business associate compliance requirements under HIPAA Security, Breach Notification Rules, and HIPAA Privacy as appropriate to the service performed for the practice.

- Keep up to date on the latest privacy and security developments and federal and state laws and regulations.
- Coordinate privacy safeguards with security officer to ensure consistency in development, documentation and training for security and privacy requirements.
- Serve as the practice's resource to regulatory and accrediting bodies for matters relating to privacy and security.
- Coordinate any audits of the Secretary of the Department of Health and Human Services (HHS) or any other governmental or accrediting organization concerning state or federal privacy laws or regulations.
- Notify individuals when health information has been used or disclosed in violation of our privacy practices.
- Regularly communicate the status of legal complaints, risks, and sanctions imposed on workforce members with the managing partner(s) of this practice.
- Work with health information systems and portable technologies.;
- Effectively communicate technical and legal information to nontechnical and nonlegal staff for employee training.

(For a larger practice)

The privacy official will report directly to the organization's risk manager and make presentations as necessary to large audiences.

The privacy official will meet the following qualifications:

- Bachelor's degree in management, information systems, human resources, health administration, or other relevant field;
- Minimum five years experience in health care;
- Familiar with regulatory development and compliance, including federal and state laws and regulations concerning information security and privacy;
- Familiar with business functions and operations of a larger institution;
- Ensure devices containing electronic protected health information (ePHI) are encrypted as required by HIPAA Security and Breach Notification Rules.
- Have strong organizational and problem-solving skills, and work in a team environment.
- Have the ability to communicate with clarity both orally and in writing.

2. Establish qualifications. The privacy official must be familiar with the clinical and administrative functions of the office; be willing to take on new responsibility, including fast-track learning of HIPAA content; highly ethical; exhibit strong organizational and communication skills; and work well with management and staff.
3. Establish a reporting structure. The office manager and privacy official, even though they may be one and the same person, may report to two different supervisors.

4. Discuss salary or bonuses for taking on the additional responsibilities. The salary for privacy officials in medical offices typically ranges from $40,000 to $65,000, depending on the size of the practice and the responsibilities of the position.
5. Document the level of independent decision-making given to the privacy official. The privacy official needs authority to oversee some activities but should consult the management team for approval on others.
6. Consult with an attorney on documentation that you can create and documentation that you will need to review before presenting to anyone outside the practice. Much of HIPAA compliance is about documentation, but keep in mind that your documentation could become evidence in a criminal or civil enforcement proceeding. Be careful what you put into writing.
7. Privacy officials may wish to obtain a privacy designation offered through URAC, also known as the American Accreditation HealthCare Commission (www.urac.org), or through the American Health Information Management Association (www.ahima.org).

Designate a Privacy Team

The privacy official cannot handle privacy implementation independently. There is too much work to be done. In addition, the privacy official cannot be the "privacy watchdog" for the office. Privacy is a team activity and requires support from many levels. Consider the following as candidates for the privacy team: your head nurse, billing supervisor, receptionist, management, and insurance clerk.

Develop a Budget and Time-and-Task Chart

But how big should your budget be? That depends on when you started and how fast you moved through the compliance process. If you've been working on compliance since 2003, most of your work on privacy has been completed. But if you have not kept accurate records of HIPAA forms, such as Authorizations, Accounting of Disclosures, and Sanctions, these may take time to build.

Include costs for legal counsel to review your Notice of Privacy Practices and business associate agreements to determine how and/or whether the Breach Notification Rule affects them. You'll learn more about that in Step 2, Step 7, and also in Chapter 4 on HIPAA Security.

Step 1B: Revisit your Notice of Privacy Practices

Standard	Code of Federal Regulations	Privacy Management
Notice of privacy practices	45 CFR 164.520; 45 CFR 164.530(i)(4)	Notice of privacy practices for PHI; changes to privacy practices stated in the notice

What to Do:

Revisit your Notice of Privacy Practices (NPP) to determine whether it needs to be updated with copies provided to patients. Your legal counsel can advise you whether updates from the Breach Notification Rule, Security and Privacy Rules are significant to warrant a new NPP.

New patient rights include the following new rights discussed in Chapter 1:

a. The right to restrict disclosure of protected health information (PHI) to a health plan for a specific treatment that the patient has paid in full and out of pocket.

b. If your organization adopts electronic health records (EHR), the patient can now request an accounting of electronic disclosures, including those for treatment, payment, and health care operations.

How to Do It:

Your Notice of Privacy Practices (NPP) is a legal document and should be developed under the advice of legal counsel. You are required to provide an NPP to individuals the first time they seek health care from providers in your organization. Required elements in your NPP include the following:

- Describe how you may use and disclose protected health information (PHI).
- State your duty to protect privacy, provide a notice of privacy practices, and abide by the terms of the current notice.
- Describe the individual's rights, including the right to complain to HHS's Office for Civil Rights and to the covered entity.

Every workforce member should understand the content in your NPP. This will help field complaints internally so that you can mitigate privacy concerns before they go outside the organization, such as to HHS.

The HITECH Act provided for updates that your attorney may identify as "material change" and thus warrant a revised NPP.

When providing the NPP to patients, you are required to:

- Provide the NPP upon the patient's first visit to your facility
- Provide the patient with an Acknowledgement of the Notice of Privacy
- Provide the NPP to any individual or a personal representative acting on behalf of a patient who requests it.

If you maintain a Web site, you may provide the NPP via e-mail, only if the individual agrees to an electronic notice and that notice has not been withdrawn.

Step 1C: Consistent with Other Documentation

Standard	Code of Federal Regulations	Privacy Management
Consistent with notice of privacy practices	45 CFR 164.502(i)	Uses and disclosures of protected health information: general rules

What to Do:

Your NPP must be consistent with other documents, including your Privacy and HIPAA Security Policies and Procedures, Breach Notification Rules, and HITECH Rules. If state privacy laws conflict with HIPAA, more stringent state laws take precedence.

How to Do It:

In small organizations, the privacy and security officials may be the same person. In larger organizations, responsibilities for privacy and security officials are significantly expanded so officials must tightly coordinate documentation to avoid conflict and confusion.

In updating or rebuilding your privacy and security policies and procedures including those that reflect state laws, your Notice of Privacy Practices (NPP), and the breach notification rule, consult a health law attorney and/or compare your documentation so that the language in one does not conflict with language in other documents.

Step 1D: Develop Policies and Procedures

Standard	Code of Federal Regulations	Privacy Management
Policies and procedures	45 CFR 164.530(i)	Administrative requirements

What to Do:

A covered entity must develop and implement written privacy policies and procedures that are consistent with the HIPAA Privacy Rule and the Breach Notification Rule.

How to Do It:

All covered entities must update policies and procedures to reflect the changes in the Privacy Rule and Breach Notification Rule. Security Rule updates are provided in Chapter 4.

As a covered entity, your organization must develop and implement written policies and procedures that are consistent with the HIPAA Privacy Rule, the Breach Notification Rule, and state law.

While the privacy official is responsible for development of policies and procedures, the task can be daunting if completed by one person. Therefore, privacy policies and procedures can be simplified using one of three strategies:

1. Form a team to review the Privacy Rule published in the Federal Register and build your policies and procedures.
2. Purchase a set of policies and procedures from a reputable organization and customize them according to the size of your organization.
3. Consult with a privacy expert or attorney and contract with them to customize your policies and procedures for your organization.

Provide hard copy or electronic access of your policies and procedures to all workforce members with an additional copy to be placed in your library.

As liability can now be extended to employers and individuals, each workforce member must also receive a copy of your updated policies and procedures and sign an acknowledgement form[1] that he or she understands the policies and procedures, and will comply with them. Retain these forms for six years.

Step 1E: Documentation

Standard	Code of Federal Regulations	Privacy Management
Documentation	45 CFR 164.530(j)	Administrative requirements

What to Do:

Maintain HIPAA documentation for six years after whichever comes later: the date of their creation or last effective date. Documents to maintain include, but are not limited to:

- Privacy policies and procedures
- Privacy practices notices
- Disposition of complaints and documentation of other actions
- Activities and designations that the Privacy Rule requires to be documented.

How to Do It:

For practices moving to an electronic format, you will find storing HIPAA forms to be part of your scanning workflow.

1. See Appendix A for sample form: Acknowledgement of Receipt of HIPAA Privacy Policies and Procedures.

Maintain all signed acknowledgements by workforce members and patients.

Maintain all hard copy documentation in a secure storage facility, and back up offsite any electronic documentation.

Permit an agent of the Secretary of HHS to access your facilities, books, records, accounts, and other information during your practice's normal business hours in response to a compliance audit or complaint investigation. If the Secretary determines that special circumstances warrant, such as in the case of hidden or destroyed files, your practice must allow HHS access at any time.

Storage and Access to Documentation

Privacy documents may be maintained in hard or electronic copy provided they are in a secure storage facility.

Step 1F: Training

Standard	Code of Federal Regulations	Privacy Management
Training	45 CFR 164.530(b); 45 CFR 160.103	Administrative requirements; definition of *workforce member*

What to Do:

Train all workforce members on Privacy and Breach Notification policies and procedures, as necessary and appropriate for them to carry out their functions.

You must apply appropriate sanctions against workforce members[2] who violate privacy policies and procedures or the Privacy Rule. No one wants to apply sanctions against fellow colleagues, but sanctions are required to be applied by the privacy official. Should you be audited by the HHS or a State's Attorney General, or required to post notice of a breach, you may be required to produce sanctions documentation.

Business associates of covered entities have certain compliance responsibilities under Breach Notification Rule,[3] with enforcement by the HHS Office for Civil Rights (OCR) commencing February 22, 2010 for incidents on or after that date.

2. Workforce members are employees, volunteers, trainees, and other persons whose conduct, in the performance of work for a covered entity, is under the direct control of such entity, whether or not they are paid by the covered entity. 45 CFR § 160.103.

3. Department of Health and Human Services, Office of the Secretary, "45 CFR Parts 160 and 164: Breach Notification for Unsecured Protected Health Information; Interim Final Rule," *Federal Register*, v.74, n.162, August 24, 2009, pp. 42739–42770.

You are not required to train business associates, as they now must train their own workforce on their HIPAA Security Rule,[4] and Breach Notification compliance policies and procedures, as well as train workforces to safeguard the PHI that they manage or transmit on behalf of a covered entity.

How to Do It:

Privacy, Security and Breach Notification training must be completed both formally (once yearly) and in an ongoing and informal way. Retraining must be part of your sanctions policy as a method to remediate workforce members needing reminders of your privacy policies and procedures.

All workforce members, including physicians, must participate in retraining on privacy policies and procedures related to the HITECH Act and the Breach Notification Rule, as well as new security regulations related to the safeguarding of PHI.[5]

Your privacy official will determine who needs additional training, the type of training that is appropriate, and the frequency with which such training will occur. New employees will participate in training within 30 days following their first date of service.

Privacy topics to be included in updated training include:

- New patient rights
- Accounting of electronic disclosures
- The right to restrict disclosures if specific service is paid in full
- Penalties imposed on individuals and employers
- New business associate requirements
- New enforcement activities, including
    - State attorneys general now empowered to also investigate privacy violations
    - Increased financial penalties
    - Office for Civil Rights audits
- Coordination of administrative, physical, and technical safeguards with your security official for training content included in the Breach Notification Rule, such as your encryption policy (discussed in Chapter 4).

Upon completing training, each member of your workforce will sign an acknowledgement form[6] that he or she participated in training and is aware of and understands our practice's privacy policies and procedures.

If retraining is the result of a sanction, maintain a copy of the workforce member's acknowledgement form in your records.

4. See Chapter 4 for discussion of business associate compliance with the Security Rule.
5. Consult Appendix A for a month-to-month sample training calendar.
6. See Appendix A for sample form: Acknowledgement of Participation in Workforce Training.

Step 1G: Sanctions

Standard	Code of Federal Regulations	Privacy Management
Sanctions	45 CFR 164.530(e)	Administrative requirements

What to Do:

A covered entity must have and apply appropriate sanctions against workforce members who violate its privacy policies and procedures or the Privacy Rule.

How to Do It:

Be cautious about applying sanctions without first researching details to verify what really happened.

The privacy official or another person designated by the privacy official must first review the privacy violation.

For repeat privacy violations, consider the following sanctions:

First violation: Privacy official provides a verbal reminder.

Second violation: Reminder and workforce member required to participate in privacy retraining.

Third violation: Reminder placed in employee's personnel file with warning that repeat offense will result in time off without pay; additional retraining.

Fourth violation: Suspension for three days without pay.

Fifth violation: Workforce member employment terminated.

Your policies and procedures also must indicate the practice reserves the right to skip steps, repeat steps, or impose other sanctions, as it deems appropriate.

No sanctions are to be imposed against workforce members whose reason for conduct is in good faith and in accordance with HIPAA Privacy Rule provisions; for example:

A whistleblower reporting to a government agency

A workforce member crime victim reporting to a law enforcement official.

Step 1H: Mitigation

Standard	Code of Federal Regulations	Privacy Management
Mitigation	45 CFR 164.530(f)	Administrative requirements

What to Do:

Mitigate, to the extent practicable, any harmful effect that is known to the covered entity of a use or disclosure of PHI in violation of its policies and procedures or requirements of the Privacy Rule by the covered entity or its business associate.

How to Do It:

Praise the workforce member who brings a complaint to the privacy official because that gives the organization an opportunity to take action to resolve the complaint before it goes to a higher level.

To mitigate something is to make it less harsh, less painful, or less severe. The Privacy Rule does not specify what steps you must take to resolve or mitigate harm to a patient from a privacy breach, but the rule does require the practice to try to resolve a complaint if the patient believes it has caused harm.

The normal human reaction is to try to mend a breach before the complaint goes to a supervisory level, but the best answer is to go directly to your privacy official with any complaint.

If a patient files a complaint with your privacy official and has chosen you as the person to blame, don't say, "She's out of her mind. That didn't happen." And don't say, "I'm really tired of hearing his whining."

Do say, "Let's talk about what happened. My view may be different from the individual's."

Once you've presented the patient's complaint to the privacy official, step out of the picture. The privacy official is usually the only employee who can make mitigation recommendations.

For the privacy official:

- Document your conversation with the individual making a complaint.
- Do not offer any immediate solutions, but do promise to look into the event. The Breach Notification Rule requires a 30-day response time. Consult Chapter 4 on how to respond to an electronic breach.
- Consult the practice leaders to determine resources required to mitigate the violation.
- In accordance with the *Guidance* contained in the August 24, 2009, Breach Notification Rule,[7] consult with legal counsel about any public notice that is required to be posted, and ensure encryption of server connections, portable computers, and all mobile devices to NIST standards specified in the *Guidance*.
- In the event of a breach of unsecured protected health information, evaluate the breach and follow requirements of the Breach Notification Rule and your policies and procedures for mitigation of harm.
- Depending on the nature of the complaint, mitigation responses may include:

7. *Guidance Specifying the Technologies and Methodologies that Render Protected Health Information Unusable, Unreadable, or Indecipherable to Unauthorized Individuals*, published in the *Federal Register* on August 24, 2009, as part of the Interim Final Rule on "Breach Notification." Department of Health and Human Services, Office of the Secretary, "45 CFR Parts 160 and 164: Breach Notification for Unsecured Protected Health Information; Interim Final Rule," *Federal Register*, v.74, n.162, Monday, August 24, 2009, pp. 42739 and 42770.

- ☐ An apology in writing
- ☐ Retrieving the protected health information from where it was sent accompanied by a letter notifying the individual of corrective actions
- ☐ Adopting policies and procedures that clarify a situation that wasn't addressed before this incident
- ☐ Retraining workforce members
- ☐ Sanctioning an employee.

- New Privacy Rules allow state attorneys general to investigate privacy violations and also prosecute individuals and/or employers. Be sure your workforce is aware of the state's expanded enforcement capabilities.
- Breaches, such as accessing a patient record of a public figure without authorization or selling health information to a news media, are subject to criminal penalties.

Most privacy violations are not intentional, but they do need to be corrected. If the violation was intentional, mitigation procedures can get complicated.

CRITICAL POINT

Demonstrating genuine concern about a possible privacy breach and responding with a plan to mitigate any harm may disarm an individual's more potent complaints filed against your organization to the HHS Office for Civil Rights.

Step 1I: Refraining from Intimidating or Retaliatory Acts

Standard	Code of Federal Regulations	Privacy Management
Refraining from intimidating or retaliatory acts	45 CFR 164.530(g)	Administrative requirements

What to Do:

A covered entity may not intimidate, threaten, coerce, discriminate against, or take other retaliatory action against any individual, who exercises his or her right to file a complaint either with the HHS Office for Civil Rights or to the privacy official.

How to Do It:

Train workforce members who retaliate against an individual filing a complaint that they will be subject to sanctions, retraining, or immediate termination of employment.

Step 1J: Waiver of Rights

Standard	Code of Federal Regulations	Privacy Management
Waiver of rights	45 CFR 164.530(h)	Administrative requirements

What to Do:

A covered entity may not require an individual to waive his or her rights under the Privacy, Security or Breach Notification Rules as a condition for obtaining treatment, enrollment in a health plan, or eligibility for benefits.

How to Do It:

The privacy official will confirm that the practice does not require patients to sign waivers of any of the following rights as a condition of receiving treatment, payment, enrollment in a health plan, or eligibility for benefits:

- Their rights to file a complaint with our practice or with the Secretary of HHS.
- Their rights under the Security Rule.
- Their rights under the Privacy Rule.
- Their rights under the Breach Notification Rule.

The privacy official must train workforce members not to request any patient to sign a waiver as a condition for obtaining treatment, payment, enrollment in a health plan, or eligibility for benefits. Workforce members who make such a request will be subject to the practice's sanctions policy, up to and including termination of employment.

Step 1K: Establish Minimum Necessary Limits for Use and Disclosures of PHI

Standard	Code of Federal Regulations	Protected Health Information Special Permissions
Minimum necessary	45 CFR 164.502(b); 45 CFR 164.514(d)	Uses and disclosures of PHI; other requirements relating to uses and disclosures of PHI

What to Do:

A covered entity must develop and implement policies and procedures to reasonably limit uses and disclosures of PHI to the minimum amount necessary to complete a task.

As it applies to a use or disclosure, a covered entity may not use, disclose, or request the entire medical record for a particular purpose unless it can specifically justify why it needs the whole record.

How to Do It:

Identify roles of workforce members and the appropriate amount of PHI that will be made available to each of them. Make reasonable efforts to limit the access of workforce members to the appropriate amount of PHI.

Implement policies and procedures for routine disclosures (which may be standard protocols) that limit the PHI disclosed to the amount reasonably necessary to achieve the purpose of the disclosure.

HIPAA did not offer well-defined direction for "Minimum Necessary," but the HITECH Act offers some clarification: The entity disclosing the PHI (as opposed to the person or organization requesting the PHI) must make responsible determination for what is the minimum amount necessary.

The HITECH Act requires the Secretary of HHS to issue guidance on what constitutes minimum necessary no later than August 17, 2010.

EHR software automatically limits medical necessary according to roles within the organization. An administrator would have to override those permissions to change medically necessary uses and disclosures.

A practice might assign access to PHI for purposes such as those listed in Table 3.1.

TABLE 3.1

Minimum Necessary Assignments

Name	Billing	Clinical		Administrative Access	Scheduling
		Vitals	Full		
(Physician)					
(Physician)					
(Nurse Practitioner)					
(Nurse)					
(Medical Assistant)					
(Receptionist)					
(Lab Technician)					

Step 2: Identify Permissions for Use and Disclosure of Protected Health Information (PHI)

Most laws allow you to do anything you want, unless there is a provision against it. HIPAA is just the opposite. You can use and disclose patient information, but you have to find a reason for each use or disclosure.

The core of the Privacy Rule is that you must identify permissions, even those that come with special requirements to use or disclose patient information.

CRITICAL POINT

To use or disclose PHI, you must first identify the permission (or a reason).

Protected Health Information Permissions: Under certain circumstances, HIPAA may permit or require a covered entity to use or disclose PHI without an individual's authorization. Under other circumstances a valid authorization from the individual is required.

Itemized steps here provide how-to guidance when obtaining valid authorizations situations where a covered entity may use and disclose patient information without the individual's authorization.[8]

In Step 2, we'll discuss the following permitted disclosures:

- Required Disclosures
  - To HHS
  - To the patient or personal representative
- Permissible Disclosures:
  - Treatment, payment, and health care operations
  - Another covered entity's treatment, payment, and health care operations
  - Family, friends, and disaster relief agencies
  - Incidental to a use or disclosure otherwise permitted or required
  - Uses and disclosures for which an authorization or opportunity to agree or object is not required
- Uses and disclosures of De-identified PHI
- Limited data set for purposes of research, public health, or health care operations

FIGURE 3.2

Required Disclosures

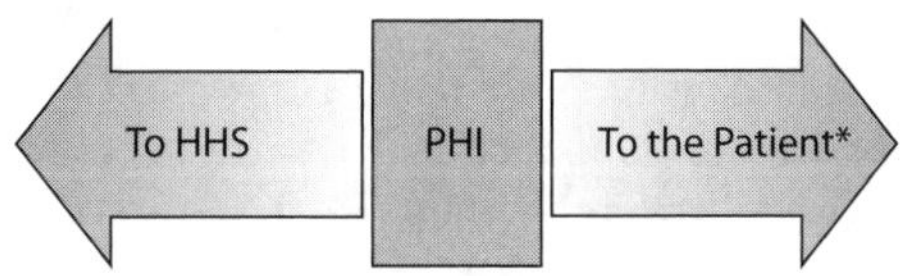

*Exceptions to patient disclosures are discussed in Step 6.

8. 45 CFR § 164.502(a)(1).

FIGURE 3.3

Permitted Disclosures

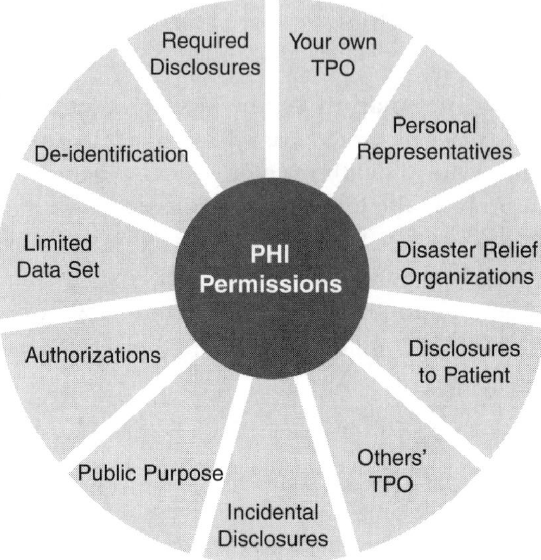
Eleven Permissions for PHI
Required Disclosures
Your own TPO
Personal Representatives
Disaster Relief Organizations
Disclosures to Patient
Others' TPO
Incidental Disclosures
Public Purpose
Authorizations
Limited Data Set
De-identification
PHI Permissions

TPO indicates treatment payment and health care operations.
Reprinted with permission from Carolyn Hartley.

Step 2A: Required Disclosures

Standard	Code of Federal Regulations	Protected Health Information Permissions
Required disclosures	45 CFR 164.502(a)(2)	Uses and disclosures of protected health information: general rules

What to Do:

Unless a use or disclosure is required or permitted by HIPAA Privacy, as a covered entity, you must disclose PHI in only two situations:

1. To individuals (or their personal representatives) specifically when they request access to, or an accounting of disclosures of, their protected health information. However, there are circumstances where you would deny this.
2. To state attorney general or HHS when it is undertaking a compliance investigation or review or enforcement action. In both situations, verify credentials.

How to Do It:

Your privacy official will determine whether a request for disclosure is required, permitted, if it requires special permission, or if an authorization is required.

The Privacy Official's Response to Request for PHI from a Patient:

First: If you do not know the person, obtain a photo ID. If this is a regular patient of the practice whom you recognize, then you are not required to obtain a photo ID.

Second: Ask what information is being requested. For example, is the request for a summary of a recent visit? Copies of radiographs or digital images? Payment history?

Third: Document the request in a log and in the patient's file.

Fourth: Provide requested information to the patient. If you are entitled to impose a fee in connection with the request, ask for payment.[9]

(a) Request from a patient's personal representative.

First: Evaluate the relationship between the patient and personal representative, referring to the discussion of "personal representative" on this page below, and examining and copying any applicable credentials or other documentation. Obtain a photo ID.

Second: Document the personal representative's request in the patient's record. If you provide the requested information, document your provision of the requested protected health information and your basis for doing so. If you refuse to provide the requested information, document your refusal and your basis for refusing (eg, your reasonable belief that the personal representative did not provide necessary credentials and/or your belief that the personal representative might endanger the patient).

A personal representative[10] is legally responsible for the individual's care and general condition. A personal representative can be named in accordance with state or federal law. For example, the personal representative of a minor child is usually the child's parent or legal guardian.

In the case of a custody decree, the personal representative is the parent who can make health care decisions for the child under the decree. If you do not know the patient or parent, you should ask to see a copy of the divorce decree and a photo ID.

---

9. A covered entity may impose a reasonable, cost-based fee when an individual requests a copy of his or her protected health information or agrees to a summary or explanation of such information, provided the fee includes ***only*** the cost of:
   (1) Copying (including the cost of supplies for and labor of copying the protected health information requested by the individual),
   (2) Postage (when the individual has requested the copy, or summary or explanation, be mailed), and
   (3) Preparing an explanation or summary of the protected health information, if the individual has agreed in advance to the preparation of a summary or explanation and to any fees imposed by the covered entity for such summary or explanation. 45 CFR § 164.524(c)(4).

10. Consult the Office for Civil Rights for more details on what is a personal representative at: www.hhs.gov/ocr/privacy/hipaa/understanding/consumers/personalreps.html.

The personal representative may also present documentation including a health care power of attorney. Make a copy of this document and include it in the patient's health record. Upon death of the individual, the personal representative for the deceased is the executor or administrator of the deceased individual's estate, and also is legally authorized by a court and/or state law to act on behalf of the deceased or the estate.

If you reasonably believe the personal representative might endanger the patient, such as in cases of domestic violence, abuse, or neglect, you can refuse to provide protected health information. Be sure to document your decision. If you suspect the patient is a victim of abuse, neglect, or domestic violence, you may as a covered entity disclose protected health information to appropriate government authorities regarding victims of abuse, neglect, or domestic violence.

Third: Document the request in a log and in the patient's file.

Fourth: Provide requested information to the personal representative. If you are entitled to impose a fee in connection with the request, ask for payment.

Request from an agent of the Secretary of HHS or from a law enforcement official:

Step 1: Politely request to see the agent or official's credentials and inform the privacy official and the physician, who should determine whether the practice's attorney should be involved.

Step 2: Verify the agent or official's credentials and determine the nature of the inquiry. Consult with the practice's attorney to determine the practice's rights and obligations with respect to its response to the inquiry and the timeframe for responding to the inquiry. Document all actions, times, and personnel involved that pertain to the inquiry and the practice's response.[11]

Step 2B: Permissible Disclosures: Treatment, Payment and Health Care Operations

Standard	Code of Federal Regulations	Protected Health Information Permissions
Permissible disclosures: treatment, payment, and health care operations	45 CFR 164.506(c)	Uses and disclosures to carry out treatment, payment, or health care operations

What to Do:

A covered entity may use and disclose PHI for its own treatment, payment, and health care operations activities. A covered entity also may disclose PHI for the treatment activities of another health care provider, the payment activities of another covered entity and of another health care provider, or the health care operations of another covered entity involving either quality or competency

11. The HHS Office for Civil Rights provides guidance on the compliance and enforcement process for Privacy and Security Rules at its Web site, www.hhs.gov/ocr/privacy/hipaa/enforcement/process/index.html.

assurance activities or fraud and abuse detection and compliance activities, if both covered entities have or had a relationship with the individual and the PHI pertains to the relationship.

How to Do It:

In accordance with your Notice of Privacy Practices (NPP), you may use PHI for treatment, payment, and health care operations without obtaining authorization from the patient, except for cases where HIPAA authorization, state law, or other special requirements apply.

Note Patient Rights:

- An individual may request that his or her health information not be submitted to a health plan for purposes of payment or health care operations. Consult Chapter 5 on Patient Rights on the decision to restrict. If the patient has paid in full and out of pocket for the services included in the restriction, you must comply with this restriction.The patient must complete the Request to Restrict Disclosure[12] prior to making a decision whether to restrict the disclosure. In all cases, the privacy official shall determine whether to refuse or honor the request.

The privacy official is designated to be the contact person for questions, suggestions, or complaints relating to use or disclosure of protected health information for our treatment, payment, and health care operations.

Step 2C: Permissible Disclosures: Another Covered Entity's Treatment, Payment, and Health Care Operations

Standard	Code of Federal Regulations	Protected Health Information Permissions
Permissible disclosures: another covered entity's treatment, payment, and health care operations	45 CFR 164.506(c)	Uses and disclosures to carry out treatment, payment, or health care operations

What to Do:

A covered entity also may disclose PHI for the treatment activities of any health care provider, the payment activities of another covered entity and of any health care provider, or the health care operations of another covered entity involving either quality or competency assurance activities or fraud and abuse detection and compliance activities, if both covered entities have or had a relationship with the individual and the protected health information pertains to the relationship.

12. 45 CFR§ 164.512(a), (b)(1)(ii), and (c).

How to Do It:

Disclose PHI for treatment, payment, and health care operations of another health care provider if that request complies with the list below or is approved by our privacy official.

There are several reasons for agreeing to such a disclosure:

1. For treatment activities of another physician or health care provider
2. To another covered entity or health care provider for payment activities of the entity receiving the protected health information
3. To another covered entity for its health care operations, as long as the other covered entity also has or had a relationship with the patient, the PHI pertains to that relationship, and the disclosure has one of the following purposes:
   (a) Quality assessment and improvement, including outcomes evaluation and developing clinical guidelines (but not primarily to obtain general knowledge)
   (b) Population-based activities related to improving health or reducing health care costs
   (c) Protocol development
   (d) Case management and care coordination
   (e) Contacting health care providers and patients with information about treatment alternatives
   (f) Functions not including treatment that are related to the purposes listed above
   (g) Performance evaluation, including reviewing the competence or qualifications of health care professionals
   (h) Evaluating practitioner or provider performance
   (i) Health plan performance
   (j) Conducting training programs in which health care students, trainees, or practitioners learn under supervision to practice or improve their skills
   (k) Training nonhealth care professionals
   (l) Accreditation, certification, licensing, or credentialing activities
   (m) Detecting health care fraud or abuse, or for compliance if they are not listed above.

Step 2D: Permitted Disclosures: Family, Friends, and Disaster Relief Agencies

Standard	Code of Federal Regulations	Protected Health Information Permissions
Permissible disclosures: family, friends and disaster relief agencies	45 CFR 164.510	Use and disclosure requiring an opportunity for the individual to agree or to object

What to Do:

A covered entity may use or disclose PHI, provided that the individual is informed in advance of the use or disclosure and has the opportunity to agree to or prohibit or restrict the use or disclosure.

How to Do It:

Either in verbal or written form, obtain the individual's agreement or objection to a use or disclosure requested by a friend, family member, or disaster relief agency.

CRITICAL POINT

Covered entities have frequently asked the Office for Civil Rights (OCR) about the rules for providing PHI to family, friends, and disaster relief. OCR has prepared a document, Communicating with a Patient's Family, Friends, or Others Involved in the Patient's Care, which is available online,[13] and is included in Appendix A.

Disclose PHI to friends and family if:

- The patient is able to agree to or prohibit use or disclosure.
- The patient is incapacitated, and the disclosure is in his or her best interest.
- The patient is present and has the capacity to make decisions, as to whether to share PHI with friends, family members, or disaster relief agencies.

If in your professional opinion, such as in cases of abuse, neglect, or domestic violence, you believe the disclosure is not in the patient's best interest, do not disclose PHI to friends or family members.

You may use or disclose PHI to a public or private disaster relief agency for the purpose of helping such entity notify a patient's family member, personal representative, or another person responsible for the patient's care, of the individual's location, general condition, or death. You should comply with the procedures discussed above regarding communicating with family members and friends if in your professional judgment you determine that doing so will not interfere with the ability to respond to the emergency circumstances.

To assist providers determine what PHI can be shared with friends, family, or other caregivers, the Office for Civil Rights has released a guidance, Communicating with a Patient's Family, Friends, or Others Involved in the Patient's Care, to provide PHI disclosure guidance to providers in an emergency.

---

13. Requests from law enforcement officials are treated in numerous sections of the HIPAA regulations. It is likely to be necessary to consult legal counsel in connection matters that involve law enforcement officials. Refer to: www.hhs.gov/ocr/privacy/hipaa/understanding/coveredentities/provider_ffg.pdf.

- An emergency room doctor may discuss a patient's treatment in front of the patient's friend if the patient asks that her friend come into the treatment room.
- A doctor's office may discuss a patient's bill with the patient's adult daughter who is with the patient at the patient's medical appointment and has questions about the charges.
- A doctor may discuss the drugs a patient needs to take with the patient's health aide who has accompanied the patient to a medical appointment.
- A doctor may give information about a patient's mobility limitations to the patient's sister who is driving the patient home from the hospital.

Step 2E: Incidental Uses or Disclosures

Standard	Code of Federal Regulations	Protected Health Information Permissions
Permissible disclosures: incident to a use or disclosure otherwise permitted or required	45 CFR 164.502(a)(1)(iii)	Uses and disclosures of PHI: general rules

What to Do:

HHS has provided guidance on what can be called an incidental use or disclosure: it cannot be a by-product of an underlying use or disclosure that violates *reasonable* Privacy Rule safeguards. *Translation*: You cannot rename a privacy violation an incidental disclosure.

How to Do It:

Put in place appropriate administrative, technical, and physical safeguards (See Step 10) that protect against uses and disclosures not permitted by the Privacy Rule and that limit incidental uses or disclosures.[14]

Ensure your organization also can meet the Privacy Rule *minimum necessary* standards.[15,16]

- Speak quietly when discussing a patient's condition with the patient, with family members in a waiting room, or other public areas.
- Avoid using patients' names in public hallways and elevators.
- Post signs in the facility to remind workforce members to protect patient confidentiality.

---

14. See 45 CFR 164.530(c).

15. 45 CFR § 164.502(b) and 45 CFR § 164.514(d).

16. See Office of Civil Rights (OCR) document, *Incidental Uses and Disclosures,* which is available at: www.hhs.gov/ocr/privacy/hipaa/understanding/coveredentities/incidentalusesanddisclosures.html.

- During the transition to an electronic office, store records in locked file cabinets until you are nearly paperless.
- Do not share passwords.
- Turn computer monitors away to avoid public viewing access
- Enforce sanctions against workforce members who do not keep voices low when discussing protected health information in public areas.

Step 2F: Other Uses or Disclosures in Which Authorization Is Not Required

Standard	Code of Federal Regulations	Protected Health Information Permissions
Other uses or disclosures for which authorization is not required	45 CFR 164.512	Uses and disclosure for which an authorization or opportunity to agree or object is not required

What to Do:

The HIPAA Privacy Rule provides details on specific circumstances in which a covered entity may be permitted to use or disclose PHI without the individual's authorization, including certain situations involving:

- Public health activities
- Victims of abuse, neglect, or domestic violence
- Health oversight activities
- Judicial and administrative proceedings
- Law enforcement purposes
- Decedents
- Organ and tissue donation
- Research
- Averting a serious threat to health or safety
- Specialized government functions (such as military and veterans, national security and intelligence, and correctional institutions)
- Workers' compensation.

How to Do It:

Each of the permitted uses and disclosures involves detailed requirements that must be met prior to use or disclosure. In most cases, you should consult an attorney as necessary prior to using or disclosing PHI under these circumstances to be sure the requirements have been met.

Consult Appendix A for guidance on building other permitted uses and disclosures into your policies and procedures. Also consult Appendix C for AMA Guidances on Uses and Disclosures in Step 2F.

Step 2G: Uses and Disclosures of De-identified Protected Health Information

Standard	Code of Federal Regulations	Protected Health Information Permissions
Uses and disclosures of de-identified PHI	45 CFR 164.502(d)(2); 45 CFR 164.514(a)-(c)	Uses and disclosures of PHI: general rules; other requirements relating to uses and disclosures of PHI

What to Do:

There are no restrictions on the use or disclosure of de-identified health information.

How to Do It:

De-identified health information is not protected health information and therefore does not require an authorization for use or disclosure.

Follow one of the two following processes to de-identify PHI:

1. Work with a credentialed statistician to de-identify PHI
2. Remove the following identifiers of the individual, the individual's relatives, household members, and employers:
   (a) Names
   (b) All geographic subdivisions smaller than a state, including street address, city, county, precinct, zip code, and their equivalent geocodes, except for the initial three digits of a zip code if, according to the current publicly available data from the Bureau of Census:
      i. The geographic unit formed by combining all zip codes with the same three initial digits contains more than 20,000 people; and
      ii. The initial three digits of a zip code for all such geographic units containing 20,000 or fewer people is changed to 000;
   (c) All elements of dates (except year) for dates directly related to the individual, including birth date, admission date, discharge date, date of death; and all ages over 89 and all elements of dates (including year) indicative of such age, except that such ages and elements may be aggregated into a single category of age 90 or older
   (d) Telephone numbers
   (e) Fax numbers
   (f) Electronic mail addresses
   (g) Social Security numbers
   (h) Medical record numbers
   (i) Health plan beneficiary numbers
   (j) Account numbers
   (k) Certificate/license numbers
   (l) Vehicle identifiers and serial numbers, including license plate numbers
   (m) Device identifiers and serial numbers

(n) Web Universal Resource Locators (URLs)
(o) Internet Protocol (IP) address numbers
(p) Biometric identifiers, including finger and voice prints
(q) Full face photographic images and any comparable images
(r) Any other unique identifying number, characteristic, or code, except as permitted for re-identification purposes provided certain conditions are met.

If you develop a code or other means of re-identifying the information, you cannot derive the code using information about the individual.

The code must not be otherwise capable of being translated so as to identify the individual.

Do not disclose the code or other means of re-identification for any other purpose or the mechanism for re-identification.

Step 2H: Limited Data Set[17] for Purposes of Research, Public Health, or Health Care Operations

Standard	Code of Federal Regulations	Protected Health Information Permissions
Limited data set for purposes of research, public health, or health care operations	45 CFR 164.514(e)	Other requirements relating to uses and disclosures of PHI

What to Do:

If your organization enters into a "data use agreement" with the recipient of your limited data set as required by HIPAA, you may only use or disclose a limited data set for purposes of research, public health, or health care operations (as defined by HIPAA) if you remove the identifiers specified in this step.

How to Do It:

If you participate in research, public health reporting (other than those required by law), or health care operations (as defined by HIPAA), your privacy official, in consultation with our practice's attorney, must either draft or review the data use agreement that safeguards protected health information. Require any limited data set recipient to sign the appropriate data use agreement.

To meet the requirements of a limited data set, remove the following 16 identifiers from protected health information.

1. Names;
2. Postal address information, other than town or city, state and zip code;

17. De-identified PHI removes 18 direct identifiers. A limited data set removes 16 identifiers, permitting only elements of dates, such as dates of birth, and town or city, state, and zip code to remain in the limited data set.

3. Telephone numbers;
4. Fax numbers;
5. Electronic mail addresses:
6. Social Security numbers;
7. Medical record numbers;
8. Health plan beneficiary numbers;
9. Account numbers;
10. Certificate/license numbers;
11. Vehicle identifiers and serial numbers, including license plate numbers;
12. Device identifiers and serial numbers;
13. Web Universal Resource Locators (URLs);
14. Internet Protocol (IP) address numbers;
15. Biometric identifiers, including finger and voice prints;
16. Full face photographic images and any comparable images.

Limited Data Set and the Breach Notification Rule

The Breach Notification Rule, discussed in Chapters 1 and 4, applies to limited data set. A limited data set is considered "unsecured" PHI under the Breach Notification Rule. If information in a limited data set is breached, you may be required to provide notification of the breach. To determine whether notification is required, you must assess the breach using a breach notification risk assessment. The risk assessment of a breach of information in a limited data set may indicate that breach notification is not required (for example, because it is so unlikely that a particular individual could be identified that disclosure does not pose a significant risk of harm). The assessment must be completed and documented nevertheless. Prior to engaging in a Limited Data Set Agreement, consult pages 42745 amd 42746 of the Breach Notification Rule. What follows is an excerpt of that discussion.

> decided against including the limited data set in the *[Guidance]* as a method for rendering protected health information unusable, unreadable, or indecipherable to unauthorized individuals due to the potential risk of re-identification of this information. … Through a risk assessment, a covered entity or business associate may determine that the risk of identifying a particular individual is so small that the use or disclosure poses not significant risk of harm to any individuals. For example, it may be determined that an impermissible use or disclosures of a limited data set that includes zip codes, based on the population features of those zip codes, does not create a significant risk that a particular individual can be identified. Therefore, there would be no significant risk of harm to the individual. If there is no significant risk of harm to the individual, then no breach has occurred and no notification is required. If, however, the covered entity or business associate

determines that the individual can be identified based on the information disclosed, and there is otherwise a significant risk of harm to the individual, then breach notification is required, unless one of the other exceptions discussed below applies. We have provided a narrow, explicit exception to what compromises the privacy or security of protected health information for a use or disclosure of protected health information that excludes the 16 direct identifiers ... as well as dates of birth and zip codes. Thus, we deem an impermissible use or disclosure of this information to not compromise the security or privacy of the protected health information, because we believe that impermissible uses or disclosures of this information—if subjected to the type of risk assessment described above—would pose a low level of risk. ... If, for example, the information does not contain birth dates but does contain zip code information or contains both birth dates and zip code information, then this narrow exception would not apply, and the covered entity or business associate would be required to perform a risk assessment to determine if the risk of re-identification poses a significant risk of harm to the individual.[18]

Step 3: Identify Uses and Disclosures that Require Authorizations

An authorization is written permission to disclose PHI to another person or entity. The authorization must be written in plain language so that the individual understands what is being disclosed and to whom.

Step 3A: Identify Uses and Disclosures that Require Authorizations

Standard	Code of Federal Regulations	Protected Health Information Permissions
Authorizations	45 CFR 164.508	Uses and disclosures for which an authorization is required

18. Department of Health and Human Services, Office of the Secretary, "45 CFR Parts 160 and 164: Breach Notification for Unsecured Protected Health Information; Interim Final Rule," *Federal Register*, v.74, n.162, August 24, 2009, pp. 42745-42746. *Guidance* referred to in the excerpt is found on pp. 42742-42743. The Breach Notification Rule, including *Guidance*, is discussed in Chapter 1.

What to Do:

If the use or disclosure is not permitted or required (Steps 1 through 2G), a covered entity must obtain a written "valid authorization" from the patient.[19] What constitutes a "valid authorization"?

FIGURE 3.4

Special Requirements for Disclosing Protected Health Information (PHI)

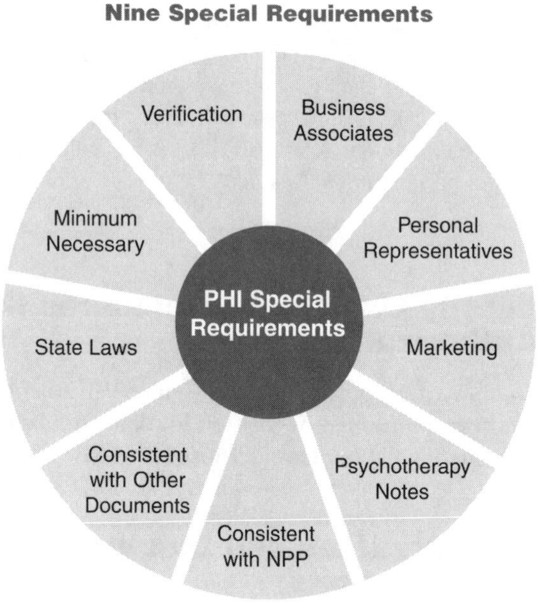

Nine Special Requirements

NPP indicates notice of privacy practices.
Reprinted with permission from Carolyn Hartley.

- It must be in plain language.
- It must contain certain "core elements" and required statements.
  - ☐ A description of the protected health information to be used or disclosed
  - ☐ The name of the person authorized to make the use or disclosure[20]

19. See the sample Authorization form in Appendix A.

20. Be sure to request and verify positive identification of the individual requesting the authorization, especially if that individual is not known to your practice.

- ☐ The name of person(s) to whom the requested use or disclosure may be made
- ☐ The purpose for the use or disclosure (if the patient has requested an authorization the privacy official may write "at the request of the individual")
- ☐ An expiration date or expiration event
- ☐ (Also see the Authorization form in Appendix A.)

- It must be signed and dated by the patient.
- You must make a copy of the authorization for the patient.

How to Do It:

Your privacy official will determine uses and disclosures that require authorization. A sampling of these may include:

- Posting pictures of patients on the wall
- Providing protected health information for a long-term care application
- Providing protected health information for health benefits plan.

Authorizations Overview

Using photos of patients as an example of treatment provided, such as before and after photos for plastic surgery, weight loss, or skin treatments. Photos of body sections that do not include the face are not de-identified and require authorization.

An authorization cannot be combined with another document. "Compounded authorizations" are prohibited.

With certain exceptions, a covered entity may not place conditions on the individual for treatment, payment, enrollment in a health plan, or eligibility for benefits on the provision of an authorization (this is referred to as a *conditional authorization*). Consult an attorney before placing any conditions on an authorization.

The patient may revoke the authorization at any time, provided the revocation is in writing. However, an authorization cannot be revoked if the practice has already taken action, relying on information provided in the authorization.

Use the workflow in Figure 3.5 to obtain an individual's authorization prior to using or disclosing PHI, which requires the individual's permission. Authorizations may be completed in person or via fax.

An authorization is defective and not valid if:

- It has expired;
- It has not been filled out completely;
- Our practice is aware that the authorization has been revoked;
- It is an impermissible *compound authorization*;
- It is an impermissible *conditional authorization*; and/or
- Our practice knows that material information in the authorization is false.

FIGURE 3.5

Authorization Workflow

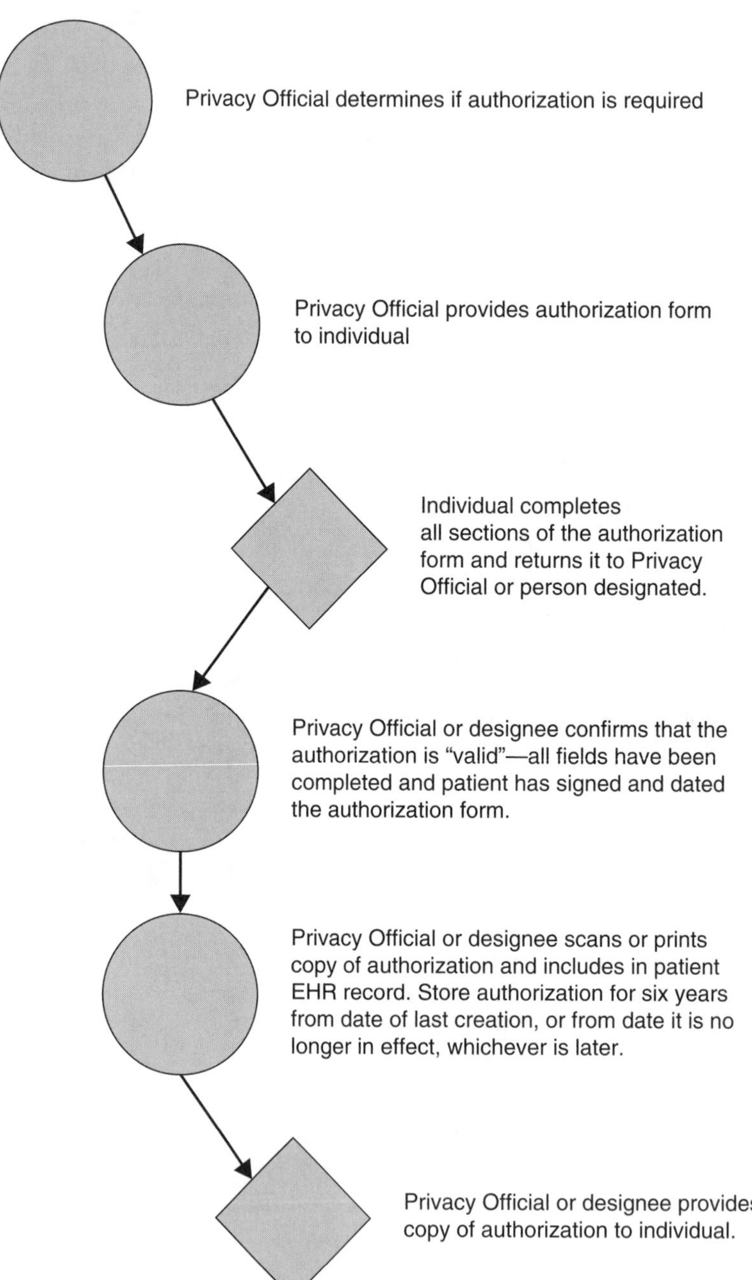

Privacy Official determines if authorization is required
Privacy Official provides authorization form to individual
Individual completes all sections of the authorization form and returns it to Privacy Official or person designated.
Privacy Official or designee confirms that the authorization is "valid"—all fields have been completed and patient has signed and dated the authorization form.
Privacy Official or designee scans or prints copy of authorization and includes in patient EHR record. Store authorization for six years from date of last creation, or from date it is no longer in effect, whichever is later.
Privacy Official or designee provides copy of authorization to individual.

CRITICAL POINT
If the use or disclosure is not for one of the following procedures (1–3), it will require an authorization.

1. Treatment, payment, or health care operations, which may include:
   - Quality assurance and quality reporting
   - Credentialing and licensing verification
   - Practitioner and provider evaluations
   - Insurance contracting and underwriting
   - Audits
   - Legal services
   - Compliance programs
   - Business planning and development
   - Management and general administration.
2. Request by the patient or his or her personal representative. (See reasons to deny requests in Step 6.)
3. Required by HIPAA, including uses or disclosures required by the Department of Health and Human Services for compliance audit or complaint investigation (See Step 2.)

Step 3B: Psychotherapy Notes

Standard	Code of Federal Regulations	Protected Health Information Permissions
Psychotherapy notes	45 CFR 164.508(a)(2)	Uses and disclosures for which an authorization is required

What to Do:
Psychotherapy notes receive special protection under HIPAA's Privacy Rule. A medical practice may not use or disclose psychotherapy notes for any purpose, including most treatment, payment, or health care operations, without a written authorization signed by the patient. However, as with all laws, there are exceptions.

How to Do It:
Obtain an authorization from the individual prior to releasing any psychotherapy notes.

Authorizations are not necessary for the following purposes:

- The originator of the notes wants to review them.
- The medical practice can use or disclose psychotherapy notes to defend itself in a legal action or other proceedings brought on by the patient.

- The Secretary of HHS wants to review them or law requires the use or disclosure.
- You need to avert a serious threat to health or safety. Consult an attorney on the release of psychotherapy notes.

"*Psychotherapy notes* excludes medication prescription and monitoring, counseling session start and stop times, the modalities and frequencies of treatment furnished, results of clinical tests, and any summary of the following items: Diagnosis, functional status, the treatment plan, symptoms, prognosis, and progress to date."[21]

Step 4: Identify Protected Health Information (PHI) Special Permissions

Standard	Code of Federal Regulations	Protected Health Information Special Permissions
Verification requirements	45 CFR 164.514(h)(2)	Other requirements relating to uses and disclosures of PHI

What to Do:

Verify the identity of a person requesting PHI. If you do not know the person making the request, request documentation that verifies who he or she is.

How to Do It:

Providers pride themselves in knowing patients and families, including details about the children, grandchildren, pets, and other relevant connections. However, you may not recognize everyone coming into the practice.

Before releasing any PHI to an individual or personal representative, ask for verification documents if you don't know the individual or if you aren't sure of the patient's name; and/or verify the identity and authority of that person using the following processes:

For New Patients:

- Upon entering the practice, each new patient is required to provide at least two forms of ID, with one being a photo ID.
- Verify that the name on a credit card is the same as the name on the photo ID.
- Make an electronic copy of the photo ID and scan it into the patient's chart. If you are still using paper charts, attach the photo to the inside of the patient record.
- Using a digital camera, take a photo of the patient and upload it into the patient's electronic chart.
- Return both cards to the individual.

21. 45 CFR 164.501

For Existing Patients:

To verify the identity and authority of an existing patient who requests PHI, we will proceed using the following steps:

- Determine whether verification is needed (do we know this person?). If we do not know the person, then proceed to Step 2.
- If you don't know the person, then follow the if-then procedures in Table 3.2.

TABLE 3.2

If-Then Verification Procedures If You Do NOT Know the Individual

If-Then Procedures	
IF	**THEN**
It's the patient in the practice or clinic.	Request a photo ID and one other credit card. You may also request an address or date of birth for verification.
It's the patient, but on the phone.	Ask the individual to provide details that would help identify the patient. This may include last name, date of birth, address, or approximate date last seen in your practice.
It's a friend or family member.	Request a photo ID; require signature from the person requesting PHI. When identity has been verified, see Step 2C regarding disclosures to friends or family members.
It's a personal representative.	If a personal representative accompanies the individual, exercise professional judgment to verify that this person is acting on behalf of the individual and verify his or her identity. If you are unsure of the representative, request a copy of the power of attorney or other document, such as legal guardianship, and request a photo ID. When identity has been verified, see Section Step 2A regarding disclosures to personal representatives.
It's a public official.	Contact the privacy official. Request to see the identification badge or other official credentials. If the request is in writing, review the appropriate government letterhead, insignia, address, and credentials. When identity has been verified, see Step 2E, "Uses and Disclosures for which an Authorization or Opportunity to Agree or Object is not Required," for more information regarding permissible disclosures to public officials.

When to Decline to Recognize Identity and Authority

If, in your professional opinion, you have followed verification procedures, and in your professional opinion, you doubt the requester's credentials, politely tell the requestor that you are unable to release the PHI. Document your decision in the verification log. If the person persists, he or she may request a meeting with our privacy official.

Require all persons receiving PHI to acknowledge receiving it by signing a Verification of Identity form.[22] This form will be scanned and saved in the patient's record or copied and placed in the patient's paper chart.

22. See Appendix A for sample form: Verification of Identity.

Step 5: Update your HIPAA Privacy Safeguards

Standard	Federal Register	HIPAA Privacy Safeguards
Administrative requirements	45 CFR 164.530(c)	Safeguards

What to Do:

A covered entity must have in place administrative, technical, and physical safeguards to protect the privacy of PHI. These safeguards must reasonably safeguard PHI from any intentional or unintentional use or disclosure that is in violation of the Privacy Rule.

How to Do It:

Create, train and implement policies and procedures, including sanctions, which safeguard PHI in oral, hard copy (paper and other physical documentation such as dental films), and electronic formats.[23]

Tables 3.3, 3.4, and 3.5 provide examples of administrative, physical, and technical safeguards for your practice.

Within the Privacy Rule, there is a sub-security rule. The following tables provide safeguards addressed in HIPAA's Privacy Rule.

TABLE 3.3

Sample Administrative Safeguards

Privacy Rule Safeguards	Required Actions
Sign-in Sheets	Patients sign in using last name only and time of arrival.
Communications	Avoid unnecessary disclosures of PHI by monitoring voice levels. Conduct dictation and telephone conversations in private areas.
Telephone Messages	Telephone messages and appointment reminders may be left on answering machines and voicemail systems unless the patient has requested he or she be contacted by alternative means, or you suspect abuse or neglect.
Faxes	Only the PHI necessary will be faxed. Use a cover sheet that includes a confidentiality notice.
Mail	PHI mailed will be concealed and sent via first class mail to the patient's primary address or the patient's alternative address.
Copies	Copies of records containing PHI will be stamped "Copy" in a color other than black.

23. The HIPAA Security Rule covers the administrative, physical, and technical safeguard implementation specifications for electronic protected health information. The security safeguards are discussed in Chapter 4.

TABLE 3.4

Sample Physical Safeguards

Privacy Rule Safeguards	Required Actions
Facility Access Controls	Outline procedures that allow facility access and support data restoration in a disaster or emergency. Control access daily.
Facility Security Plan	Outline procedures that safeguard the facility and the equipment inside from unauthorized physical access, tampering, and theft.
Access Control and Validation	Outline procedures that control and validate an individual's access to facilities based on their role or function.
Maintenance Records	Document repairs and modifications to the facility that may have an impact on security such as changes in walls, hardware, doors, and locks.
Workstation Use	Determine the functions to be performed for each workstation in the facility, the manner these functions are performed, and the physical attributes of the surroundings.
Workstation Security	Outline physical safeguards for all workstations in the facility that allow access to PHI and restrict access to authorized users.
Device and Media Controls	**For disposal**, use software that completely overwrites the magnetic area of the media that stores the data. **Media Reuse:** Treat media to be reused as PHI that is being disposed. **Accountability:** Outline procedures for documenting movements of either hardware or the electronic media containing PHI.
Patients and Visitors	Visitors and patients will be appropriately monitored during their visits at the practice. Patients will not be allowed to access other patient's records or other PHI.

TABLE 3.5

Sample Technical Safeguards

Privacy Rule Safeguards	Required Actions
Computer Controls	Determine types of information that should be made available to workforce members. EHRs are typically role-based, but the system administrator, with written justification, may modify access.
Emergency Access	Develop emergency operations procedures in the event of, and during, a disaster or emergency. At least two individuals should be designated to have responsibility for emergency access

(continued)

TABLE 3.5 (continued)

Sample Technical Safeguards

Privacy Rule Safeguards	Required Actions
Data Integrity Controls	Put security mechanisms in place and keep in working order to ensure transmission or receipt of PHI is completed securely.
Audit Controls	Review system configurations and mechanisms for tracking access to and use of networks, workstations, and information.
Encryption	Encrypt data that could be accessed on a portable device, desktop computer, server and Internet connection by an unauthorized user.
Data Authentication	Review system configuration and conduct audits to ensure data can only be created or modified by authorized users.

Step 6: Update New Patient Rights, Including Rights Provided in the HITECH Act

The HITECH Act added patient rights that will change your policies and procedures, which also may change your Notice of Privacy Practices. Consult your health law attorney to determine if a change to the NPP also must be made.

In Steps 6A through 6F, we will provide an overview of those changes, as well as updates to patient rights.

Step 6A: Right to Access Protected Health Information (PHI)

Standard	Code of Federal Regulations	Patients Rights
Access a copy of PHI	45 CFR 164.524	Individuals' access to PHI

What to Do:

Unless a covered entity has grounds to deny an individual access, an individual has a right to access, inspect, and obtain a copy of the PHI about the individual in a designated record set for as long as the PHI is maintained in the designated record set. Right to access does not include:

1. Psychotherapy notes
2. Information compiled in reasonable anticipation of, or for use in, a civil, criminal, or administrative action or proceeding
3. PHI maintained by a covered entity that is either (a) exempt from the Clinical Laboratory Improvements Amendments of 1988 (CLIA), or that is (b) subject CLIA, to the extent the provision of access to the individual would be prohibited by law.

How to Do It:

According to your internal policies and procedures, a patient's request to access PHI should be directed to the privacy official or a person designated to act in the privacy official's absence, such as the security official, if a different individual.

Verify the patient's identity. If you know the patient, you are not required to obtain verification documentation. If you do not know the patient, ask for at least two forms of identification, with one being a photo ID. If the photo ID and second piece of identification do not match, the request must be denied. In most cases, your practice can honor the patient's request for access to PHI.

Ask the patient to complete the "Patient Request to Access Protected Health Information."[24] In completing this form, ask the patient to define the information requested, such as:

- Status of accounts payable
- Lab, imaging, or pathology results from last patient visit
- A record of a child's immunization dates.

Record the request in a Request to Access PHI log.

You may charge a reasonable cost-based fee as permitted by HIPAA, unless a more stringent state law applies. These may include:

a. Charges for hard copies:
   i. Copying, including the cost of supplies for the labor of copying the requested information.
   ii. Postage, when the individual has requested the copy or a summary or explanation (see below) to be mailed.
b. A charge for preparing the summary or explanation, but only if:
   i. The individual has agreed in advance to such a summary or explanation, and
   ii. The individual has agreed in advance to the fees for preparing the summary or explanation.
c. A fee for providing an individual with an electronic copy (or an electronic summary or explanation of electronic protected health information). The fee may not be greater than the labor costs in responding to the request for the electronic copy (or summary or explanation).

Place a copy of the Request for Access to PHI in the patient's file.

Provide the requested PHI to the patient or send via US Postal Service. You may send the PHI electronically, only if the patient has signed an authorization to provide information electronically.

HIPAA Privacy Rule allows the privacy official 30 days to respond to the request.

If you are using electronic health record (EHR) software, individuals also may request that PHI be provided to them in an electronic format, such as on a USB drive, a CD, on a SIM card, or to a secure patient portal. While it is wise to advise the patient to provide safeguards to the patient-owned USB drive, security of the USB drive is the responsibility of the patient.

---

24. A Patient Request to Access Protected Health Information form is provided for you in Appendix A.

Establish protocols on what you will and will not download from your electronic patient record to a patient's electronic personal health record. Note that in such instances, state laws also may apply, which are more stringent than HIPAA. For example, some states limit a minor's access to PHI.

Reasons to deny access:

- You determine the individual making the request is not the patient.
- You do not hold information requested in a designated record set.
- In your professional judgment, the patient's access is reasonably likely to endanger the life or physical safety of the individual or another person.
- The PHI makes reference to another person (unless the other person is a health care provider) and in your professional judgment, the access requested is reasonably likely to cause substantial harm to that other person.
- The request is made by a personal representative, and in your professional judgment, the personal representative is reasonably likely to cause substantial harm to the individual or another person.

In some cases, the individual may request that your denial be reviewed.[25] Unreviewable grounds for denial include the following:

- The covered entity does not hold the requested information in its designated record set.
- The information was compiled in reasonable anticipation of or for use in a civil, criminal, or administrative action or proceeding.
- Information was obtained from someone other than your clinicians under a promise of confidentiality, and access would reveal the source of the information.

Denial procedures:

If your practice denies the request, put the reason for denial in a plain language letter to the patient. The letter must include:

a. A plain language reason for the denial. If the denial is based on "reviewable" grounds, the denial must state that the individual may request a review of the denial and describe how the individual may exercise such review right.[26]

---

25. See 45 CFR. 164.524(a)(2) for the full list of unreviewable grounds for denial, which also includes certain provisions relating to psychotherapy notes, the Clinical Laboratory Improvements Amendments of 1988 (42 USC 263a), inmates of correctional institutions, research, and the Privacy Act (5 USC 552a).

26. In general, if an individual requests a review, the covered entity must designate a licensed health care professional who was not directly involved in the denial to review the decision and must promptly refer the request for review to such professional. The professional must determine, within a reasonable period of time, whether or not to deny access. The covered entity must promptly provide written notice to the individual of the determination and must take any action required to carry out the determination. Reviewable grounds for denying access are listed at 45 CFR 164.524(a)(3). The procedure for responding to a review of a denial of access are found in 45 CFR 164.524(a)(4) and 164.524(d)(4).

b. A description of how the individual may complain to the practice (including the name or title and telephone number of the contract person or office that have designated to receive complaints)[27] or to the Secretary of HHS.

If your practice does not maintain the PHI but knows where it can be located, inform the patient where to redirect his or her request for access.

Document your decision to deny access to the patient's record, and keep a denial of access log. Consult a health law attorney, if the individual requests a review of your denial and you are uncertain how to proceed.

Figure 3.4 outlines the access and denial decision paths for your practice.

FIGURE 3.6

Access and Denial Decision Paths

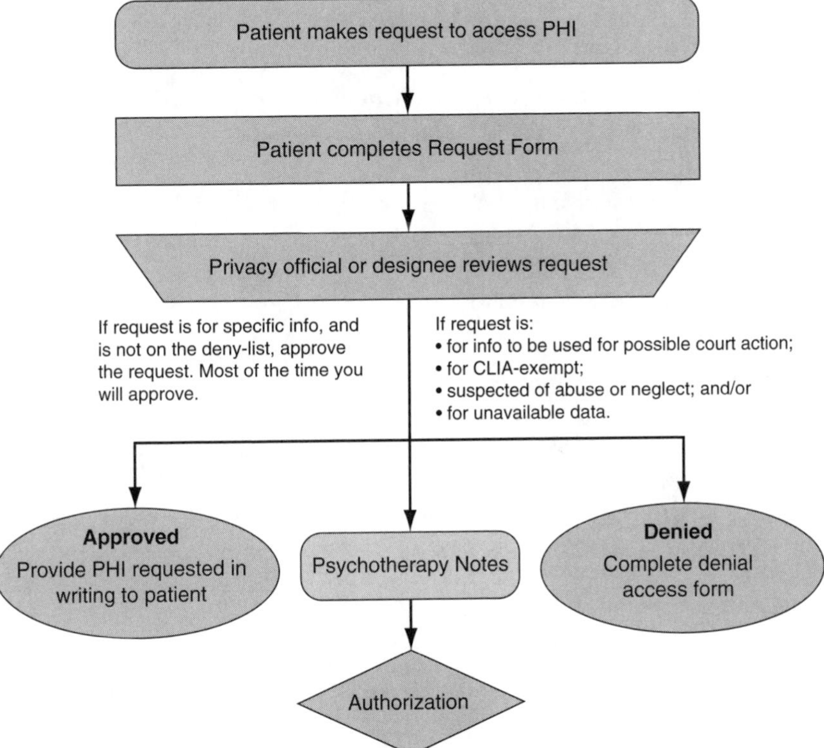

CLIA indicates clinical lab improvement amendment

Step 6B: Patient's Right to Request an Amendment to Content in Patient Record

Standard	Code of Federal Regulations	Patients Rights
Request to amend	45 CFR 164.526	Amendment of PHI

27. See Section 2.4.6, "Complaints."

What to Do:

You must allow an individual to request an amendment to content included in the patient's record. You may deny the individual's request to make the amendment, but if you agree with the request, then you must amend the record.

How to Do It:

In your Notice of Privacy Practices, you have stated that an individual may request in writing that you amend information in the individual's medical record if that information is incorrect.

Ask the patient to provide the amendment request in writing. If you agree to the amendment, you must amend the PHI in your designated record set(s). If you deny the request, notify the individual in writing why you are denying the request.

Complete the amendment within 60 days of receipt. You are entitled to one 30-day extension, if you explain the delay to the individual in writing.[28]

Maintain documentation of each amendment request, [29] including a log of amendment requests.[30]

Reasons to Deny Request for an Amendment

The information or record that is the subject of the request:

1. Is accurate and complete;
2. Would not be available for access by the individual;[31]
3. Was not created by our practice (unless the individual provides a reasonable basis to believe the originator is no longer available); or
4. Is not part of the designated record set.[32]

If your practice grants a request to amend the patient's PHI, complete the following:

1. Inform the patient of your decision;
2. Identify the affected records and make the amendment;
3. Inform parties whom the patient identifies as requiring the newly amended information;
4. Make reasonable efforts to provide the amendment to identified and designated individuals in the amendment request (including your business associates).

28. 45 CFR 164.526(b)(2)(ii).

29. See Appendix A for sample form: Patient Request for Amendment of Patient's Protected Health Information.

30. See Appendix A for sample form: Amendment Request Log.

31. See section 2.4.1 "Access Request" in this chapter or 45 CFR 164.524 for more information about when information is available for access by the individual.

32. *Designated record set* generally includes medical records, billing records, health plan enrollment, payment, claims adjudication, and case management records, or other records that we use to make decisions about individuals. For purposes of defining a *designated record set*, the word "record" includes any item, collection, or grouping of information that includes protected health information that is maintained, collected, used, or disseminated by or for the practice. For the complete definition, see 45 CFR 164.501 or Glossary.

Step 6C: Accounting of Disclosures

Standard	Code of Federal Regulations	Patient Rights
Accounting of disclosures	45 CFR 164.528	Accounting of disclosures of PHI

What to Do:

An individual has a right to receive an accounting of the disclosures of PHI made by a covered entity in the six years prior to the date in which the accounting is requested with certain exceptions. This accounting of disclosures does not include those for treatment, payment, and health care operations.

New If your practice is using an EHR system, the individual also may now request an electronic accounting of disclosures, including those for treatment, payment, and health care operations, which were made up to three years prior to the request. Consult the Guidance for Electronic Accounting of Disclosures in this step for a description of compliance dates.

Consult your EHR software company to ensure it will be ready to provide these electronic accountings of disclosures.

How to Do It:

Take all requests for an accounting of disclosures to the privacy official or person designated by the privacy official. Ask the patient to put the request for an accounting of disclosures in writing using the Request for Accounting of Disclosures form provided in Appendix A. You have 60 days from the date of receipt of the request to provide an accounting, with a one time 30-day extension, if you provide the individual with a written statement of the reasons for the delay and the date on which you will provide the accounting.[33]

What to Do:

Use the Accounting of Disclosures Log provided in Appendix A. Maintain documentation of content provided in each disclosure, and the title of the person or office responsible for receiving and processing requests for an accounting for six years from the date of its creation, or the date when it was last in effect, whichever is later.

You must provide the first accounting to the patient in any 12-month period without charge, but you may charge a reasonable cost-based fee for subsequent requests within the 12-month period if:

- you have informed the patient in advance of the cost, and
- you have provided the patient with an opportunity to withdraw or modify the request to avoid or reduce the fee.

An individual has the right to request an accounting of disclosures made up to 6 years prior to the date of request, but not prior to April 14, 2003.

33. 45 CFR § 164.528(c)(1)(ii).

Guidance for Electronic Accounting of Disclosures

If a covered entity uses an EHR, an individual has the right to receive an accounting of disclosures for treatment, payment, and health care operations, which the covered entity made during the 3 years prior to the date of the request. The effective date of this requirement depends on when the EHR was adopted. An entity that adopted an EHR before January 1, 2009, must comply on January 1, 2011. A practice that adopted an EHR on or after January 1, 2009, must comply by January 1, 2014. The Secretary of HHS may extend these dates.

For a discussion with your EHR software vendor, ask about forthcoming updates and functionalities that will allow you to generate an accounting of the following:

- Disclosures to individuals of protected health information
- Disclosures made incident to a disclosure otherwise permitted or required under HIPAA privacy
- Disclosures that were authorized by the individual[34]
- Appropriate disclosures to family and friends (see Step 2C of this chapter)
- Certain disclosures for national security or intelligence[35] or to correctional institutions or law enforcement officials[36]
- Disclosures of information as part of a limited data set (see Step 2H of this chapter).

The accounting of disclosures must include the following information regarding disclosures made by a practice or by one of the business associates during the applicable time period:

- Date of disclosure.
- Name of the entity or person who received the information, and if known, the address of the entity or person.
- A brief description of the PHI disclosed.
- A brief statement of the purpose of the disclosure, or if applicable, a copy of the written request for disclosure.[37]

Under certain circumstances, our practice may be required to suspend a patient's right to receive an accounting of his or her disclosures made to health oversight agencies or law enforcement officials.[38]

---

34. 45 CFR 164.508.

35. 45 CFR 164.512(k)(2).

36. 45 CFR 164.512(k)(5).

37. A copy of the written request for disclosure may be provided instead of a brief statement of the purpose of the disclosure if the disclosure was made to HHS in connection with an investigation or determination of HIPAA Privacy compliance 45 CFR 164.528(b)(2)(iv) and 45 CFR §164.502(a)(2)(ii) or if the disclosure was required by law, for public health activities, about victims of abuse, neglect, or domestic violence, for health oversight activities, for judicial and administrative proceedings, for law enforcement purposes, about decedents, organ or tissue donation, research, to avert a serious threat to health or safety, specialized government functions (such as military and veterans activities, and government programs providing public benefits), and workers compensation (see 45 CFR 164.512).

38. 45 CFR 164.528(a)(2).

Step 6D: Confidential Communications Requirements

Standard	Code of Federal Regulations	Patient Rights
Confidential communications requirements	45 CFR 164.522 (b)	Rights to request privacy protection for PHI

What to Do:

A covered entity health care provider must permit individuals to request and must accommodate reasonable requests by individuals to receive communications of PHI from the covered entity by alternative means or at alternative locations. For example, an individual may request to be contacted on a mobile phone rather than the home phone for any calls from the provider's office, including appointment reminder calls, test results, or other communications. You may set conditions for Alternative Communications to ensure an address for billing purposes is included in your records.

How to Do It:

Upon signing in as a new patient, require the patient to complete a "Confidential Communications Information Sheet," which indicates that you communicate with him or her at a specific telephone number or address, if the alternative means or location is different from the primary address.

When making appointments for existing patients, ask if contact information has changed in the last year.

Step 6E: Right of an Individual to Request Restriction of Uses and Disclosures

Standard	Code of Federal Regulations	Patient Rights
Right of an individual to request restriction of uses and disclosures	45 CFR 164.522(a)	Rights to request privacy protection for PHI

What to Do:

A covered entity must permit an individual to request that the covered entity restrict (1) uses or disclosures of PHI about the individual for treatment, payment, or health care operations[39]; and (2) permitted disclosures involving the individual's care and notification purposes.[40]

As a covered entity, you are not required to agree to a restriction, but if you agree to the restriction, you must comply, except for the following reasons:

39. See Step 2B: Permissible Disclosures: Treatment, Payment, and Health Care Operations.

40. See Step 2C: Permissible Disclosures: Another Covered Entity's Treatment, Payment, and Health Care Operations.

1. ***Emergency Treatment:*** If the individual, who requested the restriction, needs emergency treatment and, the restricted PHI is needed for such treatment, you may use the restricted information or may disclose the information to a health care provider to provide emergency treatment. The covered entity must request that the emergency care provider not further use or disclose the information.
2. ***HHS Investigation:*** A covered entity is required to disclose PHI when required by the Secretary of HHS in connection with an investigation or to determine compliance with HIPAA Privacy.
3. ***Permitted Uses and Disclosures:*** An agreement to restrict disclosure is not effective to prevent uses or disclosures for which an authorization or opportunity to agree or object is not required.[41]

New As of February 18, 2010, a covered entity must comply with an individual's request to restrict the disclosure of his or her PHI to a health plan for payment or health care operations (as defined by HIPAA), if the PHI pertains solely to a health care item or service for which the health care provider has been paid out of pocket in full.[42]

This restriction may adjust reimbursement workflows. For example, if a patient receives two or more services in one visit, pays for one of the services in full out of pocket, and requests that you not disclose information about the second service, you must determine how best to appropriately maintain the PHI in relation to the procedures to comply with the request.

Other than the out-of-pocket payment-in-full provision, the covered entity is not required to agree to a requested restriction. In general, most covered entities agree to restrictions only when exceptional circumstances exist and when they can reasonably accommodate them.

The privacy official should determine whether or not to agree to the request.

Document the decision if you agree to a restriction request. You may use and disclose PHI for treatment, payment, and health care operations, except as noted for the out-of-pocket payment-in-full provision, and as required or permitted by HIPAA for emergency treatment, HHS investigation, and/or permitted uses and disclosures.

To terminate a restriction:

1. The patient agrees to, or requests the termination in writing.
2. The patient orally agrees to the termination, and the oral agreement is documented.
3. Inform the individual that you are terminating the restriction agreement, but the termination is effective only to PHI created or received after you have informed the patient that the restriction has been terminated.

---

41. See 45 CFR 164.512, covering certain uses and disclosures required by law and certain uses and disclosures pertaining to public health activities, victims of abuse, neglect or domestic violence, health oversight activities, judicial and administrative proceedings, law enforcement purposes, decedents, organ or tissue donation, research purposes, averting a serious threat to health or safety, specialized government functions, and workers' compensation.

42. 42 USC 17935(a).

Step 6F: Right to File a Complaint

Standard	Code of Federal Regulations	Patients Rights
Complaints	45 CFR 164,530 (a)(ii); 45 CFR 164.520(b)(1)(vi); 45 CFR 164.530(d); 45 CFR 164.530(g)	Notice of Privacy Practices for PHI; administrative requirements

Since April 14, 2003, when HIPAA Privacy Rule became enforceable, complaints filed with the Office for Civil Rights have grown from 3,743 in 2003 to 8,526 in 2008.

TABLE 3.8

Top Five Issues in Investigated Cases Closed with Corrective Action, by Calendar Year[43]

	Issue 1	Issue 2	Issue 3	Issue 4	Issue 5
Partial Year 2003	Safeguards	Impermissible Uses and Disclosures	Access	Notice	Minimum Necessary
2004	Impermissible Uses and Disclosures	Safeguards	Access	Minimum Necessary	Mitigation
2005	Impermissible Uses and Disclosures	Safeguards	Access	Minimum Necessary	Notice
2006	Impermissible Uses and Disclosures	Safeguards	Access	Minimum Necessary	Notice
2007	Impermissible Uses and Disclosures	Safeguards	Access	Minimum Necessary	Notice
2008	Impermissible Uses and Disclosures	Safeguards	Access	Minimum Necessary	Amendments
2009	Impermissible Uses and Disclosures	Safeguards	Access	Minimum Necessary	Complaints to Covered Entity

What to Do:

Designate the contact person or office responsible for receiving complaints and for providing further information about the Notice of Privacy Practices. To accommodate complaints, provide a process to receive and mitigate complaints.

Include a statement in your Notice of Privacy Practices that individuals may complain to the practice's privacy official and the Secretary of HHS, if they

43. Office for Civil Rights,

believe their privacy rights have been violated. Provide a brief description of how the individual may file a complaint with the privacy official and a statement that the individual will not be retaliated against for filing a complaint.

New The Privacy Rule and Breach Notification Rules require that a process be put in place to receive complaints. A covered entity may not intimidate or take retaliatory action against an individual for filing a complaint.

The Breach Notification Rule requires extensive communications for an electronic breach of PHI. Consult Chapter 4 for more information on this rule.

Train all workforce members on the contents of the Notice of Privacy Practices and how to enter the time, date, and a brief description of the complaint into a log.[44]

The privacy official's next step includes the following:

- Listen to the individual's complaint, and then ask the individual to document the details of the complaint to make sure that the practice has a common understanding of the nature of the complaint and a record of the complaint;
- Make inquiries into the nature of the complaint to determine what has occurred, and whether it constitutes a HIPAA privacy breach of PHI and/or a violation of the practice's policies and procedures;
- Put a response in writing to the complainant, either describing how the practice will address and resolve the complaint, or explaining why the practice's action did not violate any policies or procedures and/or breach of PHI; and
- Remind the individual that, *at no time,* will the practice retaliate against an individual for filing a privacy complaint.

Step 7: Disclosures to Business Associates

Standard	Code of Federal Regulations	Protected Health Information Special Permissions
Disclosures to business associates	45 CFR 164.502(e); 45 CFR 164.504(e)	Uses and disclosures of PHI: general rules

What to Do:

A covered entity may disclose PHI to a business associate, and may allow a business associate to create or receive PHI on its behalf, if the covered entity obtains satisfactory assurance that the business associate will appropriately safeguard the information.

CRITICAL POINT

Effective February 17, 2010, business associates are required to comply with the Security Rule and Breach Notification Rule. Consult with your vendors, including your EHR vendor, to determine if a risk analysis to determine the threats and vulnerabilities of their products and services has been conducted.

44. See Appendix A for sample form: Complaint Log.

Effective February 17, 2010, business associates are required to comply with the Security Rule and Breach Notification Rule, with the latter being enforced for covered entities and business associates on February 22, 2010, for breaches occurring on or after that date. According to the HITECH Act, covered entities and business associates must create new or amend existing business associate agreements to incorporate relevant obligations for each party to the agreement.[45]

In a Business Associate Agreement, a covered entity and its business associates provide satisfactory assurances that PHI will be secure and that each develops and implements policies and procedures to safeguard the PHI. Effective February 17, 2010, business associates will be regulated directly by the federal government for the first time in the same manner that covered entities are regulated under HIPAA.

A covered entity is not in compliance with the Business Associate Agreement standard if it knows of a pattern of activity, or practice of the business associate that constitutes a material breach or violation of the business associate's obligation under the contract unless the covered entity takes reasonable steps to cure the breach or end the violation, as applicable. If such steps are unsuccessful, the covered entity must terminate the contract, if feasible, or if termination is not feasible, report the problem to the Secretary of HHS. Effective February 17, 2010, this obligation works both ways: a business associate thereafter must report a violation of the covered entity for which the covered entity has not taken reasonable steps to cure the breach.

How to Do It:

The privacy official will work with the practice's attorney to identify business associates and to develop an updated business associate agreement form for our practice, or with another covered entity acting in a business associate role.

Develop a policy that says effective February 17, 2010, no member of the workforce is permitted to disclose PHI to a business associate unless your practice has an updated executed agreement with that business associate.

"Business associate" is defined by HIPAA:[46]

- A "business associate" means an entity, or a person who is not a member of a covered entity's workforce, that performs, on behalf of a covered entity, a function or activity involving the use or disclosure of PHI.
- Examples of business associates include claims processing or administration, data analysis, processing or administration, utilization review, quality assurance, billing, benefit management, practice management, and repricing. Entities and persons are also business associates if they provide a covered entity legal, actuarial, accounting, consulting, data aggregation, management, administrative, accreditation, or financial services to the covered entity, in

45. See 42 USC 17931 (security obligations) and 42 USC 17934 (privacy obligations).

46. See Appendix A for the regulatory definition of *business associate*, or see 45 CFR§ 160.103.

which the provision of the service involves the disclosure of individually identifiable health information from such covered entity or arrangement, or from another business associate of the covered entity.

- A covered entity may be a business associate of another covered entity.
- Any organization that provides electronic data transmission services of PHI to a covered entity or its business associate and that requires access on a routine basis to such PHI will be treated as a business associate. Examples of such organizations include Health Information Exchange Organizations (HIEOs), Regional Health Information Organizations (RHIOs), E-prescribing Gateways, and certain vendors whose contracts with covered entities involves EHR, practice management, or personal health record systems.[47]

Any business associate requesting access to PHI must first consult the privacy official.

The privacy official ensures that new business associate agreements incorporating privacy and security provisions of the HITECH Act are in place with each of our business associates before February 17, 2010.

The privacy official must train the workforce members to report any pattern of activity or practice of a business associate that constitutes a material breach or violation of the business associate's obligation under the contract.

If you discover such a pattern of activity or practice, it is the privacy official's duty to take reasonable steps to cure the breach or end the violation, as applicable.

If corrective steps are unsuccessful, the practice may terminate the contract, if feasible, or if termination is not feasible, report the problem to the Secretary of HHS.

Step 8: Revise and Protect Marketing Activities

Standard	Code of Federal Regulations	Protected Health Information Special Permissions
Marketing	45 CFR 164.508	Uses and disclosures for which an authorization is required

What to Do:

New Providing PHI for marketing purposes may only be completed after obtaining a "valid authorization" in connection with a marketing communication. This applies irrespective of whether the communication is made by your practice or by another entity. The marketing authorization must also contain additional provisions. This determination is a complex matter with many provisions and

47. 42 USC 17938.

exceptions, and it becomes even more complicated as the HITECH Act takes effect. HIPAA, as amended by the HITECH Act, regulates the types of authorization that is required, which is listed in the following type of situations:

- A covered entity uses PHI (such as patients' names and addresses, and/or information about their health conditions) to make a marketing communication about the covered entity's own products and services;
- A covered entity uses PHI to make a marketing communication in exchange for payment from an outside entity;
- A covered entity discloses PHI so that a business associate can make a marketing communication; and
- A covered entity exchanges PHI for payment or other remuneration so that another entity can send a marketing communication.

How to Do It:

The HIPAA marketing communication regulations will change over time as the HITECH Act becomes effective and as the HHS adopts new HITECH regulations.

Keep up to date on HITECH developments and consult with your practice's legal counsel about how your practice handles marketing communications.

As a general rule, a covered entity may not use or disclose PHI for communication about a product or service that encourages the recipient of the communication to purchase the product or service unless the covered entity has obtained a certain form of "valid authorization"[48] from the individual.

An authorization is not required when communication is face to face with an individual or when communication is in the form of a promotional gift of nominal value.

Examples of marketing activities that require authorization include, but are not limited to:

- A company that wants to send a marketing communication to all your patients with diabetes offers to give you direct or indirect remuneration or payment in exchange for these patients' names and addresses. You must obtain prior valid authorization from these patients. The authorization must state that remuneration is involved. As of 2011, the authorization is required to specify if the company receiving the data can further exchange it for remuneration; and/or
- A company offers to pay you to send a communication to all your patients encouraging them to purchase one of the manufacturer's products. You will require authorization before sending such communications, and the communication must state that such remuneration is involved.

Examples of communications that do not require authorizations include, but are not limited to:

- You send out a notice to your patients that your office is relocating;
- You announce the arrival of a new physician or nurse practitioner;
- You recommend case management or care coordination for the individual, or direct or recommend alternative treatments, therapies, health care providers, or settings of care to the individual, and you do not receive direct or indirect payment for making such communication;

48. 45 CFR. § 164.508.

- A pharmacy sends out a refill reminder for a medication that you prescribed for a patient; and/or
- A pharmaceutical company offers to pay you to send a marketing communication to certain of your patients, and the communication describes only a drug or biologic that is currently being prescribed for the recipients of the communication, and any payment that you receive in exchange for making the communication is reasonable in amount (HHS will adopt regulations regarding what is reasonable).

Step 9: Train Your Staff on New Issues and Provide Refreshers for Privacy Policies and Procedures

The most dynamic privacy training sessions occurred in April 2003 when the Privacy Rule became enforceable. Informal training in most practices has continued as reactive measures, primarily as issues come up.

In February 2009, when President Obama signed the American Recovery and Reinvestment Act, allocating billions of dollars to reimburse health care providers for adopting EHR, the privacy safeguards and enforcement penalties escalated dramatically. Consumers needed additional confidence that taxpayer dollars would be used to benefit health information exchange and improved coordination of care, and that their PHI would be used and exchanged securely.

More information is provided about the Enforcement Rule in Chapters 1 and 4, but in a nutshell, it includes the following:

- Compliance is no longer voluntary, but driven by well-funded compliance officers hired to conduct random privacy and security audits.
- State attorneys general are authorized to conduct independent investigations into privacy and security breaches. On January 13, 2010, the state of Connecticut filed a historic lawsuit against Health Net for failing to secure patient medical records and financial information involving 446,000 Connecticut enrollees, and to promptly notify customers endangered by the security breach.[49]
- The Office for Civil Rights has been named the enforcement agency for both privacy and security breaches, effective July 27, 2009.
- The Breach Notification Rule obligates covered entities and business associates to provide an expanded notice-of-incidents, using specific language to "prominent media outlets," including HHS, if more than 500 residents in one state are affected by the breach. The privacy official, in

49. *Attorney General Sues Health Net for Massive Security Breach Involving Private Medical Records and Financial Information on 446,000 Enrollees.* Press Release on the Connecticut Attorney General's Office Web site, January 13, 2010. Available at: www.ct.gov/ag/cwp/view.asp?Q=453916&A=3869.

collaboration with the security official, is required to notify patients of breaches of security that involve their medical information. Guidance on how to manage a breach is provided in Chapters 1 and 4. Because of the complexity of the Breach Notification Rule, physicians are strongly encouraged to create a breach notification plan that also includes consultation with legal counsel.

- A comprehensive document, "What You Need to Know About the New HIPAA Breach Notification Rule" from the AMA is included in Appendix C. Before building your training program, read the guidance in Appendix C and send a copy to your health law attorney. For training purposes, include at a minimum.
  1. An overview of the Breach Notification Rule, including penalties;
  2. What the practice must do to inform patients of a security breach and the projected costs and reputation outcomes of those communications. Specific guidance is provided in detail in Appendix C;
  3. Policies and procedures about encrypting portable devices and sanctions imposed against violators of that policy;
  4. Possible devices to track the location of portable and stationery devices, including paper records; and measures to disengage access to medical information in the event a device is lost.
- Covered entities must annually report all unsecured security breaches to HHS.[50]
- Covered entities, business associates, employers, and individuals may be subject to criminal liabilities if they use or disclose PHI without valid authorization.

In light of these additional enforcement approaches, let's take a look at the HIPAA Privacy Rule training requirements.

HIPAA Privacy Rule Training Requirements:

- Workforce members, including employees, volunteers, trainees, and may also include other persons whose conduct is under the direct control of the entity (whether or not they are paid by the entity).[51]
- A covered entity must train all workforce members on its privacy policies and procedures, as necessary and appropriate, for them to carry out their functions. New workforce members must be trained

---

50. In January 2010, according to the HHS Office for Civil Rights, "there have been 35 reports of breaches affecting 500-plus individuals, resulting in 712,000 notices. Most of the reports were ePHI contained in lost or stolen unencrypted media or portable devices. There were more than 300 reports of smaller breaches." See Dom Nicastro, "Business Associates Can Pay Directly for Breaches," *Health Leaders Media*, February 5, 2010, which is available at: www.healthleadersmedia.com.

51. 45 CFR 160.103.

within a reasonable amount of time after they have been hired. Anytime someone is promoted or changes job position, you must provide privacy training according to the new job responsibilities.[52]

- A covered entity must have and must apply appropriate sanctions against workforce members who violate its privacy policies and procedures or the Privacy Rule.[53]

HIPAA and HITECH Training: Time to Double Down

By Edward Shay, Partner, Post and Schell

As the healthcare industry continues to digest profound HITECH changes to HIPAA Privacy and Security rules, two observations already are apparent and indisputable for covered entities and their business associates. First, time and resources spent on a workforce that is well-trained on the Privacy and Security rules will be an investment of exponential value. Second, enforcement of those same rules will make negligent and uncorrected errors very costly. A well-trained workforce makes fewer mistakes, and identifies and fixes those that it makes. A workforce that violates the rules because it does not know them or does not care to know them makes an inviting target for HITECH's new enforcement initiatives. The lesson seems clear: train on HITECH and re-train on existing HIPAA rules—or pay some new and onerous penalties for workforce mistakes.

Here are three hard truths about the HITECH amendments. First, after HITECH, penalties for each violation of HIPAA can now exceed civil penalties for violating the anti-kickback statute. Second, HITECH mandates much more enforcement by HHS, including compliance audits, and allows enforcement by state Attorneys General. Third, under the recently adopted breach notification rules, covered entities are required to submit annually logs of protected health information (PHI) breaches to the Secretary of HHS. Because by definition each of those reported "breaches" involves a violation of the Privacy Rule, covered entities also will be informing the Secretary of their Privacy Rule violations. You won't have to worry about possible whistleblowers; you are the whistleblower.

One major piece of good news in HITECH is that Congress provided that unless a violation is caused by willful neglect, penalties for the violation may be avoided by taking corrective action within 30 days. This is where training comes in, and where training pays off. A vigorous training program enables the workforce of a covered entity to identify violations quickly because the workforce knows what are proper PHI uses and disclosures and what are not. For example, if workforce members do not understand the concept of "minimum necessary," they will not know that sending an entire medical record to a third party payer is highly likely to violate the Privacy Rule. If workforce members know what the "minimum necessary" disclosure is, they will either avoid an improper disclosure or move to correct it within the thirty-day corrective action grace period.

As with so many other areas of HIPAA, HITECH introduces many new concepts. New regulations have been published on unsecured breaches and more regulations are coming on privacy, security, and enforcement. Making these rules

52. 45 CFR 164.530(b).

53. 45 CFR 164.530(e).

comprehensible to your workforce members (including management) and applicable to your environment requires training—and some re-training on the existing HIPAA Privacy and Security rules and how they all fit together.
This article was posted as a blog on HIPAA.com and is reprinted with permission.

Quick Training Tips:

- Training keeps your workforce from making costly mistakes.
- Proof of attendance, such as signing a training attendance roster, verifies the practice provided training in the event of an incident or breach.
- Don't let the fear of breaches drive your training program. Fear usually results in confused thinking and knee-jerk responses.
- Use a combination of media resources for training, including onsite sessions, group discussions, online training resources, and email reminders.
- Training must be provided to the extent that is necessary for each employee to carry out his or her work functions.

No single training medium works all the time and/or for all employees, but privacy should always be the top priority. Determine how extensive your training should be by dividing your staff into three categories (see Table 3.7).

TABLE 3.7

Training by Job Category

Patient Contact Category	Amount of Training Needed
Employees with direct patient contact: physicians, nurses, office manager, privacy official	Extensive training, with regular updates and reminders throughout the year
Employees with some patient contact: receptionist, billing and insurance clerks, medical-records staff, lab technicians, volunteers, coders	Awareness training, with regular updates and reminders throughout the year
Employees with little or no patient contact: maintenance and housekeeping staff	Awareness training, with reminders or posters where employees can and will see them

A good training program, whether you develop it yourself or use an outside resource, should include the following topics:

- **Part I: HIPAA awareness (30 minutes to 1 hour)**
  - ☐ Overview of new HIPAA Privacy and Breach Notification Rules
  - ☐ The practice's approach to protecting patient privacy
  - ☐ New and expanded patient rights, including a refresher on previous rights. Define how the practice will honor those rights.
  - ☐ The role of the privacy official

- ☐ How the practice plans to enforce the Privacy and Breach Notification Rules
- ☐ Any updates that may be required.

- **Part II: Your HIPAA policies and procedures (2 hours)**
  - ☐ Key terms
  - ☐ Permissions for use and disclosure of protected health information
  - ☐ Special requirements for use and disclosure of PHI
  - ☐ Patient rights
  - ☐ Privacy management.
- **Part III: Year-round training (15 to 30 minutes, once a month)**
  - ☐ Include training exercises and contingency scenarios as part of monthly staff meetings.
  - ☐ You'll find a comprehensive training program, including year-round topics for discussion, and an action approach to changing behavior in Appendix A.

As part of each training session, you should also:

- Test for understanding and keep records of each person's test;
- Have employees sign an attendance register and maintain records and date(s) of attendance;
- Ask employees and volunteers to sign a confidentiality agreement at the end of the HIPAA training; and
- Review confidentiality provisions with employees as part of the training, at least once a year.

Note: In Appendix B, you'll find a detailed month-by-month schedule of training topics, which can be very helpful as you build a privacy program in your medical practice.

Step 10: Implement Your Plan and Evaluate Your Compliance Status

No office can avoid all privacy violations, but show good faith that you are trying to make the office violation-free.

What to Do:

Safeguard your valued relationships with patients by implementing new Privacy and Breach Notification Rules.

How to Do It:

- Reinvigorate your privacy official and show up for privacy training.
- The privacy official's job has escalated, and if your privacy official also is your security official, the practice leaders must show support by also participating in privacy training, which also is required under the Privacy Rule.

It may save your practice significant embarrassment in the public media, as well as save the trust you've earned with patients.

- Evaluate the privacy official's workload. Should some of this work be delegated or reassigned?
- Remind all clinicians that safeguards for incidental disclosures include keeping voices low when talking about patients in public areas.
- Using NIST standards (discussed in Chapter 4) to encrypt portable devices that contain, or are used to access PHI.
- Implement sanctions! You must demonstrate through the HIPAA documentation requirements that you are following your policies and procedures. Failure to document is tantamount to noncompliance.
- Communicate with everyone on staff about how they are doing.
- Tell your patients how you are managing patient privacy. Keep in mind that your patients and your staff have different approaches to privacy, but both desire the same outcome. Physicians and their staff have always believed that they practiced confidentiality. Patients may believe what they read, hear, or see in the media, particularly stories about celebrities having their medical records looked at by unauthorized individuals, or the loss of a laptop with tens of thousands of sensitive financial or medical records that are not encrypted for security. If patients are informed about how you protect their PHI, they will trust and believe you. If they see that you are taking measures to protect their PHI, they will have more faith and believe you as well. Nothing can derail your privacy goals faster than announcing a privacy or security breach in a 30-second sound bite on the evening news. Trustful patients make for good customer satisfaction, which also strengthens your foundation for successful HIPAA privacy procedures and the stability of your practice as a business.
- Evaluate your training status. Do you have new employees? Have current employees taken on new responsibilities that require retraining? Have your policies and procedures or HIPAA rules changed?
- Build new policies and procedures to accommodate updates to the Privacy and Breach Notification Rules. Retrain the workforce on updated rules and changes.
- Conduct a monthly privacy check. Are you using your new documentation procedures? Are patients signing valid authorizations? Are you honoring patient requests that you have agreed to?

During the transition to EHR, security measures will become more prominent and gain increasing momentum. In Chapter 4, we present HIPAA Security requirements effective 2004 and include encryption implementation specifications.

chapter 4

HIPAA Security: Tougher, but with Safe Harbors

The purpose of this chapter is to provide you with a basic understanding of the final HIPAA Administrative Simplification Security Rule that was published in the *Federal Register* on February 20, 2003.[1] For covered entities, compliance was required by April 21, 2005.[2] For business associates, compliance was required by February 17, 2010, as required by the Health Information Technology for Economic and Clinical Health Act (HITECH Act), which was enacted as part of the American Recovery and Reinvestment Act of 2009 (ARRA).[3]

In this chapter you will learn:

- The basic structure of the Security Rule
- The basic foundation of the Security Rule
- How the Security Rule relates to the Privacy Rule and to the Breach Notification Rule
- Why the Security Rule is technologically neutral and scalable

---

1. Department of Health and Human Services, Office of the Secretary, "45 CFR Parts 160, 162, and 164—Health Insurance Reform: Security Standards; Final Rule," *Federal Register*, v.68, n.34, February 20, 2003, pp. 8333-8381. Citations to this document hereafter are in the standard reference format of 68 *Federal Register* <page(s)>: (eg, 68 *Federal Register* 8333).
2. Small health plans had an additional year to comply by April 21, 2006.
3. ARRA is available at: www.gpo.gov:80/fdsys/pkg/PLAW-111publ5/pdf/PLAW-111publ5.pdf. The HITECH Act is comprised of two titles in ARRA: Title XIII (Health Information Technology) in Division A (Appropriations Provisions), pages 226-279; and Title IV (Medicare and Medicaid Health Information Technology; Miscellaneous Medicare Provisions) in Division B (Tax, Unemployment, Health, State Fiscal Relief, and Other Provisions), pages 467-496. Further references to the HITECH Act in this chapter are in the format: *HITECH Act* <page(s)>. For example, privacy is discussed in Subtitle D of Title XIII: *HITECH Act* 258-279, and *Application of Security Provisions and Penalties to Business Associates of Covered Entities* (42 USC 17931) is on page 260.

- How the Security Rule is designed to provide scalability and flexibility
- How to conduct a risk analysis
- What the difference is between *required* and *addressable* implementation specifications that underpin the security standards, and how to manage those terms when implementing the Security Rule
- Why reasonable and appropriate actions provide the framework for the Security Rule, irrespective of size, complexity, or environment in which the covered entity or business associate operates
- What the characteristics are of administrative, physical, and technical security safeguards
- Why cost is a consideration in exercising responsibility to comply with the Security Rule, but that "cost is not meant to free covered entities from this responsibility."[4]

Key Terms

Addressable
Administrative safeguards
Availability
Breach
Confidentiality
Covered entity
Electronic protected health information (ePHI)
Electronic media
Encryption
Guidance
Implementation specification
Integrity
Physical safeguards
Protected health information (PHI)
Security incident
Required
Technical safeguards
Unsecured protected health information

ABOUT HIPAA'S SECURITY RULE

The Security Rule was effective April 21, 2003, and required compliance no later than April 21, 2005, for most covered entities: health plans, health care clearinghouses, and health care providers who transmit any health information in electronic form in connection with a standard transaction.[5]

4. 68 *Federal Register* 8343.
5. 68 *Federal Register* 8334.

The Privacy Rule, which required compliance by covered entities by April 14, 2003,[6] also required that administrative, technical, and physical safeguards of protected health information in oral, hard copy, and electronic forms be in effect as of that date.[7] As a result, the Privacy Rule accelerated the need for implementation of security provisions, and the final Security Rule provided guidance for the "appropriate" (security) safeguards required under the Privacy Rule.

Unlike the Privacy Rule, which applies to PHI in oral, hard copy, and electronic form, the Security Rule applies only to *electronic* protected health information (ePHI). Both rules cover protected health information *in use* (creation, retrieval, revision, and deletion), *at rest* (database), and *in motion* (transmission).

The Privacy rule defines authorized and required uses and disclosures of protected health information and the rights patients have with respect to it. The Security Rule defines safeguards for such information. Three key properties[8] are the foundation of privacy and security working together:

- ***Confidentiality*** is the property that protected health information is "not made available or disclosed to unauthorized persons or processes."
- ***Integrity*** is the property that protected health information "has not been altered or destroyed in an unauthorized manner."
- ***Availability*** is the property that protected health information "is accessible and useable upon demand by an authorized person."

These properties, and other security attributes, are embodied in three types of security standards: administrative safeguards, physical safeguards, and technical safeguards.

Within administrative, physical, and technical safeguard categories are standards and implementation specifications that are examined in detail in this chapter. Covered entities, since April 21, 2005, and business associates, since February 17, 2010, have been required to comply with the standards and to follow the implementation specifications, which define what needs to be done to achieve compliance with the Security Rule. Compliance is designed to provide "a floor of protection of all electronic protected health information" but takes into consideration that covered entities and business associates are of different sizes and complexities, and, thus, likely to require different means to achieve protection of such information. As a result, the Security Rule is considered "technologically neutral."[9]

---

6. Small health plans had an additional year to comply.

7. 45 CFR 164.530(c)(1).

8. 45 CFR 164.304.

9. "The standards do not allow organizations to make their own rules, only their own technology choices." 68 *Federal Register* 8343. As we shall see in the discussion of *encryption* in technical safeguards later in this chapter, the one exception to technology neutrality is the specification of acceptable encryption

CRITICAL POINT
HIPAA's Security Rule is technologically neutral. The Security Rule does not tell your organization what technology choices (inputs) to make, just what protections (outputs) to achieve.

The foundation of the Security Rule is that security protections must be "reasonable and appropriate," as assessed in a required risk analysis and study of risk-management measures. The Security Rule is designed to be "scalable and flexible." As a result, a small physician practice will have a different array of security protections than a large practice, clinic, or hospital, with the selection of security protections determined by the risk analysis. Many of these protections will be reflected and documented in written policies and procedures that your organization must keep current. Documentation may be in hard copy or electronic form and retained for six years from the date of creation or the date last in effect, whichever is later. Your organization also must similarly document "actions, activities, and assessments" related to its Security Rule policies and procedures. Both types of documentation must be made available to your organization's workforce[10] members who are responsible for or affected by the Security Rule.

CRITICAL POINT
Your organization must document its Security Rule policies, procedures, actions, activities, and assessments, and retain such documentation in hard copy or electronic form for six years from its date of creation or the date last in effect, whichever is later.

General Rules

There are five general rules in HIPAA's Security Rule:

- general requirements
- flexibility of approach

(continued)

technologies to "secure" electronic protected health information in the August 24, 2009, *Guidance Specifyng the Technologies and Methodologies that Render Protected Health Information Unusable, Unreadable, or Indecipherable to Unauthorized Individuals*, pp. 42742–42743 in Department of Health and Human Services, Office of the Secretary, "45 Parts 160 and 164: Breach Notification for Unsecured Protected Health Information; Interim Final Rule," *Federal Register*, v.74, n.162, August 24, 2009, pp. 42739–42770.

10. "*Workforce* means employees, volunteers, trainees, and other persons whose conduct, in the performance of the work for a covered entity, is under the direct control of such entity, whether or not they are paid by the covered entity." 45 CFR 160.103.

- standards
- implementation specifications
- maintenance.

General Requirements

There are four general requirements:

- Ensure the confidentiality, integrity, and availability of all electronic protected health information that the covered entity creates, receives, maintains, or transmits.
- Protect against any reasonably anticipated threats or hazards to the security or integrity of such information.
- Protect against any reasonably anticipated uses or disclosures of such information that are not permitted or required under Privacy of Individually Identifiable Health Information.
- Ensure compliance with the Security Rule by the practice's workforce.[11]

These requirements serve as the foundation for the administrative, physical, and technical safeguards.

Flexibility of Approach

The general rules provide for flexibility of approach in complying with the Security Rule. Because of its importance in providing a foundation for the scalability of administrative, physical, and technical safeguards, the two parts of this rule are reproduced here:

1. Covered entities may use any security measures that allow the covered entity to reasonably and appropriately implement the standards and implementations specifications as specified in Security Standards for the Protection of Electronic Protected Health Information.
2. In deciding which security measures to use, a covered entity must take into account the following factors:
   a. The size, complexity, and capabilities of the covered entity.
   b. The covered entity's technical infrastructure, hardware, and software security capabilities.
   c. The costs of security measures.
   d. The probability and criticality of potential risks to electronic protected health information.[12]

CRITICAL POINT

To determine what are reasonable and appropriate security measures for your organization, you must take factors *a–d* into account in your risk analysis.

11. 68 *Federal Register* 8376.

12. 68 *Federal Register* 8376-8377.

Standards

This part of the general rules requires that covered entities must comply with the security standards with respect to all electronic protected health information. Under the HITECH Act, business associates of covered entities were required to comply with those standards on February 17, 2010.[13] Failure to comply leads to liability for civil sanctions[14] and potential loss of business.

Implementation Specifications

There are two types of implementation specifications, *required* and *addressable*, and each implementation specification is so designated. If an implementation specification is designated *required*, a covered entity must implement the specification. The term *addressable* is more complicated and gives the covered entity options. These options are outcomes of the risk analysis that the practice conducts. When analyzing a particular addressable implementation specification for a standard, the practice must determine "whether each implementation specification is a *reasonable and appropriate* safeguard in its environment, when analyzed with reference to the likely contribution to protecting the entity's electronic protected health information."[15] For example, in a large physician practice, you likely would conduct a detailed background investigation of a person seeking employment (clearance implementation specification). In a solo practice with only the physician's spouse as the "workforce," a common occurrence, such a clearance procedure likely would not be considered reasonable or appropriate.

In this and other addressable implementation specifications, the covered entity must balance the safeguard specification with the degree of risk mitigation the specification affords, taking into consideration its analysis of risk, strategy for risk mitigation, security protections already in place, and cost of implementation. If the covered entity determines that the implementation specification is a reasonable and appropriate safeguard, it must implement the specification.

---

13. *HITECH Act* 260 (42 USC17931).

14. The HITECH Act increased civil financial penalties, with the maximum for each category of violation increasing 60-fold to $1.5 million for repeat of an identical violation in a calendar year. See Department of Health and Human Services, Office of the Secretary, "45 CFR Part 160—HIPAA Administrative Simplification: Enforcement; Interim Final Rule," *Federal Register*, v.74, n.209, October 30, 2009, pp. 56123-56131. Categories of violations and respective penalty amounts appear on p. 56127.

15. 68 *Federal Register* 8377.

If your practice determines that the implementation specification is not reasonable and appropriate, you have two options, and for each of them you must document why the implementation specification is not reasonable and appropriate. First, you must document why it is not reasonable and appropriate and implement one or more alternative equivalent measures, or a combination of such measures, if reasonable and appropriate. Second, if you can otherwise document that the standard can be met, you may choose to implement neither the implementation specification nor alternative equivalent measure(s). In either circumstance, written documentation of the decision is critical.

Maintenance

This part of the general rules requires that covered entities review their security measures periodically and make modifications as necessary to ensure that they continue to provide "reasonable and appropriate protection of electronic protected health information."

Security Standards and Implementation Specifications Overview

Table 4.1 outlines the 18 administrative, physical, and technical safeguard standards of the Security Rule, which are defined as follows.[16]

- Nine administrative safeguard standards are "administrative actions, and policies and procedures, to manage the selection, development, implementation, and maintenance of security measures to protect electronic protected health information and to manage the conduct of the covered entity's workforce in relation to the protection of that information."
- Four physical safeguard standards are "physical measures, policies, and procedures to protect a covered entity's electronic information systems and related buildings and equipment from natural and environmental hazards, and unauthorized intrusion."
- Five technical safeguard standards are "the technology and the policy and procedures for its use that protect electronic protected health information and control access to it."

There are 36 defined implementation specifications for the safeguard standards, which can be *required* or *addressable*. Six standards do not have defined implementation specifications, and for these standards, the language of the standard explains what is *required* to be implemented.

16. 68 *Federal Register* 8376.

TABLE 4.1

Security Safeguard Standards and Implementation Specifications

Standards	Code of Federal Regulations (CFR) Section	Implementation Specification (IS)	Required (R) or Addressable (A)
Administrative Safeguards[17]			
Security management process	164.308(a)(1)	A. Risk analysis	R
		B. Risk management	R
		C. Sanction policy	R
		D. Information system activity review	R
Assigned security responsibility	164.308(a)(2)		R
Workforce security	164.308(a)(3)	A. Authorization and/or supervision	A
		B. Workforce clearance procedure	A
		C. Termination procedures	A
Information access management	164.308(a)(4)	A. Isolating health care clearinghouse functions	R
		B. Access authorization	A
		C. Access establishment and modification	A
Security awareness and training	164.308(a)(5)	A. Security reminders	A
		B. Protection from malicious software	A
		C. Log-in monitoring	A
		D. Password management	A
Security incident procedures	164.308(a)(6)	Response and reporting	R
Contingency plan	164.308(a)(7)	A. Data backup plan	R
		B. Disaster recovery plan	R
		C. Emergency mode operation plan	R
		D. Testing and revision procedures	A
		E. Applications and data criticality analysis	A

(continued)

17. See 68 *Federal Register* 8346–8353 for discussion of Administrative Safeguards (45 CFR 164.308) in the preamble of the Final Security Rule.

TABLE 4.1 (continued)

Security Safeguard Standards and Implementation Specifications

Standards	Code of Federal Regulations (CFR) Section	Implementation Specification (IS)	Required (R) or Addressable (A)
Evaluation	164.308(a)(8)		R
Business associate contracts and other arrangements	164.308(b)(1)	Written contract or other arrangement	R
Physical safeguards[18]			
Facility access controls	164.310(a)(1)	i. Contingency operations	A
		ii. Facility security plan	A
		iii. Access control and validation procedures	A
		iv. Maintenance records	A
Workstation use	164.310(b)		R
Workstation security	164.310(c)		R
Device and media controls	164.310(d)(1)	i. Disposal	R
		ii. Media re-use	R
		iii. Accountability	A
		iv. Data backup and storage	A
Technical Safeguards[19]			
Access control	164.312(a)(1)	i. Unique user identification	R
		ii. Emergency access procedure	R
		iii. Automatic logoff	A
		iv. Encryption and decryption	A
Audit controls	164.312(b)		R

(continued)

18. See 68 *Federal Register* 8353–8354 for discussion of Physical Safeguards (45 CFR 164.310) in the preamble of the Final Security Rule.

19. See 68 *Federal Register* 8354–8358 for discussion of Technical Safeguards (45 CFR 164.312) in the preamble of the Final Security Rule.

TABLE 4.1 (continued)

Security Safeguard Standards and Implementation Specifications

Standards	Code of Federal Regulations (CFR) Section	Implementation Specification (IS)	Required (R) or Addressable (A)
Integrity	164.312(c)(1)	Mechanism to authenticate ePHI	A
Person or entity authentication	164.312(d)		R
Transmission security	164.312(e)(1)	i. Integrity controls	A
		ii. Encryption	A

In the sections that follow, we outline administrative, physical, and technical standards and implementation specifications. For each standard, we identify the implementation specifications and references. References have three components:

- Relevant location in Title 45 (Public Welfare), Subtitle A (Department of Health and Human Services), Subchapter C (Administrative Data Standards and Related Requirements), Part 164 (Security and Privacy), Subpart C (Security Standards for the Protection of Electronic Protected Health Information) of the Code of Federal Regulations (CFR)[20]
- The National Institute of Standards and Technology (NIST) document, *An Introductory Resource Guide for Implementing the Health Insurance Portability and Accountability Act (HIPAA) Security Rule*, Special Publication (SP) 800-66 Revision 1, October 2008[21]
- Language of each standard and implementation specification as it appears in the final Security Rule.[22]

For sample policies and procedures for each security implementation specification, which is beyond the scope of this book, see our book *Policies and Procedures for the Electronic Medical Practice*.[23]

20. The most up-to-date CFR source is the electronic CFR, which is available at: http://ecfr.gpoaccess.gov/cgi/t/text/text-idx?c=ecfr&tpl=%2Findex.tpl.

21. Page references refer to key activities, sample questions, and a description of activities relevant to each standard. http://csrc.nist.gov/publications/nistpubs/800-34-rev1/sp800-34-rev1.pdf. Accessed August 18, 2010.

22. 68 *Federal Register* <page(s)>.

23. Jones, ED and Harley, CP, *Policies and Procedures for the Electronic Medical Practice*. Chicago, IL: AMA, 2010.

ADMINSTRATIVE SAFEGUARD STANDARDS AND IMPLEMENTATION SPECIFICATIONS

Security Management Process

Standard	Implementation Specifications	References
Security management process	A. Risk analysis (R) B. Risk management (R) C. Sanction policy (R) D. Information system activity review (R)	45 CFR 164.308(a)(1)(i) NIST SP 800-66, pp. 17–19 68 Federal Register 8377

What the Standard Requires

Implement policies and procedures to prevent, detect, contain, and correct security violations.

This standard and the four required implementation specifications "form the foundation upon which an entity's necessary security activities are built."[24] In essence, a covered entity is to evaluate and manage its security risks, provide sanctions as a disincentive for or deterrent to noncompliant behavior, and review periodically its security controls. "Covered entities have the flexibility to implement the standard in a manner consistent with numerous factors, including such things as, but not limited to, their size, degree of risk, and environment."[25] A covered entity can find guidance for implementing these specifications from the Computer Security Resource Center (CSRC) of the National Institute of Standards and Technology (NIST).[26]

CRITICAL POINT

"Your first priority is to develop a way to quantify and evaluate risk. You need to know what you are protecting and how much it's worth before you can decide how to protect it."[27]

24. 68 *Federal Register* 8346.

25. *Ibid.*

26. See NIST Special Publication (SP) 800-30, "Risk Management Guide for Information Technology Systems," July 2002, especially chapters 3 (Risk Assessment) and 4 (Risk Mitigation). This document is available at: http://csrc.nist.gov/publications/nistpubs/800-30/sp800-30.pdf.

27. Al Berg, "6 Myths About Security Policies: Leave Your Preconceptions Behind and Write Policies That Work in the Real World," *Information Security*, October 2002, p. 49.

Risk Analysis

Implementation Specification	Standard	Reference
A. Risk analysis (R)	Security management process	164.308(a)(1)(ii)(A)

What to Do:

Conduct an accurate and thorough assessment of the potential risks and vulnerabilities to the confidentiality, integrity, and availability of electronic protected health information held by the covered entity.

How to Do It:

We recommend that you consult Appendix E of NIST Special Publication 800-66 Revision 1, cited earlier, and NIST Special Publication 800-30, *Risk Management Guide for Information Technology Systems*, July 2002.[28] There are nine steps to conduct during a risk analysis:

- Define the scope of the risk analysis pertaining to your practice's electronic systems[29] that contain ePHI.
- Identify and compile relevant information.
- Identify realistic threats.
- Identify potential vulnerabilities.
- Assess current security controls in your practice.
- Determine the likelihood and impact of a threat exercising a vulnerability that would affect your electronic systems containing ePHI.
- Determine levels of risk to your practice's electronic systems that contain ePHI.
- Recommend security controls to mitigate such risk levels.
- Document the risk assessment findings.

CRITICAL POINT

Your practice's risk analysis is the foundation of your practice's risk mitigation strategy and the source of guidance for implementing administrative, physical, and technical safeguards to protect your practice's electronic systems that contain ePHI.

Risk Management

Implementation Specification	Standard	Reference
B. Risk management (R)	Security management process	164.308(a)(1)(ii)(B)

28. This document is available at: http://csrc.nist.gov/publications/nistpubs/800-30/sp800-30.pdf.

29. Be sure to include stationary, portable, and mobile electronic devices and media in your risk analysis.

What to Do:

Implement security measures sufficient to reduce risks and vulnerabilities to a reasonable and appropriate level to comply with the general requirements of the Security Rule.[30]

How to Do It:

These are threat-management outcomes of the risk analysis that you will conduct. They will provide the foundation of your practice's policies and procedures. Your practice is unique, so you must evaluate your practice's threats and vulnerabilities to be able to implement an effective security strategy to safeguard your electronic systems that contain ePHI.

Sanction Policy

Implementation Specification	Standard	Reference
C. Sanction policy (R)	Security management process	164.308(a)(1)(ii)(C)

What to Do:

Apply appropriate sanctions against workforce members who fail to comply with the security policies and procedures of the covered entity.

How to Do It:

Your practice must determine appropriate internal penalties for violations of your practice's security policies and procedures by the practice workforce. Such penalties should be an incentive to comply with your practice's policies and procedures and deter noncompliant actions (for example, posting passwords on computer terminals or desktops). Your sanction policies and procedures will be an outcome of your practice's risk analysis and should be related to the practice's determination of harm pertaining to a particular security incident.

Information System Activity Review

Implementation Specification	Standard	Reference
D. Information system activity review (R)	Security management process	164.308(a)(1)(ii)(D)

30. The *general requirements* were outlined earlier in this chapter.

What to Do:

Implement procedures to regularly review records of information system activity, such as audit logs, access reports, and security incident tracking reports.

How to Do It:

Ask your practice-management system vendor for help in setting up system audit logs, access reports, and security incident tracking reports. As part of your security-management process, identify all reporting requirements and establish procedures for compiling requisite information, creating log entries, safeguarding the documentation, and maintaining the documentation for "6 years from the date of its creation or the date when it last was in effect, whichever is later."[31]

Assigned Security Responsibility

Standard	Implementation Specifications	References
Assigned security responsibility		45 CFR 164.308(a)(2) NIST SP 800-66, p. 20 68 Federal Register 8377

What the Standard Requires

Identify the security official who is responsible for the development and implementation of the policies and procedures required by the Security Rule for the entity.

The implementation specification is reflected in the language of the standard and, as such, is required.

The HIPAA Security Rule requires that "[f]inal security responsibility must rest with one individual to ensure accountability within each covered entity"[32] for the security of the electronic systems that contain ePHI. The role of the Security Official may be combined with the role of the privacy official in a small practice.

Qualifications of the Security Official should include the following:

- Knowledgeable about technological and business applications in the practice
- Good oral and written communication skills with ability to discuss technical terms in plain language
- Ability to compile, update, and maintain documentation of policies, procedures, actions, and assessments pertaining to implementation specifications of the security standards
- Good people management skills inside the practice and with business associates such as electronic system vendors

31. 45 CFR 164.316(b)(2)(i).

32. 68 *Federal Register* 8347.

- Ability to enforce security policies, procedures, and sanctions in the practice
- Ability to lead risk analysis processes and training programs in the practice.

Security Official Job Description

The Security Official will have overall responsibility in the practice for compliance with the Security Rule generally and, in particular, for implementing policies and procedures that ensure the confidentiality, integrity, and availability of the practice's electronic protected health information.

The Security Official may already be an employee who will work closely with the Privacy Official. The Security Official may delegate tasks and responsibilities but is ultimately responsible for compliance with the Security Rule.

Tasks

- Prepare and manage the budget allocated to the practice's security program and be responsible for protecting the practice's information system assets, including an up-to-date record of inventory of hardware and software.
- Develop and implement security policies, procedures, and guidelines to direct and carry out the objectives of the practice's security program; research and recommend new security measures for the practice; and monitor and test the practice's security program for effectiveness.
- Ensure that the following policies and procedures are in place: security policies and procedures; baseline security safeguards; security risk management; security administration; security of the computer network; security of servers; security of personal computers; physical security; disaster recovery plan; security awareness training.
- Maintain documentation regarding levels of access granted to each information system user in the practice and review these levels of access periodically and when the status of a workforce member changes—controlling access, as appropriate.
- Investigate, respond to, and remedy security incidents.
- Supervise personnel of vendors or business associates who perform technical system maintenance activities in the practice and provide and document that such personnel have security awareness training, as appropriate.
- Document and maintain system access authorization records, which would be signed by personnel of vendors or business associates who perform technical system maintenance activities in the practice.

Workforce Security

Standard	Implementation Specifications	References
Workforce security	A. Authorization and/or supervision (A) B. Workforce clearance procedure (A) C. Termination procedures (A)	45 CFR 164.308(a)(3)(i) NIST SP 800-66, pp. 21–22 68 Federal Register 8377

What the Standard Requires

Implement policies and procedures to ensure that all members of its workforce have appropriate access to electronic protected health information, as provided under [the Information Access Management Standard], and to prevent those workforce members who do not have access under [the Information Access Management Standard] from obtaining access to electronic protected health information.

This standard requires your practice to control access to ePHI in your practice. Simply put, you must have controls in place to allow appropriate access to ePHI for workforce members to perform their job responsibilities and to preclude such access to workforce members who do not need such information for conduct of their job responsibilities. The latter also includes workforce members whose job responsibilities may have changed and those who have left the practice or have been terminated from employment.

The three implementation specifications for this standard illustrate the concept of addressability, especially with regard to risk analyses pertaining to small physician practices. For example, in designing a clearance procedure, the "need for and extent of a screening process is normally based on an assessment of the risk, cost, benefit, and feasibility as well as other protective measures in place. ... For example, a personal clearance may not be reasonable or appropriate for a small provider whose only assistant is his or her spouse."[33] Similarly, with regard to termination procedures, "in certain circumstances... in a solo physician practice whose staff consists only of the physician's spouse, formal procedures may not be necessary."[34] Finally, "the purpose of termination procedure documentation is to ensure that termination procedures include security-unique actions to be followed, for example, revoking passwords and retrieving keys when a termination occurs."[35] Certainly, the procedures would be different in the solo practice example above from a multi-physician, large-workforce practice. In each case, however, given addressable implementation specifications, it is required that the standard compliant policies and procedures be documented in writing.

Authorization and/or Supervision

Implementation Specification	Standard	Reference
A. Authorization[36] and/or supervision (A)	Workforce security	164.308(a)(3)(ii)(A)

33. 68 *Federal Register* 8348.

34. Ibid.

35. 68 *Federal Register* 8349.

36. Authorization refers to "permission given to a user to access the computing resources, programs, process, and/or data of an entity." See Amatayakul, M, et al. *Handbook for HIPAA Security Implementation*. Chicago, IL: American Medical Association (AMA) Press, 2004, p. 206.

What to Do:

Implement procedures for the authorization and/or supervision of workforce members who work with electronic protected health information or in locations where it might be accessed.

How to Do It:

As part of your practice's risk analysis, determine which workforce members have need for access to ePHI as part of their job responsibilities. Describe such needs, corresponding authorization, and supervision responsibilities in job descriptions. Ensure that each member of the workforce understands those responsibilities.

Workforce Clearance Procedure

Implementation Specification	Standard	Reference
B. Workforce clearance procedure (A)	Workforce security	164.308(a)(3)(ii)(B)

What to Do:

Implement procedures to determine that the access of a workforce member to electronic protected health information is appropriate.

How to Do It:

Clearance will be an outcome of the risk analysis and elaboration of authorization in job descriptions. As part of the risk analysis, the practice should consider criteria for a background check for each workforce member candidate.

Termination Procedures

Implementation Specification	Standard	Reference
C. Termination procedures (A)	Workforce security	164.308(a)(3)(ii)(C)

What to Do:

Implement procedures for terminating access to electronic protected health information when the employment of a workforce member ends or as required by determinations made as specified in [the Workforce Clearance Implementation Specification of this Standard].

How to Do It:

Establish an exit-interview format in which passwords are invalidated, inform terminated workforce members that any authorizations are denied, outline federal penalties for unauthorized access to ePHI in the practice, and have the terminated employee acknowledge in writing the receipt and understanding of the information conveyed in the exit interview.

Information Access Management

Standard	Implementation Specifications	References
Information access management	A. Isolating health care clearinghouse functions (R) B. Access authorization (A) C. Access establishment and modification (A)	45 CFR 164.308(a)(4)(i) NIST SP 800-66, p. 23–24 68 Federal Register 8377

What the Standard Requires

Implement policies and procedures for authorizing access to electronic protected health information that are consistent with the applicable requirements of [the HIPAA Privacy Rule].

This standard is analogous to other HIPAA Administrative Simplification standards in the Privacy Rule that restrict access to PHI to authorized users. It requires that your practice have a management system in place to authorize workforce members to have access to ePHI through a "workstation, transaction, program, process, or other mechanism."[37] Today, another mechanism could be a mobile device such as a personal data assistant (PDA) that was a technology in its infancy when the HIPAA Security Rule was promulgated.

Isolating Health Care Clearinghouse Functions

Implementation Specifications	Standard	Reference
A. Isolating health care clearinghouse functions (R)	Information access management	164.308(a)(4)(ii)(A)

What to Do:

If a health care clearinghouse is part of a larger organization, the clearinghouse must implement policies and procedures that protect the electronic protected health information of the clearinghouse from unauthorized access by the larger organization.

How to Do It:

This is not an implementation specification that a practice will have to address directly, but the practice needs to know about it if the practice engages a health care clearinghouse as a business associate. As a result of the HITECH Act, enacted as part of the American Recovery and Reinvestment Act (ARRA) on February 17, 2009, which we discussed in Chapter 1, a business associate of a covered entity must comply with the Security Rule no later than February 17, 2010. In addition, the business associate agreement between the covered entity and the business

37. 68 *Federal Register* 8377 and 45 CFR 164.308(a)(4)(ii)(B).

associate must incorporate the additional security requirements of the HITECH Act.[38] Prior to February 17, 2010, the business associate provided "satisfactory assurances" in the business associate agreement that it would comply with appropriate safeguards of PHI. Now, it must be stated explicitly that the business associate is in compliance with the Security Rule, along with other privacy obligations that relate primarily to the August 24, 2009, Breach Notification Rule that also was discussed in Chapter 1. Accordingly, with respect to this implementation specification, your practice, if it engages a clearinghouse as a business associate, must determine if the clearinghouse is part of a larger organization.[39] If it is, your practice must make sure that the workforce outside of the clearinghouse operation understands security and confidentiality of ePHI and sanctions for unauthorized access to such information, that the business associate documents such understanding as part of its compliance with the Security Rule, and your business associate agreement incorporates those considerations.

Access Authorization

Implementation Specifications	Standard	Reference
B. Access authorization (A)	Information access management	164.308(a)(4)(ii)(B)

What to Do:

Implement policies and procedures for granting access to electronic protected health information, for example, through access to a workstation, transaction, program, process, or other mechanism.

How to Do It:

Determine through the risk analysis which workforce members have need for access to ePHI. Reflect the need for such access in job responsibilities incorporated in job descriptions. Ask for help from your business associate electronic systems vendors about system capacities for setting access controls and address such capacities as part of your practice's risk analysis. In addition, determine which business associates need access to your electronic systems containing ePHI, and consider the implications of such access authorization in your risk

38. "The additional requirements of this title that relate to security and that are made applicable with respect to covered entities shall also be applicable to such a business associate and shall be incorporated into the business associate agreement between the business associate and the covered entity." See Section 13401(a): Application of Security Provisions, p.260 in the American Recovery and Reinvestment Act, Public Law 111-5, February 17, 2009, which is available at: www.gpo.gov:80/fdsys/pkg/PLAW-111publ5/pdf/PLAW-111publ5.pdf.

39. This required implementation specification relating to a health care clearinghouse that is part of a larger business organization illustrates the need to restrict access to only those persons with authorized access to electronic protected health information.

analysis.[40] Your practice privacy and security officials jointly should develop policies and procedures related to access that are consistent with the access authorization provisions of the Privacy and the Security Rules.

Access Establishment and Modification

Implementation Specification	Standard	Reference
C. Access establishment and modification (A)	Information access management	164.308(a)(4)(ii)(C)

What to Do:

Implement policies and procedures that, based upon the entity's access authorization policies, establish, document, review, and modify a user's right of access to a workstation, transaction, program, or process.

How to Do It:

Establish procedures for periodically reviewing and modifying access based on a change in an authorized workforce member's modified job responsibilities. Document and maintain access authorization records according to the HIPAA documentation standard. Such records should include changes in authorization due to modification of job responsibilities relating to grants of access, levels of access, times of access, and place(s) or system(s) of access, as applicable.

CRITICAL POINT

The addressable *Access Authorization* and *Access Establishment and Modification* implementation specifications recognize that there are alternatives to complying with this standard that may be based on a practice's size and degree of electronic system automation.

Security Awareness and Training

Standard	Implementation Specification	References
Security awareness and training	A. Security reminders (A) B. Protection from malicious software (A) C. Log-in monitoring (A) D. Password management (A)	45 CFR 164.308(a)(5)(i) NIST SP 800-66, pp. 25–26 68 Federal Register 8377

40. For example, does a member of the workforce accompany authorized business associate representatives when they are performing system maintenance? Are such representatives given background checks by the covered entity? Are such representatives' actions with regard to the electronic systems audited or tracked, and are audit logs or tracking reports examined to ensure that such actions conform to your practice's policies and procedures?

What the Standard Requires

Implement a security awareness and training program for all members of its workforce (including management).

Training is an ongoing internal process for safeguarding PHI from unauthorized use or disclosure as business policies and procedures evolve and regulatory standards are initiated or modified.

Further, training requires that workforce members, including management, demonstrate awareness and understanding on an ongoing basis and that covered entities and business associates document that their workforce members have been trained. As examples, the first implementation specifications of the Security Rule "Security Awareness and Training" standard is "Security reminders (addressable). Periodic security updates." One part of the implementation specification for the Privacy Rule "Training" standard states that a "covered entity must provide training... [t]o each member of covered entity's workforce whose functions are affected by a material change in the policies or procedures required by the Privacy Rule, within a reasonable period of time after the material change becomes effective. ..."[41]

Whether it is Privacy, Security, or Breach Notification Rule training, each member of the workforce must participate in training, including the management of the practice. It is important that training be coordinated across each of the rules as they are interrelated. It also is important that each member of the workforce receive the same training so that workforce members reinforce one another in safeguarding PHI in the practice in any form: oral, hard copy, or electronic.

Your practice must make your business associates aware of your security policies and procedures. As of February 17, 2010, business associates must comply with the Security Rule and so must have their own security awareness and training programs in place. It would be prudent business practice to determine how your practice's business associates are training their workforce members to safeguard your ePHI.

As a business that generates revenue on a transactional basis during the business day, it may be costly and inconvenient to take time away from patients to conduct training. Your practice may wish to consider online training programs that your workforce members can take outside of the business day at their convenience, such as in the evening or on weekends. Be sure to document your training programs, including the time, curriculum, and results for each workforce member.

Each of the four implementation specifications is addressable. Even though the implementation specifications are addressable, "[s]ecurity awareness training is a critical activity, regardless of an organization's size."[42] While training is required, content and method are addressable.

---

41. 45 CFR 164.530(b)(2)(c).

42. 68 *Federal Register* 8350.

That the implementation specifications are addressable reflects several considerations discussed in the preamble to the Security Rule, namely, that training is "[d]ependent upon an entity's configuration and security risks," and "[a]n on-going, evolving process as an entity's security needs and procedures change."[43]

Each person with access to ePHI must be knowledgeable about and understand the appropriate security measures to reduce the risk of improper access, uses, and disclosures. Awareness is the first goal of training. Awareness is not a one-time outcome for the workforce, though, but rather a continuing responsibility as technology changes, new technology is introduced into the practice,[44] and as policies and procedures change in response to possible modifications of HIPAA standards, as occurred with the HITECH Act that was enacted on February 17, 2009.[45] The practice is not responsible for providing training to anyone outside of its workforce, but the practice is responsible for ensuring that business associates are aware of the practice's security policies and procedures and for informing the covered entity of any discovered breaches of ePHI for which they are responsible. This level of awareness of policies and procedures also should be imparted to individuals who may be at your practice facility or facilities for a limited period of time, such as vendors, maintenance personnel, and others. Such individuals can be made aware of the covered entity's safeguard policies and procedures by giving them pamphlets or copies of the safeguards for which compliance is required.

The National Institute of Standards and Technology (NIST) highlights the importance of awareness and training programs:

---

43. 68 *Federal Register* 8350.

44. An example of this is the growing use of mobile technologies and portable computers in the medical practice. Such devices with electronic protected health information therein are at a different risk level of being mislaid, stolen, or lost if used outside of the practice than stationary workstations in the practice under physical safeguards. Retraining on the use of these devices is critical to avoid the consequences of breach.

45. Training is a dynamic process. Although the comment in the preamble of the January 16, 2009, Final Rule pertaining to HIPAA Electronic Transaction Standards (that we discussed in Chapter 2) refers to "administrative transactions," it may be instructive in the context of training as well: "HHS does not recognize certification of any systems or software for purposes of HIPAA compliance." [74 *Federal Register* 3310] The burden on a covered entity or business associate is to conduct and periodically review its risk assessment, implement policies and procedures to safeguard protected health information, conduct awareness training for all workforce members based on those policies and procedures, update that training if policies and procedures change or HIPAA privacy and security regulations are initiated or modified, and document in writing those activities. Certification, which relates only to a static point in time, is not a requirement in that process.

"Awareness programs set the stage for training by changing organizational attitudes to realize the importance of security and the adverse consequences of its failure. "The purpose of training is to teach people the skills that will enable them to perform their jobs more effectively."[46]

This quotation highlights two important attributes of a successful awareness and training program: a change in corporate culture is required, and the payoff can be greater workforce productivity. When the practice's workforce pulls together to conduct a risk analysis, each member has a stake in the inputs and in the security safeguards. Management plays an important role in effecting change and in realizing the risk mitigation payoff. Quite simply, that is reflected in the language of the standard.

CRITICAL POINT

All members of your practice workforce, including management, are required to participate in security awareness and training. When the practice workforce pulls together to conduct a risk analysis, each member has a stake in the inputs and in the security safeguards, and the practice can effect change and realize risk mitigation payoffs.

Security Reminders

Implementation Specification	Standard	Reference
A. Security reminders (A)	Security awareness and training	164.308(a)(5)(ii)(A)

What to Do:

[Implement] periodic security reminders.

How to Do It:

Post security reminders in work areas, and periodically broadcast security reminders via e-mail to workforce members. At meetings of workforce members, be sure to include at least one security safeguard topic on the agenda.

Protection from Malicious Software

Implementation Specification	Standard	Reference
B. Protection from malicious software (A)	Security awareness and training	164.308(a)(5)(ii)(B)

46. National Institute of Standards and Technology, *Information Technology Security Training Requirements: A Role- and Performance-Based Model*, NIST SP 800-16, April 1998, which is available at: http://csrc.nist.gov/publications/nistpubs/800-16/800-16.pdf. See Chapter 4, "Training Development Methodology," from which the quotation is derived (p. 52).

What to Do:

[Implement] procedures for guarding against, detecting, and reporting malicious software.

How to Do It:

Discuss technologies for guarding against, detecting, and reporting malicious software with your systems vendor(s). Install commercially available virus detection and firewall software programs on all of the practice's electronic devices and media. Apply sanctions to any workforce member who is noncompliant with the practice's procedures relating to safeguarding ePHI from malicious software.

Log-in Monitoring

Implementation Specification	Standard	Reference
C. Log-in monitoring (A)	Security awareness and training	164.308(a)(5)(ii)(C)

What to Do:

[Implement] procedures for monitoring log-in attempts and reporting discrepancies.

How to Do It:

Discuss with your practice management-software vendor how to monitor and track log-in attempts and report discrepancies. Check the documentation of your operating system to determine its capability for tracking authorized log-ins and unauthorized log-in attempts. Implement either the operating system capability or acquire and activate a commercially viable software program for doing so. Maintain log-in activity reports according to the HIPAA documentation standard.

Password Management

Implementation Specification	Standard	Reference
D. Password management (A)	Security awareness and training	164.308(a)(5)(ii)(D)

What to Do:

[Implement] procedures for creating, changing, and safeguarding passwords.

How to Do It:

Develop a policy and corresponding procedures for password management. The practice's designated system administrator and security official should be the only persons with access to passwords of other workforce members.[47] Passwords should

47. In the discussion of the administrative safeguard standard *Contingency Plan*, we recommend that the security official have a sealed envelope of passwords of key workforce members who would be responsible for disaster recovery, along with an emergency password for use in emergency mode operations.

be changed periodically based on threat exposures (eg, every 30, 60, or 90 days, with timing an output of the practice's risk analysis). Implement and carry out sanctions for any workforce member posting of a password on a workstation terminal or desktop, or sharing of passwords with workforce members.

Security Incident Procedures

Standard	Implementation Specification	References
Security incident procedures	Response and reporting (R)	45 CFR 164.308(a)(6)(i) NIST SP 800-66, pp. 27–28 68 Federal Register 8377

What the Standard Requires

Implement policies and procedures to address security incidents.

A security incident is defined as "the attempted or successful unauthorized access, use, disclosure, modification, or destruction of information or interference with system operations in an information system."[48] Your practice must consider the wide variety of risks that this definition encompasses as you assess threats and vulnerabilities in your risk analysis.

The HITECH Act, discussed in Chapter 1, provided for breach notification, the requirement of which was embodied in an enabling regulation published in the *Federal Register* on August 24, 2009. If your practice fails to encrypt ePHI in your practice database(s) (data at rest) or in your transactions (data in motion), and there is a breach of your *unsecured* ePHI, then your practice is subject to the new response and reporting requirements of the Breach Notification Rule discussed in Chapter 1.

Response and Reporting

Implementation Specification	Standard	Reference
Response and reporting (R)	Security incident procedures	164.308(a)(6)(ii)

What to Do:

Identify and respond to suspected or known security incidents; mitigate, to the extent practicable, harmful effects of security incidents that are known to the covered entity; and document security incidents and their outcomes.

How to Do It:

Prior to enactment of the HITECH Act, this required implementation specification did not mandate reporting security incidents to outside authorities. The Security Rule indicated that such decisions should be based upon "business and

48. 68 *Federal Register* 8376 and 45 CFR 164.304.

legal considerations."[49] Then, as now, your practice had an obligation to respond and report, keeping track of your practice's actions, in writing, if your practice experienced a security incident. Your practice also was required then, as now, to mitigate harms arising from the incident and to put in place more effective safeguards to mitigate the risk of the incident occurring again. Then, as now, your practice was required to update its risk analysis. With the HITECH Act, there are requirements for responding to a security breach of unsecured ePHI, which we discussed in Chapter 1. We recommend, here as elsewhere in this chapter, that your practice encrypt its ePHI at rest and in motion in order to avoid the consequences of a security incident in which unsecured ePHI is potentially exposed to unauthorized individuals. With significantly increased civil penalties for a security violation, which became effective with enactment of the HITECH Act on February 17, 2009, and with federal enforcement effective on February 22, 2010, for discovered breaches occurring on or after that date, the consequences of a security incident could be costly. Use the content of the sample Security Incident Report in Figure 4.1 and sample Security Incident Log in Figure 4.2 to document and maintain records of any security incidents that your practice experiences.

CRITICAL POINT
Your practice is required to respond to and mitigate any harmful effects of security incidents and to document and maintain a log of all security incidents.

Contingency Plan

Standard	Implementation Specifications	References
Contingency plan	A. Data backup plan (R)	45 CFR 164.308(a)(7)(i)
	B. Disaster recovery plan (R)	NIST SP 800-66, pp. 29–30
	C. Emergency mode operation plan (R)	68 Federal Register 8377–8378
	D. Testing and revision procedures (A)	
	E. Applications and data criticality analysis (A)	

What the Standard Requires

Establish (and implement as needed) policies and procedures for responding to an emergency or other occurrence (for example, fire, vandalism, system failure, and natural disaster) that damages systems that contain electronic protected health information.

As your practice comes to rely increasingly on electronic systems to conduct business, it is vital to create, test, and update plans to respond and

49. 68 *Federal Register* 8350.

FIGURE 4.1

Sample Security Incident Report

Description of Attempted or Actual Security Incident: ______________________

____

____

Date: ____________ Time: ____________ Location: ______________________

Who Discovered Security Incident: ____________________________________

How Was Security Incident Discovered: ________________________________

____

____

Evidence of Incident: ____

____

____

Actions Taken to Minimize Damages to Practice's Systems and Electronic Data:

____

____

____

____

Policy and Procedural Changes Implemented to Avoid Recurrence: ___________

____

____

____

Security Official Name ________________ Signature _________ Date ________

FIGURE 4.2

Security Incident Log

Date	Location	Description	Severity Level of Incident 1 → 5 Least Serious … Most Serious

recover from a contingency that impairs your ability to access electronic systems that contain ePHI. Those systems and the protected health information therein are the lifeblood of your business as a medical practice. Part of your strategy for response and recovery is to develop data backup, disaster recovery, and emergency mode operation plans. Your practice needs to develop contingency plans around answers to these questions:

- How will the practice's patients be affected?
- What practice resources could be lost?
- What costs are associated with any loss?
- What efforts, costs, resources, and time are required to achieve recovery?
- What is the overall effect on the viability of the business as a medical practice?

There are five implementation specifications for this standard, with three required and two addressable.

Data Backup Plan

Implementation Specification	Standard	Reference
A. Data backup plan (R)	Contingency plan	164.308(a)(7)(ii)(A)

What to Do:

Establish and implement procedures to create and maintain retrievable exact copies of electronic protected health information.

How to Do It:

Check with your practice management-software vendor to determine if your software accommodates backup with exact-copy capability. If you are a small practice, you might consider using a daily tape, CD, DVD, or external hard drive backup and maintain that electronic media off-site in a secure location.[50] If you are a large practice, you might consider using a more complex procedure, such as a real-time, online, encrypted data stream or periodic batch duplicate data download to a secure off-site location. Maintaining the integrity of your ePHI is paramount, and, in fact, a technical safeguard standard.

Disaster Recovery Plan

Implementation Specification	Standard	Reference
B. Disaster recovery plan (R)	Contingency plan	164.308(a)(7)(ii)(B)

50. If you do so, be sure that the electronic media is encrypted to prevent a breach of unsecured electronic protected health information if the electronic media is mislaid, lost, or stolen in transit to a secure location.

What to Do:

Establish (and implement as needed) procedures to restore any loss of data.

How to Do It:

Disaster recovery planning will be an outgrowth of the identification of threats in the risk analysis. Your practice will need to determine outcomes of threats and the effect on the operations of the practice. Plan for the worst outcome! Develop safeguards to mitigate those outcomes, and identify key workforce members in the practice to take responsibility for recovery should those outcomes become a reality. "The final rule calls for covered entities to consider how natural disasters could damage systems that contain electronic protected health information and develop policies and procedures for responding to such situations. We [HHS] consider this to be a reasonable precautionary step to take since in many cases the risk would be deemed to be low."[51]

With regard to preparing a disaster recovery plan, we recommend that your practice consult the following document from the National Institute of Standards and Technology:

Contingency Planning Guide for Federal Information Systems, NIST Special Publication 800-34 Revision 1, May 2010.[52]

Emergency Mode Operation Plan

Implementation Specification	Standard	Reference
C. Emergency mode operation plan (R)	Contingency plan	164.308(a)(7)(ii)(C)

What to Do:

Establish (and implement as needed) procedures to enable continuation of critical business processes for protection of the security of electronic protected health information while operating in emergency mode.

How to Do It:

This plan will be a component part of your disaster recovery plan. It is important to get input from each workforce member as to duties and workflow in order to establish a workable emergency mode operation plan. Use that information to prepare a workflow map of how your practice operates, which will prove to be useful in normal operations as well. Even though you are in an emergency mode, your practice must still safeguard ePHI. Develop the plan to securely access electronic systems (including servers and workstations) that

51. 68 *Federal Register* 8351.

52. This document is available online at: http://csrc.nist.gov/publications/nistpubs/800-34-rev1/. See Appendix I: Resources (2 pages) for an updated list of print and Web resources related to contingency and disaster recovery planning.

contain an exact copy of your practice's most current ePHI. Select and maintain an alternative site to perform the practice's data processing functions if a disaster seriously disrupts access and availability of ePHI at your practice facility. Ensure hardware and software compatibility at primary and backup sites. Provide backup power and communications in the event of an emergency. Appoint personnel to the emergency mode operations team. Train all personnel in the emergency mode operation plan, with emphasis on whom and under what circumstances a key workforce member initiates emergency mode operations. Test the emergency mode operation plan and make modifications as necessary. Document all plans and actions, including test results, in writing and maintain the documentation according to the HIPAA documentation standard.

CRITICAL POINT

Do not forget to consider in your disaster recovery planning that loss of electricity in your practice curtails your access to electronic systems that contain ePHI, thereby triggering an emergency mode operation plan.

Testing and Revision Procedures

Implementation Specification	Standard	Reference
D. Testing and revision procedures (A)	Contingency plan	164.308(a)(7)(ii)(D)

What to Do:

Implement procedures for periodic testing and revision of contingency plans.

How to Do It:

After the disaster recovery plan is created, it is important to test the plan by creating a disaster scenario and going through the recovery steps in the plan. This test should be planned in advance and conducted at a time when the practice is not open for business, such as a weekend afternoon. Be sure to document the successful provisions in the plan test, response times, and, most importantly, any failures that require correction. Make corrections to the plan as soon as possible, and make sure all workforce members know the new procedures and why they are being implemented. Test the plan at least annually, making sure that any deficiencies from the preceding test are evaluated to ensure that they have been corrected.

Applications and Data Criticality Analysis

Implementation Specification	Standard	Reference
E. Applications and data criticality analysis (A)	Contingency plan	164.308(a)(7)(ii)(E)

What to Do:

Assess the relative criticality of specific applications and data in support of other contingency plan components.

How to Do It:

Determine the applications and data that are most critical to the operation of your business as a medical practice. Prioritize decisions and actions, starting with answers to these questions that will inform your practice's risk analysis:

- What are the most important considerations in safeguarding the practice's electronic systems that contain ePHI?
- What are the practice's biggest security threats?
- Where are the areas that the practice is most vulnerable from a security perspective?
- What steps should be taken first and in what order thereafter in the event of a contingency in order to recover critical business functions?

Remediation will be part of determining risk mitigation strategies. As your practice experiences growing use of electronic business processes, it is prudent to have in place the three required implementation specifications relating to contingencies: data backup, disaster recovery, and emergency mode operation plans. "Contingency planning will be scalable based upon other factors, office configuration, and risk assessment."[53]

CRITICAL POINT

Some scenarios that might invoke a disaster recovery and emergency mode operation plan for a covered entity would be just a contingency or an inconvenience in other businesses. Again, loss of electricity is critical to a covered entity such as a medical practice, whereas it might just be an inconvenience to another type of business.

Evaluation

Standard	Implementation Specifications	References
Evaluation		45 CFR 164.308(a)(8) NIST SP 800-66, pp. 31–32 68 Federal Register 8378

53. 68 *Federal Register* 8351. Also, "[w]hen the Department of Health and Human Services' Office for Civil Rights will conduct audits of organizations' compliance with the HIPAA security rule, a comprehensive business continuity contingency plan is one of many pieces investigators will be looking for.... That means data back-up and disaster recovery plans are required." See Goedert, J. "OCR: We Want to See Contingency Plans," *HDM Breaking News*, May 13, 2010. Available at: www.healthdatamanagement.com/news/ocr-disaster-recovery-contingency-hipaa-security-40277-1.html.

What the Standard Requires

Perform a periodic technical and nontechnical evaluation, based initially upon the standards implemented under this rule and subsequently in response to environmental or operational changes affecting the security of electronic protected health information, that establishes the extent to which an entity's security policies and procedures meet the requirements of [the HIPAA Security Rule].

The implementation specification is reflected in the language of the standard, and, thus, is required.

Your practice should design an evaluation format, establish an evaluation committee chaired by the security official and comprised of workforce members, and set up a schedule for evaluating security systems, risk mitigation, and compliance with Security Rule safeguard standards. While your practice must perform periodic evaluation, you have the option of conducting the evaluation internally using your own workforce or using an external accreditation agency. The preamble to the Security Rule recognizes that cost may be a consideration for an external evaluation, especially for some entities such as small physician practices. Good sources of information and guidance pertaining to evaluation of standards under the Security Rule are the following:

- National Institute of Standards and Technology[54]
- URAC[55]
- Electronic Healthcare Network Accreditation Commission (EHNAC)[56]
- Workgroup for Electronic Data Interchange (WEDI).[57]

Your practice is required under the Security Rule to maintain acceptable levels of risk. If risks are not acceptable, your practice is required to effect changes in its policies and procedures to move to acceptable levels of risk. In an evaluation of the cost of attaining acceptable levels of risk, be sure to include consideration of the civil monetary penalties for violations of the Security Rule. Note that the HITECH Act significantly increased the penalties, with the maximum fine for repeated incidence of a single violation increasing 60-fold to $1.5 million per calendar year. Also, note that the 2009 cost per customer record for a breach was estimated by survey to be $208, which was based on a combination of "legal fees, disclosure expenses related to customer contact and public response;

54. www.csrc.nist.gov.

55. www.urac.org.

56. www.ehnac.org.

57. www.wedi.org. WEDI is charged in the HIPAA legislation and enabling regulations as a consultant to the Secretary of HHS and as an advisor to the National Committee on Vital and Health Statistics (NCVHS) on matters related to HIPAA Administrative Simplification.

consulting help; and remediation expenses such as technology and training."[58]

Business Associate Contracts and Other Arrangements

Standard	Implementation Specifications	References
Business associate contracts and other arrangements	Written contract or other arrangement	45 CFR 164.308(b)(1) NIST SP 800-66, pp. 33–34 68 Federal Register 8378

What the Standard Requires

A covered entity, in accordance with Security Standards: General Rules of the HIPAA Security Rule,[59] may permit a business associate to create, receive, maintain, or transmit electronic protected health information on the covered entity's behalf only if the covered entity obtains satisfactory assurances, in accordance with the standard for business associate contracts or other arrangements of Organizational Requirements of the Security Rule,[60] that the business associate will appropriately safeguard the information.

This standard requires your practice to have appropriate written business associate agreements in place for any entity that creates, receives, maintains, or transmits ePHI on your practice's behalf. The HITECH Act changed the relationship between covered entity and business associate in four ways, which we discussed in Chapter 1. First, on February 17, 2010, business associates had to comply with the HIPAA Security Rule. Second, a business associate is required to inform its covered entity of any breach of "unsecured" ePHI that it discovers or experiences and to assist the covered entity by providing requisite information that will facilitate the covered entity's fulfillment of breach notification requirements. Third, business associates are subject to the same penalties as covered entities, and with respect to a violation of breach notification requirements, federal enforcement commenced February 22, 2010, for breaches discovered on or after that date. Finally, business associate agreements had to incorporate specific security and privacy provisions of the HITECH Act in the business associate agreement.[61]

---

58. Messmer, E. "Data breach costs top $200 per customer record: Ponemon Institute's annual study says overall organization cost per incident rises to $6.75 million," *NetworkWorld*, January 25, 2010. Available at: www.networkworld.com/news/2010/012510-data-breach-costs.html.

59. 45 CFR 164.306.

60. 45 CFR 164.314(a).

61. 42 USC 17931 (security) and 42 USC 17934 (privacy).

Before enactment of the HITECH Act, if a business associate violated the satisfactory assurances of the business associate agreement, the covered entity's recourse was to cancel the business associate agreement.[62] The covered entity was liable for civil penalties related to the violation. Under the HITECH Act, the business associate is regulated directly by the federal government for the first time, and it, too, may be liable for civil penalties in the same manner as a covered entity. It is important to note, however, that business associates are **not** covered entities.[63] Rather, the HITECH Act requires certain obligations of business associates in the same manner as they are required of covered entities.

Written Contract or Other Arrangement

Implementation Specification	Standard	Reference
Written contract or other arrangement	Business associate contracts and other arrangements	164.308(b)(4)

What to Do:

Document the satisfactory assurances required by the Business Associate Contracts and Other Arrangements standard through a written contract or other arrangement with the business associate that meets the applicable requirements of Organizational Requirements of the Security Rule.

How to do It:

The HITECH Act requires that covered entities amend their business associate agreement content to reflect new requirements and changes in the relationship between a covered entity and its business associates. As an example of an amended business associate agreement, please see the North Carolina Healthcare Information and Communications Alliance, Inc. (NCHICA) *Amended and Restated Business Associate Agreement*, which was approved for public distribution on February 1, 2010.[64] As mentioned in Chapter 1, please be alert to forthcoming HITECH Act privacy and security enabling regulations, which most likely will require compliance in mid-2011, and may require additional changes or amendments to business associate agreements.

62. If the business associate agreement included an enforceable indemnity clause, the covered entity could sue the business associate for indemnification of harms resulting from the violation.

63. There are examples of covered entities acting in a business associate role, such as a health care clearinghouse processing electronic transactions for a physician practice.

64. www.nchica.org.

PHYSICAL SAFEGUARD STANDARDS AND IMPLEMENTATION SPECIFICATIONS

Physical safeguards are designed to help you protect your investment in the facilities and electronic systems, devices, and media that contain ePHI.

Facility Access Controls

Standard	Implementation Specifications	References
Facility access controls	i. Contingency operations (A) ii. Facility security plan (A) iii. Access control and validation (A) iv. Maintenance records (A)	45 CFR 164.310(a)(1) NIST SP 800-66, pp. 35–36 68 Federal Register 8378

What the Standard Requires

Implement policies and procedures to limit physical access to its electronic information systems and the facility or facilities in which they are housed, while ensuring that properly authorized access is allowed.

There are four implementation specifications pertaining to facility access controls, each of which is addressable, which means that you may tailor your policies and procedures for controlling access to your particular physical environment. The language of the implementation specifications is straightforward. Specifications will be determined based on a covered entity's risk analysis and other factors, such as the characteristics of the practice facility itself. Several clarifications are important with respect to this standard. First, the facility access controls standard applies to a covered entity's "business location or locations," and the facility includes "physical premises and the interior and exterior of a building(s)."[65] Please note that the term *facility* includes premises for workforce members who may be authorized to work with ePHI from their homes and covers *electronic systems, devices*, and *media* that may be used in a home environment or mobile capacity. Next, a covered entity "retains responsibility for considering facility security even where it shares space with other organizations."[66]

Contingency Operations

Implementation Specification	Standard	Reference
i. Contingency operations (A)	Facility access controls	164.310(a)(2)(i)

65. 68 *Federal Register* 8354.

66. 68 *Federal Register* 8353.

What to Do:

Establish (and implement as needed) procedures that allow facility access in support of restoration of lost data under the disaster recovery plan and emergency mode operations plan in the event of an emergency.

How to Do It:

This implementation specification is related to the administrative safeguard contingency plan and outlines the procedures to be followed to restore ePHI in the event of an emergency situation. So, compliance with this standard requires coordination of the procedures here with the disaster and emergency mode operation plans that are covered by that administrative safeguard standard. The procedures will be based on outcomes of your practice's risk analysis. Questions to address might include the following examples:

- What are your procedures for recovery if your practice is damaged by fire?
- What are your procedures for recovery if your practice loses electricity supply for a prolonged period of time, say, because of a natural disaster?
- Where would your practice relocate in the event of a natural disaster?[67]

Remember, the critical outcome is re-establishing access to the practice's electronic systems that contain ePHI. Identify your software vendor(s) and key workforce members that will be responsible for achieving that outcome. Finally, it also is important to have a procedure for keeping your patients informed of your progress in restoring practice operations.

Facility Security Plan

Implementation Specification	Standard	Reference
ii. Facility security plan (A)	Facility access controls	164.310(a)(2)(ii)

What to Do:

Implement policies and procedures to safeguard the facility and the equipment therein from unauthorized physical access, tampering, and theft.

How to Do It:

Develop procedures to protect your practice's facility and electronic systems, devices, and media from "unauthorized physical access, tampering, and theft." Include policies regarding building exteriors, interiors, access, tampering, and theft. Also, include procedures for handling intrusions and deliberate impairment of systems, which may include computer systems and electricity serving

67. A home office and electronic system that had not been configured for compliance with the Security and Privacy Rules prior to an emergency is not a suitable recovery environment. Consider a hot site instead, from which you could access your exact backup copy of electronic protected health information and be back in operation in an emergency situation.

your facility location. Develop access policies and implement procedures to safeguard your practice's facility and electronic systems, using locks, alarm systems, identification systems such as pass cards, anti-intrusion systems, and similar devices that are suitable to your practice as a business environment.

CRITICAL POINT

During practice hours, the receptionist can play a key role in controlling access and ensuring only authorized individuals have access to systems containing ePHI.

FIGURE 4.3

Sample Checklist of Facility Access Controls

- ❑ Who has access to electronic systems and what is their mode of access (dial-up, modem, Internet, and so forth)?
- ❑ What are your opening and closing procedures?
- ❑ Who maintains the layout and design of the facility? Who authorizes access to the facility?
- ❑ Who has control over locks and keys?
- ❑ What are the locking mechanisms for doors, gates, windows, and other access points?
- ❑ Does staff have access badges and cards, door keys, etc?
- ❑ Do you have sign-in and sign-out procedures?
- ❑ Do you have door and window locations and security devices for each?
- ❑ Are you in a flood zone? Are there fire or water hazards on the premises?
- ❑ Who is authorized to handle contingencies?
- ❑ Are there environmental controls (heating, ventilation, and air conditioning) for electronic systems?
- ❑ Do you have a plan for monitoring and periodically evaluating the facility security plan?

Access Control and Validation Procedures

Implementation Specification	Standard	Reference
iii. Access control and validation procedures (A)	Facility access controls	164.310(a)(2)(iii)

What to Do

Implement procedures to control and validate a person's access to facilities based on [his or her] role or function, including visitor control, and control of access to software programs for testing and revision.

How to Do It:

This implementation specification typically is based on job function and need. Your practice needs to implement procedures to control access to electronic systems that contain ePHI. In accordance with the "minimum necessary" requirement of the Privacy Rule, these Security Rule access procedures should cross-reference with Privacy Rule access controls to avoid conflicting policies. Your procedures should verify authorization for any workforce member or business associate to access electronic systems that contain ePHI. In addition, your practice should control access and movement within the practice. For business associates, and any other non-patient visitor to the practice, your practice should use "Business associate" and "Visitor" sign-in and badge systems. Your practice should escort visitors in areas that contain access to ePHI, should there be a reason for them to be in such areas. The security official should be aware of and oversee business associates responsible for software testing and revision and should document all such activities as to time and result.

Maintenance Records

Implementation Specification	Standard	Reference
iv. Maintenance records (A)	Facility access controls	164.310(a)(2)(iv)

What to Do:

Implement policies and procedures to document repairs and modifications to the physical components of a facility that are related to security (for example, hardware, walls, doors, and locks).

How to Do It:

Create a log and description of repairs or modifications made to the facility's physical security components, including hardware, walls, doors, and locks. The log should document, in writing, each repair and be maintained according to the HIPAA documentation standard. Electronic documentation is permissible, but be sure to routinely back up the log after each new entry.

Workstation Use

Standard	Implementation Specifications	References
Workstation use		45 CFR 164.310(b) NIST SP 800-66, p. 37 68 Federal Register 8378

What the Standard Requires

Implement policies and procedures that specify the proper functions to be performed, the manner in which those functions are to be performed, and the physical attributes of the surroundings of a specific workstation or class of workstation that can access electronic protected health information.

The implementation specification is reflected in the language of the standard, and, as such, is required.

Note the definition of workstation in the Security Rule: "[A]n electronic computing device, for example, a laptop or desktop computer, or any other device that performs similar functions, and electronic media stored in its immediate environment."[68] Accordingly, this standard applies to workstations and electronic media that are stationary in the practice as well as those that may be portable or mobile and used outside the practice. An example of a policy and accompanying procedure pertaining to this standard would be that workforce members log off before leaving a workstation unattended. Another example would be that a receptionist has to make sure that the workstation that he or she uses to log patients into the practice for an encounter has to be shielded from the patients signing in. A third example would be that workstations used throughout the practice should not have screens visible to passersby, such as unauthorized patients and visitors. A final example would be that any workstation containing ePHI not have Internet access over an open network and that any workforce members using an authorized portable or mobile device have encryption that safeguards ePHI at rest and in motion.

Workstation Security

Standard	Implementation Specifications	References
Workstation security		45 CFR 164.310(c) NIST SP 800-66, p. 38 68 Federal Register 8378

What the Standard Requires

Implement physical safeguards for all workstations that access electronic protected health information, to restrict access to authorized users.

The implementation specification is reflected in the language of the standard and, as such, is required.

The compliance solution for this standard will be "dependent on the entity's risk analysis and risk management process."[69] All practice electronic

68. 68 *Federal Register* 8376 and 45 CFR 164.304.

69. 68 *Federal Register* 8354.

systems and workstations in the practice that contain ePHI must have authentication[70] controls to allow access to authorized users while precluding access by unauthorized individuals. In addition to this safeguard, the practice must consider in its risk analysis the physical location and working environment in the practice as further safeguard possibilities. An example is shielding the screen of the receptionist's computer from the view of a patient signing in for an encounter, as mentioned in the previous standard discussion. Another example is having automatic log-off on all workstations; an automatic log-off would activate after a period of time determined as an outcome of the practice's risk analysis. Workstation security also pertains to portable and mobile devices used inside and outside the practice, all of which should be safeguarded through authentication and encryption controls.

Device and Media Controls

Standard	Implementation Specifications	References
Device and media controls	i. Disposal (R) ii. Media re-use (R) iii. Accountability (A) iv. Data backup and storage (A)	45 CFR 164.310(d)(1) NIST SP 800-66, p. 39 68 Federal Register 8378

What the Standard Requires

Implement policies and procedures that govern the receipt and removal of hardware and electronic media that contain electronic protected health information into and out of a facility, and the movement of these items within the facility.

This standard has two required implementation specifications and two addressable implementation specifications and requires your practice to establish policies and implement procedures to account for your practice's hardware and electronic media that contain ePHI. We discussed the August 24, 2009, *Guidance Specifying the Technologies and Methodologies that Render Protected Health Information Unusable, Unreadable, or Indecipherable to Unauthorized Individuals*[71] in Chapter 1, and the provisions of that *Guidance* informs the discussion that follows on the implementation specifications. The *Guidance* applies to the two required implementation specifications: Disposal and Media Re-use.

---

70. Authentication means "corroboration that a person is the one claimed." 45 CFR 164.304.

71. 74 *Federal Register* 42742–42743. The *Guidance* is a part of the Breach Notification Interim Final Rule, published August 24, 2009.

Disposal

Implementation Specification	Standard	Reference
i. Disposal (R)	Device and media controls	164.310(d)(2)(i)

What to Do:

Implement policies and procedures to address the final disposition of electronic protected health information, and/or the hardware or electronic media on which it is stored.

How to Do It:

We repeat here the relevant portion of the *Guidance*:

> "Protected health information (PHI) is rendered unusable, unreadable, or indecipherable to unauthorized individuals if one or more of the following applies: . . .

(b) The media of which the PHI is stored or recorded have been destroyed in one of the following ways: . . .

(ii) Electronic media have been cleared, purged, or destroyed consistent with NIST Special Publication 800-88, *Guidelines for Media Sanitation,*[72] such that the PHI cannot be retrieved."

We recommend that your practice follow the *Guidance* for disposal of hardware and electronic media. By doing so, if *secured* ePHI is breached, you may not have to send breach notifications to affected parties under the Breach Notification Rule. Consult your hardware and software vendors for help on interpreting the NIST *Guidelines for Media Sanitation*, referred to above.

Media Re-use

Implementation Specification	Standard	Reference
ii. Media re-use (R)	Device and media controls	164.310(d)(2)(ii)

What to Do:

Implement procedures for removal of electronic protected health information from electronic media before the media are made available for re-use.

72. This document, dated September 2006, is from the National Institute of Standards and Technology (NIST). Available at: http://csrc.nist.gov/publications/nistpubs/800-88/NISTSP800-88_rev1.pdf.

How to Do It:

How to handle media re-use will be an outcome of your practice's risk analysis. Since this implementation specification was promulgated, electronic media have become relatively inexpensive and are becoming more so with each passing year. Accordingly, in your risk analysis, your practice needs to compare the cost of replacing rather than re-using electronic media, with the latter including expected costs (based on risk) that you might incur should a breach occur from reused electronic media. The expected costs should now include the costs and harms of having to conduct breach notification. Given how inexpensive electronic media have become, we recommend **not** re-using electronic media, but rather destroying such media according to the procedure outlined in the preceding implementation specification (disposal).

Accountability

Implementation Specification	Standard	Reference
iii. Accountability (A)	Device and media controls	164.310(d)(2)(iii)

What to Do:

Maintain a record of the movements of hardware and electronic media and any person responsible therefor.

How to Do It:

Create and maintain an inventory and track movement of electronic systems, workstations, devices, and media within your practice. The inventory should include model and serial number, date purchased, place of purchase, warranty and/or maintenance contract (if applicable), location, workforce member responsible, and any movement from one location to another (if applicable). This implementation specification "does not address audit trails within systems and/or software. Rather it requires a record of the actions of a person relative to the receipt and removal of hardware and/or software into and out of a facility that are traceable to that person. The impact of maintaining accountability on system resources and services will depend upon the complexity of the mechanism to establish accountability . . . such as receipt and removal restricted to specific persons, with logs kept."[73] Please keep in mind that this implementation specification is addressable: "[S]mall providers would be unlikely to be involved in large-scale moves of equipment that would require systematic tracking, unlike, for example, large health care providers or health plans."[74]

73. 68 *Federal Register* 8354.

74. Ibid.

Data Backup and Storage

Implementation Specification	Standard	Reference
iv. Data backup and storage (A)	Device and media controls	164.310(d)(2)(iv)

What to Do:

Create a retrievable, exact copy of electronic protected health information, when needed, before movement of equipment.

How to Do It:

Prior to moving any electronic systems, workstations, devices, or electronic media in the practice, make sure that you create an exact copy of ePHI contained therein. Maintain that copy in a separate file backed up in a secure off-site database environment. This copy must be readily retrievable in the event that hardware or electronic media are damaged in movement or if a disaster or other contingency affects the practice.

TECHNICAL SAFEGUARD STANDARDS AND IMPLEMENTATION SPECIFICATIONS

By now, more than five years after the compliance date for covered entities, your practice has implemented the security standards. As security becomes even more important with the growing use of electronic health record (EHR)[75] systems and ePrescribing[76] by health care providers, you will find the policy and procedures information in this chapter useful as your practice checks on its own policies and procedures.

Many of the technical safeguards may require information from your hardware or software vendor. Be sure to ask your vendor if you have any questions. Remember, you may use *reasonable* and *appropriate* measures to demonstrate compliance.

75. See the following publications on electronic health record (EHR) systems: Hartley CP, Jones ED III. *EHR Implementation: A Step-by-Step Guide for the Medical Practice*, Foreword by Newt Gingrich, Chicago, IL: AMA Press, 2005; Hartley, CP, Jones, ED III, Ens D, Whitt, D. *Technical and Financial Guide to EHR Implementation*. Chicago, IL: AMA, 2007.

76. Electronic prescribing (ePrescribing) was included in the Medicare Modernization Act (MMA) of 2003. The final rule pertaining to formulary and benefit transactions, medication history transactions, and fill status notifications was published in the *Federal Register* on April 7, 2008 (73 *Federal Register* 18917–18942).

Access Control

Standard	Implementation Specifications	References
Access control	i. Unique user identification (R) ii. Emergency access procedure (R) iii. Automatic log-off (A) iv. Encryption and decryption (A)	45 CFR 164.312(a)(1) NIST SP 800-66, pp. 40–41 68 Federal Register 8378

What the Standard Requires

Implement technical policies and procedures for electronic information systems that maintain electronic protected health information to allow access only to those persons or software programs that have been granted access rights as specified by the Administrative Safeguard Standard: Information Access Management.

Unique User Identification

Implementation Specification	Standard	Reference
i. Unique user identification (R)	Access control	164.312(a)(2)(i)

What to Do:

Assign a unique name and/or number for identifying and tracking user identity.

How to Do It:

The Security Official should:

- Assign unique user identification to each workforce member.
- Manage and track user identity, especially when new workforce members come on board and when current employees change jobs or names.
- Change passwords according to a timetable based on your risk analysis and policies and procedures. We recommend passwords contain at least 7 alphanumeric characters to make them difficult to decode or guess and that they be changed every 30, 60, or 90 days, depending on outcomes from your practice's risk analysis.

Emergency Access Procedure

Implementation Specification	Standard	Reference
ii. Emergency access procedure (R)	Access control	164.312(a)(2)(ii)

What to Do:

Establish (and implement as needed) procedures for obtaining necessary electronic protected health information during an emergency.

How to Do It:

The security official should:

- Determine types of situations that warrant immediate access to your practice's ePHI.
- Work with your practice's IT vendors to establish emergency access procedures to accommodate various situations.[77]
- Coordinate your practice's emergency access procedures with your practice's Administrative Safeguard Contingency Plan and Physical Safeguard Contingency Operations procedures.
- Document procedures for emergency access and train workforce members on their use.
- Develop strict "alarm" procedures to avoid abuse of emergency access, such as audit trails, and hold users accountable for their actions.

Automatic Log-off

Implementation Specification	Standard	Reference
iii. Automatic log-off (A)	Access control	164.312(a)(2)(iii)

What to Do:

Implement electronic procedures that terminate an electronic session after a predetermined time of inactivity.

How to Do It:

The security official should:

- Activate a password-protected screensaver that automatically prevents unauthorized users from viewing or accessing ePHI from unattended computer workstations.
- Establish a timeout period before the log-off capability locks the computer workstation and makes information inaccessible.[78]
- Work with your practice's IT vendor to ensure that all workstations containing ePHI have activated log-off features in place.

77. For example, you may wish to establish a special user password that allows full access to all electronic protected health information and safeguard the use of that password by creating a special audit log when it is used.

78. Workstations in high-traffic areas should have a timeout of 2 to 3 minutes. Those in protected areas with limited access, such as a laboratory or isolated office, may have a longer timeout period, say, 10 minutes. A log-off requires the user to re-enter a password to gain access to data.

Encryption and Decryption

Implementation Specification	Standard	Reference
iv. Encryption and decryption (A)[79]	Access control	164.312(a)(2)(iv)

What to Do:

Implement a mechanism to encrypt and decrypt electronic protect health information.

How to Do It:

The security official should:

- Ensure that all ePHI *at rest* in a database is encrypted.
- Ensure that all ePHI *in transit* is encrypted.

On August 24, 2009, the Department of Health and Human Services (HHS) published in the *Federal Register* an Interim Final Rule: *Breach Notification for Unsecured Protected Health Information.*[80] Section 13402 of the Health Information Technology for Economic and Clinical Health (HITECH) Act, part of the American Recovery and Reinvestment Act of 2009 (ARRA) enacted February 17, 2009, required HHS to issue interim final regulations within 180 days to require covered entities under HIPAA and their business associates to provide notification in the case of breaches of unsecured PHI. HHS included in the August 24, 2009, Interim Final Rule an update of guidance that it had earlier published in the *Federal Register* on April 27, 2009,[81] to conform with HITECH Act provisions, which explained the meaning of "unsecured protected health information." The August 24, 2009 guidance, entitled, *Guidance Specifying the Technologies and Methodologies that Render Protected Health Information Unusable, Unreadable, or Indecipherable to Unauthorized Individuals*, is reproduced[82] here:

B. Guidance Specifying the Technologies and Methodologies that Render Protected Health Information Unusable, Unreadable, or Indecipherable to Unauthorized Individuals

---

79. *Encryption* converts a message in a file or document from a readable format to an unreadable format. *Decryption* does the reverse: it allows an encrypted, or unreadable, message to be converted into a readable format.

80. Department of Health and Human Services, Office of the Secretary, "45 CFR Parts 160 and 164: Breach Notification for Unsecured Protected Health Information; Interim Final Rule," *Federal Register*, v.74, n.162, August 24, 2009, pp.42739–42770.

81. Department of Health and Human Services, Office of the Secretary, "45 CFR Parts 160 and 164:Guidance Specifying the Technologies and Methodologies That Render Protected Health Information Unusable, Unreadable, or Indecipherable to Unauthorized Individuals for Purposes of the Breach Notification Requirements Under Section 13402 of Title XIII (Health Information Technology for Economic and Clinical Health Act) of the American Recovery and Reinvestment Act of 2009; Request for Information," *Federal Register*, v.74, n.79, April 27, 2009, pp.19006–19010.

82. 74 *Federal Register* 42742–42743.

Protected health information (PHI) is rendered unusable, unreadable, or indecipherable to unauthorized individuals if one or more of the following applies:

(a) Electronic PHI has been encrypted as specified in the HIPAA Security Rule by "the use of an algorithmic process to transform data into a form in which there is a low probability of assigning meaning without use of a confidential process or key"[83] and such confidential process or key that might enable decryption has not been breached. To avoid a breach of the confidential process or key, these decryption tools should be stored on a device or at a location separate from the data they are used to encrypt or decrypt. The encryption processes identified below have been tested by the National Institute of Standards and Technology (NIST) and judged to meet this standard.

  (i) Valid encryption processes for data at rest are consistent with NIST Special Publication 800-111, Guide to Storage Encryption Technologies for End User Devices.[84]

  (ii) Valid encryption processes for data in motion are those which comply, as appropriate, with NIST Special Publications 800-52, Guidelines for the Selection and Use of Transport Layer Security (TLS) Implementations; 800-77, Guide to IPsec VPNs; or 800-113, Guide to SSL VPNs, or others which are Federal Information Processing Standards (FIPS) 140-2 validated.[85]

(b) The media on which the PHI is stored or recorded has been destroyed in one of the following ways:

  (i) Paper, film, or other hard copy media have been shredded or destroyed such that the PHI cannot be read or otherwise cannot be reconstructed. Redaction is specifically excluded as a means of data destruction.

  (ii) Electronic media have been cleared, purged, or destroyed consistent with NIST Special Publication 800-88, Guidelines for Media Sanitization,[86] such that the PHI cannot be retrieved.

We highly recommend that your practice encrypt its ePHI according to the recommendations in the *Guidance*, whether that information is *at rest* in a database or *in motion* over a communications network. It is essential that you encrypt your data, if your practice uses portable or mobile electronic devices outside of the practice that could be misplaced, lost, or stolen. In your risk analysis, be sure to compare the cost of encrypting your ePHI to make it *secure*, with the potential costs to your practice of having *unsecured* ePHI accessible to unauthorized individuals, meeting breach notification requirements, and incurring federal fines.

83. 45 CFR 164.304, definition of "encryption."

84. Available at: http://csrc.nist.gov; NIST Roadmap plans include the development of security guidelines for enterprise-level storage devices and such guidelines will be considered in updates to this guidance, when available.

85. Available at: http://csrc.nist.gov.

86. Available at: http://csrc.nist.gov.

Audit Controls

Standard	Implementation Specifications	References
Audit controls		45 CFR 164.312(b) NIST SP 800-66, pp. 42–43 68 Federal Register 8378

What the Standard Requires

Implement hardware, software, and/or procedural mechanisms that record and examine activity in information systems that contain or use electronic protected health information.

The implementation specification is reflected in the language of the standard and, as such, is required.

Audit controls allow your practice to monitor who is accessing information, when they access it, and what they do with the information. Small and large practices are required to have audit controls in place to monitor activity on their electronic systems. They must also review audit control records to ensure all activity is appropriate. This may include reviewing and monitoring log-ons and log-offs, file accesses, updates, edits, system activity, and security incidents. How your practice meets this requirement is an outcome of your risk analysis.

How to Do It

The security official should:

- Define the reason for the audit trail (eg, system troubleshooting, policy enforcement, security incident, etc.)
- Determine whether workforce member users are accessing information or performing tasks beyond the scope of their job responsibilities.
- Determine whether workforce members are sharing their user IDs. One measure of evidence that a user is sharing his or her ID is that the user is logged on to two or more computer workstations simultaneously.
- Determine if the user is logged on over a period of several days, which indicates the user does not log off at the end of a work session.[87]
- Maintain and periodically review audit trails[88] or activity logs for critical application systems, including user-written applications.
- Follow up on suspicious entries, such as unauthorized accesses and attempts, and identify and resolve inappropriate activity.

---

87. This may not be an issue if your practice has automatic log-off capabilities in place and in force.

88. Failure to regularly review audit trails may mean that a security incident goes undetected for a period of time, which may be construed as willful neglect under the October 30, 2009, enforcement Interim Final Rule, which we discussed in Chapter 1.

For larger practices:

- Determine if unauthorized users are looking at ePHI. Staff members may be curious about friends, family members, co-workers, or celebrities. Without authorization, such curiosity may provide proof of a breach of confidentiality.
- Review Internet audit trails. If employees are bored, they may be logging onto inappropriate Web sites and exposing your practice to a potential breach if unsecured ePHI is intercepted and accessed by an unauthorized individual. Check for evidence of streaming videos, audio files, or other non-business-related programs that slow your network.
- Determine if users are downloading executable files that make your practice liable for software licensing agreement violations.
- Measure the effect of auditing on system performance.

Integrity

Standard	Implementation Specifications	References
Integrity	Mechanism to authenticate ePHI(A)	45 CFR 164.312(c)(1) NIST SP 800-66, pp. 44–45 68 Federal Register 8378–8379

What the Standard Requires

Implement policies and procedures to protect electronic protected health information from improper alteration or destruction.

Integrity is "the property that data or information has not been altered or destroyed in an unauthorized manner."[89] Along with *confidentiality* and *availability*, integrity is one of the three key pillars of the security rule. It means in practice that the right person can access the right information at the right time and that the data are not altered or destroyed in any manner. Inaccurate data could result in harm to or even potential death of a patient.

Access controls and audit trails can keep individuals from breaching confidentiality, but data can become corrupt from several sources: data entry errors, hacking or tampering, mechanical errors in storage devices, transmission error, and poor data integration, such as downloading lab reports into an electronic health record or other database system. Software or programming bugs, computer viruses, and human error also can cause corruption. A practice must ensure that its ePHI has not been altered without its knowledge and approval.

89. 45 CFR 164.304.

Mechanism to Authenticate Electronic Protected Health Information

Implementation Specification	Standard	Reference
Mechanism to authenticate ePHI(A)	Integrity	164.312(c)(2)

What to Do:

Implement electronic mechanisms to corroborate that electronic protected health information has not been altered or destroyed in an unauthorized manner.

How to Do It:

The security official should:

- Verify with the practice's IT vendor that the practice's electronic systems have mechanisms to detect unauthorized intrusion and data corruption and to verify data integrity.
- Ensure that the practice's electronic systems, applications, and databases are backed up regularly, with backups tested on a routine schedule.
- Use and review daily audit trails of intrusion detection systems to identify any system hacking attempts.

Person or Entity Authentication

Standard	Implementation Specification	References
Person or entity authentication		45 CFR 164.312(d) NIST SP 800-66, p. 46 68 Federal Register 8379

What the Standard Requires

Implement procedures to verify that a person or entity seeking access to electronic protected health information is the one claimed.

The implementation specification is reflected in the language of the standard and, as such, is required.

This standard requires password management and audit trails that enable your practice to authenticate who is accessing, reading, altering, or transmitting ePHI. A person or entity authentication involves a "round trip" question and answer routine, such as with a username/password query:

- User replies to question: Who are you? User provides username.
- After reply, software states: Prove it. User provides password.

How to Do It

The security official should ensure that your practice's electronic systems certify that the user or entity seeking access to the practice's ePHI can provide verification of identity.[90]

Transmission Security

Standard	Implementation Specification	References
Transmission security	i. Integrity controls (A)	45 CFR 164.312(e)(1)
	ii. Encryption (A)	NIST SP 800-66, p. 47
		68 Federal Register 8379

What the Standard Requires

Implement technical security measures to guard against unauthorized access to electronic protected health information that is being transmitted over an electronic communications network.

Your practice's local network may have no connectivity to any entity outside your practice, but in today's electronic environment this is increasingly rare. Your IT vendors likely have some connection to your network so that they can provide your practice with IT support. Because many practices also are considering going wireless or using mobile devices, such as multifunction personal data assistants (PDAs), a poorly designed local network or communications over external open networks can threaten your information system, especially if it compromises the availability and integrity of your data.

Today's systems are more secure, but older systems likely contain unused or unnecessary programs that leave your practice exposed to open networks. Ask your practice's IT vendor or an IT consultant to help your practice identify any of your systems that can be discarded or updated to mitigate potential transmission threats.

90. Proof of identity can be authenticated in one of several ways:
- Something you know (eg, user ID, mother's maiden name, personal ID number such as a national provider identifier, or password).
- Something you have (eg, smart card, token, swipe card, or badge).
- Something you are (eg, biometric such as finger image, voice scan, or iris or retina scan).

See Hartley CP, et al. *Handbook for HIPAA Security Implementation*, Chicago, IL: AMA Press, 2004, p.90.

Integrity Controls

Implementation Specification	Standard	Reference
i. Integrity controls (A)	Transmission security	164.312(e)(2)(i)

What to Do:

Implement security measures to ensure that electronically transmitted electronic protected health information is not improperly modified without detection until disposed of.

If someone changed the telephone numbers and addresses in your personal database without your permission, you would question whether the remainder of the information was accurate. Ensuring data integrity means that ePHI has not been altered or destroyed without appropriate knowledge and approval.

How to Do It:

The security official should:

Assign a unique user ID to workforce members authorized to log onto the practice's information systems, which ensures that entries by those users can be identified and tracked appropriately.

Make sure that your audit trails track username/password entries so that your information system can track unauthorized changes to electronic records by the person making the changes.

Apply appropriate sanctions to workforce members if changes to ePHI are made without authorization.

Encryption

Implementation Specification	Standard	Reference
ii. Encryption (A)	Transmission security	164.312(e)(2)(ii)

What to Do:

Implement a mechanism to encrypt electronic protected health information whenever deemed appropriate.

How to Do It:

The Encryption and Decryption implementation specification of the Technical Safeguard standard: Access Control focuses on preventing a person or entity from deciphering ePHI should the person or entity gain entry to a database on an information system without authorization for access. This Encryption implementation specification relates to the movement of ePHI in a communication over a network.

Encryption is appropriate if the practice is using open networks such as the Internet for transmission of ePHI. As practices increasingly are using e-mail communications between physician and patient, adopting electronic health record systems, transmitting and receiving ePHI from labs and pharmacies, encryption is a must. Your vendor can assist the practice in making sure that all communications over open networks are encrypted.

Encryption also is a must for portable and mobile devices—PDAs, notebook computers, and tablet computers—that may be mislaid, lost, or stolen. The practice's notice of privacy practices should address the practice's policy and procedures regarding encryption of ePHI, especially as it relates to physician-to-patient and patient-to-physician e-mail communications.[91]

We recommend that you read carefully the boxed texts pertaining to the Encryption and Decryption implementation specification of the Technical Safeguard standard: Access Control, and discuss the encryption options therein with your practice's IT vendor.

91. It is a good idea for physician practices to use a secure e-mail server for communicating with patients that is separate from the database server containing electronic protected health information. Once a patient authorizes electronic communications, the practice should issue the patient a username/password for access to the secure e-mail server and a decryption key for reading encrypted files from that server. If the patient requests electronic protected health information from the practice, an encrypted file can be placed on the e-mail server and a message can be sent to the patient to log onto the e-mail server to retrieve the file. Even with encryption, this is the appropriate procedure as the physician is a covered entity with obligations for safeguarding electronic protected health information while the patient is not subject to those obligations.

chapter 5

Communication, Training, and Social Networking Media

What You Will Learn in This Chapter

In a book about HIPAA, why bother with communications?

Our experience tells us that training and communications go hand in hand. Good communications comes from good training. You can have bad communications from good training, but you cannot deliver good communications out of bad training.

This is especially true when it comes to the privacy and security rules that specify what you must do to protect written, oral, and electronic communications. We'll cover that in this chapter, along with a quick reference grid on permitted incidental uses and disclosures and a communications plan that will help you in a crisis.

Some people put communications into that touchy-feely category and pass it off as fluff. But ask anyone who has been the subject of an Office for Civil Rights investigation, investigated by an inquisitive reporter about the importance of good communication, or had to deal with an unsatisfied customer or patient. When carefully managed, that touchy-feely communication becomes poise and dignity.

As with the first few years into HIPAA's Privacy and Security Rules, workforce will again have reasons to express concern that may come across as scary or embarrassing. For the most part, that's nervous energy. At some time, each of will have a HIPAA Epiphany, Part II. When it happens to you, you'll be deeply grateful for a chapter on strategy, poise and dignity.

A good oral and written communications plan is the best defense if a patient files a claim against you, or if the Office for Civil Rights (OCR) launches an investigation, or if a staff member gets into a jam. Do more than develop the plan. Implement it.

In this chapter you will learn:

- What HIPAA says about oral and written communications
- The affect of social networking sites on health care
- How the staff can confidently deal with the new HIPAA and Breach Notification Rule
- What patients want to know about HIPAA
- How to customize your internal and external communications plan
- HIPAA crisis communications management.

Key terms
Health information
Physical safeguards
Administrative safeguards
Technical safeguards
Social networking

WHY TALK ABOUT COMMUNICATIONS IN A HIPAA BOOK?

Implementing HIPAA is more about changing culture (behavior, actions) than it is about accepting a law. But general guidelines on how to manage culture and behavioral change are not included in rule-making. That's because HIPAA is a law to be interpreted by lawyers.

Until now, most of us have been rushing to meet the letter of HIPAA's law. But patients think that if our offices are now HIPAA-compliant, we're culturally and behaviorally reconditioned and we take precautions to protect their confidential health information.

True, but reconditioning takes more than a one or two hour seminar. You've gone through the motions to meet the law. Now, make privacy and security happen. And that is why it's so critical for us to be straight with patients. Let patients know that the health care community is in the throes of advancing into an electronic environment. Changes aren't always easy, but privacy and security are the cornerstones of that process.

Communications start with the "Director of First Impressions"—the front-line employee (receptionist, nurse, billing clerk).

WHAT HIPAA SAYS ABOUT ORAL AND WRITTEN COMMUNICATION

Oral Communications in the Medical Office

There's a reason why HIPAA's Privacy Rule includes guidelines on how to protect oral communications.

Most people think oral communications begins when someone starts talking.

But oral communication doesn't happen unless someone is listening—even if that conversation is one person talking to himself.

People spend more time listening than any other communication activity. The communication process looks like this:

- 40% listening
- 35% talking
- 16% reading
- 9% writing.[1]

The patient-physician process begins by knowing the difference between hearing and listening. Hearing is a passive activity. You're not actively involved; you're simply allowing sound waves to penetrate your ears. When you're listening, you are an active participant determining the meaning of what you hear.

Physicians listen to patients—to the words used to describe a pain or illness, to the sounds of the body, to the heartbeat and so forth.

When patients come into a medical office, they have several incentives to be an active listener. They are likely to feel better if they listen to the nurse or physician's recommendations; and they are likely to feel better quicker if they feel someone listened to them. The point is that when patients are in the medical office, their listening quotient is very high. So, when a provider is talking in an open area about another patient, they might as well be talking into a megaphone.

When moving into an electronic environment, the physician or nurse has added a computer into the mix. At first, patients are likely to say, "she pays more attention to that computer than me."

By anticipating that response, you can tell the patient, "We're moving into the electronic age, and we're still trying to get the hang of it. But I want to capture everything you're saying. Do you mind if I record some notes in our system?"

Soon after the adoption of EHR software, the provider will settle into a new style, but don't give up on using the EHR. Doctors have long been experts at remembering details so that at the end of the day, they can dictate encounter summaries or letters. Learning to use the software can cloud that memory, so build new good habits; for example, step into your office and update the patient record between visits.

We've seen some physicians say, "I'm going to dictate the note, give me just a moment." Then he dictates the note, and says, "Did that sound right to you?"

---

1. Siress, RH, Riddle, C, and Shouse, D. *Working Woman's Communications Survival Guide.* Indianapolis, IN. Prentice Hall Trade, 1993:p.136.

Also, the process of electronically prescribing medications and being able to reconcile medications with the patient's current list can be disarming for the patient.

Tell the patient in advance that you are electronically sending a prescription. Most likely the name of the pharmacy is already in your system, but it never hurts to verify the location. You may also tell the patient during the ePrescribing process, systems check with each other for other medications in the pharmacy database that may cause an interaction. Even though the nurse probably asked for a current list of medications, most doctors ask again and then cross-check with possible alerts driven by the ePrescribing process.

Communication and Social Networking

Have you noticed who's on Facebook, YouTube, LinkedIn, Plaxo or Twitter lately? For a more peer-focused network, medical-specific networking sites also have emerged. At publication of the second edition, at least 25 social networking sites, from Microsoft HealthVault, Google Health to Trusted.MD, offer secure exchange of information for medical and healthcare professionals.[2] Patients also can blog with others managing the same disease on portals such as PatientsLikeMe.com, or rate physicians on RateMDs.com.

Today, hospitals, clinics and physician groups and emergency responders look to social media outlets and mobile phones to inform and engage people to help them live healthier lives. If you are providing health care advice, such as immunization advice or prenatal care, this can be a great tool for you.

Social media is being used not only to communicate with residents in disasters, but it is also used to spread news about generator safety in power outages or even by patients to leave testimonials about their stay or patient care experience.

But social networking is hazardous material if covered entities are exchanging protected health information via unencrypted devices.

You may say, "I wouldn't do that." But does your receptionist send a text that your 10:00 appointment is here? You look at your smart phone calendar, and there's your patient's name, phone number, and reason for visit.

Most recently, workforce members and interns either have not participated in privacy and security training, or simply haven't thought through the complications of exchanging PHI with peers.

Any protected health information electronically transmitted is subject to the Breach Notification and HIPAA Security Rules and subsequent penalties, so be sure to include social media in your risk analysis. Build a policy and procedure to manage this potential risk.

---

2. One site to preview these networking portals is Medalicious, hosted by the Medical Lab Technicians School, and is available at: http://medicallabtechnicianschool.org/2009/top-25-social-networking-sites-for-healthcare-medical-professionals/.

Be sure to include social networking training in your updated HIPAA communications.

INCIDENTAL USES AND DISCLOSURES

HHS's December 3, 2002, Guidance, *Standards for Privacy of Individually Identifiable Health Information*[3] provides *guidance* on incidental uses and disclosures. In the Guidance, the Secretary of HHS provided clarity to covered entities about what can be written and spoken. This grid gives you a basic overview of incidental uses and disclosures, but we encourage you to read the Guidance in its entirety or talk to your attorney if you have any questions about what you can do or say.

Written Incidental Uses and Disclosures	**Oral Incidental Uses and Disclosures**
You may use sign-in sheets to call out the names of patients in waiting rooms. You are permitted to leave medical charts at bedside or outside of exam rooms. But, implement safeguards to protect the individual's privacy by placing patient charts with identifying information facing the wall. In a hospital, you may display patients' names next to the door of the hospital room they occupy. Covered entities are not required to document incidental uses and disclosures provided to the individual. You are not obligated to prevent any incidental use or disclosure of protected health information (PHI). The Rule requires that you implement reasonable safeguards to limit incidental uses or disclosures.	Physicians can engage in confidential conversations with other providers, even if there is a possibility that they could be overheard. Use reasonable precautions (lowered voices or talking apart from others): ■ Health care staff orally coordinates services at nursing stations ■ Nurses or other health care professionals may discuss a patient's condition over the phone with the patient, a provider, or a family member. ■ A health care professional may discuss lab test results with a patient or other provider in a joint treatment area. ■ A physician may discuss a patient's condition or treatment regimen in the patient's semi-private room. ■ Health care professionals may discuss a patient's condition during training rounds in an academic or training institution. ■ A pharmacist may discuss a prescription over the pharmacy counter, or with a physician or the patient over the phone. Offices do not need to be retrofitted to provide soundproofed walls to avoid conversations that may be overheard.

(continued)

3. This 123-page guidance is available at: www.hhs.gov/ocr/hipaa/guidelines/guidanceallsections.pdf.

(continued)

Written Incidental Uses and Disclosures	Oral Incidental Uses and Disclosures
	Physician's offices may leave messages through the mail, on an answering machine, or with a family member to remind a patient of an appointment. But, reasonably safeguard the individual's privacy and limit the information on the message system.
	Protected health information (PHI) in group therapy settings are treatment disclosures and are allowed.

HOW THE STAFF CAN CONFIDENTLY DEAL WITH HIPAA

The first step to confidently deal with HIPAA is to understand that HIPAA is a huge law filled with standards on how to handle patient health information.

CRITICAL POINT
Talking about patient privacy for a few hours once a year will meet the training requirement, but it won't change anyone's actions unless there is a cohesive training and communications plan.

Follow this five-step plan to implement an internal process so that no one person feels he or she must carry the HIPAA burden alone. Everyone in the office must work together.

Step 1: Educate the staff. Invite conversations about privacy and security incidences.

a. Make HIPAA training a year-round process.
b. Be a team. No one can do HIPAA alone.
c. Help each other with answers, especially those that relate to updated Patient Rights, Breach Notification and HIPAA Security Rules.
d. Set aside personal differences in the best interests of the patients and the practice.
e. Build an esprit de corps around ensuring privacy and security in the practice, and the pride in your accomplishment will be noticed by your patients.

Step 2: Schedule regular training sessions.

a. Use ideas from the training calendar provided for you in Appendix B.
b. Invite staff members to take leadership roles on training topics.

c. Schedule a session on computer security. Explain why the practice can no longer allow computer games or Internet shopping on office equipment, or texting activities in the practice.
d. Do impromptu "stand up" meetings where staff comes together and stands for a quick briefing. These work if you are suddenly aware of a problem and need to inform the staff.

Step 3: Develop a line of fire.

a. The Privacy and Security and Breach Notification Rules require your practice to identify a contact person to receive patient complaints.
b. The Rules also require one person to be named the privacy official, and the same or another person the security official. These officials are delegated to represent your practice and take responsibility for learning many legal and practical HIPAA details.
c. Train a backup privacy and security team in the event the officials are not available should an incident occur. Ultimately, the official is the accountable party, but this situation highlights the need to get each staff member involved with privacy and security in the practice.

Step 4: Conquer the fear of conflict.

a. HIPAA gives patients six rights, with some more enhanced than before. Be sure your staff is aware of these expanded rights.
b. Use one of the following techniques to ease out of a trying situation:
   (1) Get out of the line of fire. You say, "I understand your position. Let's talk to the privacy official." Avoid saying words like "but" or "however." That puts you back on the firing line and negates the first part of the sentence.
   (2) Be an active listener. Repeat what you have heard the patient say so that the patient knows you are listening, and ask for a response: "What I'm hearing from you is that you're concerned about what the insurance company will see. Is that right?"
   (3) Compliment your adversary. You say, "With your ability to analyze facts, I know we'll come to a great solution."
   (4) Work together rather than separately. Resolve the concern while the patient is still in the office. It's your best chance to find a resolution.
   (5) Establish comfort. Make the other person feel at ease.
   (6) Ask for help. If the day's events are too stressful, ask for help from another staff member.

Step 5: People will make mistakes.

a. No practice can be HIPAA compliant all of the time. People will unintentionally and inadvertently make a mistake, but mistakes can be fixed before they become major incidents. If you discover you've made a mistake, tell your privacy official right away so that the practice can begin to look for a solution. Mistakes that continue unresolved become incidents, incidents cost time and money, and can damage your credibility, reputation, and business.

b. If someone in your office makes the same mistake several times and doesn't show signs of understanding the privacy or security policy, that employee may need retraining or disciplinary action, such as time off without pay, depending on how your office addresses sanctions in the policies and procedures manual.
c. Go to the regulations for clarification. The Privacy Rule and Security Rules, both of which are enforced by the HHS' Office of Civil Rights (OCR), can be found at www.hhs.gov/ocr. You also can access both rules through the Office of the National Coordinator's portal, healthit.hhs.gov.
d. Include legal counsel on your HIPAA team. If there is an error, and you feel you need legal assistance, consult your attorney.

WHAT PATIENTS WANT TO KNOW ABOUT HIPAA

For most common office visits, patients just want to know how soon they will feel better. But often, patients will want to make sure their health information is kept in strict confidence. For example,

A woman is pregnant and she doesn't want her husband or parents to know.

A teenager is experimenting with drugs and needs help.

A man tests positive for Hepatitis C and is afraid he'll lose his job.

There are thousands more like these, and patients will want to know what you're doing to protect privacy. It's doubtful patients will ask whether you lock the doors at night, but savvy patients may ask about security systems, even encryption processes. They also may ask who has access to electronic files and ask for a summary of their medical records.

We've been tracking consumer stories about patient privacy, and what we've learned is that patient rights rank highest among consumer concerns, but the Notice of Privacy Practices has been very well received as a move in the right direction. These are some of the questions you might be asked and some possible answers.

Frequently Asked Consumer Questions	Possible Answers
Why am I receiving so many privacy notices?	Every health care provider that is a covered entity is required to send an NPP to individuals who seek treatment.
I appreciate this privacy notice. Why is it coming now?	The compliance date to meet HIPAA's Privacy Rule was April 14, 2003, and our NPP is part of that process. We want you to know how we'll protect your health information.

(continued)

Frequently Asked Consumer Questions	Possible Answers
I'd like to request access to my medical record.	Please sign this form that you'd like access to your record, and I'll set up an appointment for you to talk to our privacy official.
I don't want the insurance company to know everything in my record.	They'll receive only the minimum necessary for them to make payment decisions. Or you can pay personally and in full for the service, in which case you have a right to ask us to withhold details about the service you just received.
I want you to send my medical records to another physician.	We'll be happy to do that. Just sign this authorization form, and tell us where you want it sent.
I don't want this information in my medical record, and I want to amend it.	I'll set up an appointment for you to talk to our privacy official about that.
How will I know you amended it?	If we agree to make the amendment, we'll send you a copy of the changes. Where would you like us to send it?
Don't call me at home anymore. Call me on my cell phone.	I'll acknowledge that in writing in your file, and when you're next in the office, please sign this documentation.
How did you handle my patient records before this rule?	Our office has always treated patient information confidentially. And now HIPAA's Privacy Rule requires that we document our privacy efforts. That's the biggest change.
I'd like an accounting of where your practice has sent my health records.	I'll set up a meeting with our privacy official to talk about that.
Can I still have my (spouse) pick up my prescriptions?	Yes, you may.
When I called to get my records faxed to another physician, they were told you needed me to sign something. It didn't used to be this way.	Unless we make the referral to another provider, the Privacy Rule requires that we first obtain written authorization from you before we send your medical files to another provider.
Who in your office has access to my medical records?	We follow our privacy policies and procedures regarding this question. Would you like to talk to our privacy official about that?
I want to file a complaint.	Thanks for bringing your concerns to us first. You have the right to file a complaint. Would you like to speak with our contact person about that?

(continued)

(continued)

Frequently Asked Consumer Questions	Possible Answers
What will happen to me if I file a complaint?	Our policy here is that we will not take any action against a patient who files a complaint. Would you like to speak to our privacy official?
I didn't give you authorization for this.	We keep excellent documentation here, but if you have a question about our privacy activities, you may speak to our privacy official.
What are you going to do to discipline the person who breached my confidentiality?	Any action is the decision of our privacy official and our practice's management team based upon the practice's written sanction policy.
How many of these rights apply to my children?	We follow state and federal laws when it comes to unemancipated minors. Would you like to talk to our privacy official about that?
I demand to know why my son/daughter was in here.	We follow state and federal laws that dictate when we can release patient information about a minor. Would you like to talk to our privacy official about that?

This list could go on for pages, but there's a common response formula used in the majority of the answers.

Respect the individual's request.

Refer to your policies and procedures or federal and state laws.

Ask if the individual wishes to speak to a privacy official.

CUSTOMIZE YOUR INTERNAL AND EXTERNAL COMMUNICATIONS PLAN

What to do:

Decide on one or two common communication goals, such as, "Prepare everyone on staff to know what to do and say if there are patient inquiries, complaints, privacy breaches or security incidents. Create an environment where everyone feels part of the HIPAA solution.

How to do it:

1. Develop an internal communications plan. Ask two or three people to assemble a communications committee to think this through. The most important goal in your internal communications plan is to help staff accept new privacy and security standards. Use humor or cartoons to help make a point.

Offer an incentive to encourage positive results

- Bring in lunch on Friday when the office has had a good week.
- Give an extra half day vacation for staff.
- Acknowledge someone who has helped another staff member through a difficult complaint process.

Create a Quick Reminder E-mail Program

No one has time to read long e-mails, but you can send quick one or two line reminders through your internal secure e-mail system that might actually be fun to read. Put them in multiple choice or true/false questions such as:

True or False: You can shop the Internet from your computer without putting medical records at risk.

Multiple Choice: When an individual asks for access to medical records, say:

A. Come back when we're not busy.

B. Your records are in storage and it will take us 60 days to find them.

C. Call in that request between 8:00 and 10:00 tomorrow morning.

D. I'll get the privacy official, and the two of you can talk about this.

Develop an Internal Newsletter

Do feature stories on physicians and staff, and broaden the scope of the newsletter to include subjects like computer tips, seasonal illnesses and preventions, or policies and procedures. Route the e-mail electronically or print it and put it in employee mailboxes.

Develop a Re-Act Program in your Office

When you report privacy violations to the privacy official you give that person an opportunity to analyze and fix the problem. One reporting method is to describe the incident on a 3x5 card. Then give the violation two separate ratings, using a scale of 1 to 5, with 5 being the highest risk. The first rating is your evaluation of how the Office for Civil Rights would respond. The second rating is how much attention you think this patient will give to the violation. If you identify and rate a problem, you also must determine how to manage that risk.

A sample rating system might look like this:

Office for Civil Rights (OCR) Rating

1 = OCR is likely to read this complaint and call to check out the details.

2 = OCR is likely to send an official letter.

3 = OCR is likely to send out an investigator and provide technical assistance to improve patient privacy in your office.

4 = OCR is likely to send out an investigator, request access to practice's written records pertaining to HIPAA policies and procedures, discover a preventable breach, and assign a penalty.

5 = OCR is likely to launch a major investigation that could result in penalties and fines if you don't do something to mitigate the privacy breach or security incident now. A very serious privacy breach could be referred to the Department of Justice for criminal investigation.

Patient Rating

1 = The patient will probably leave with a bad feeling about our practice.

2 = The patient will likely talk about this breach to a friend or family member.

3 = The patient will likely file a complaint with your contact person.

4 = The patient will likely call the ACLU to determine if rights have been violated.

5 = The patient will likely file a complaint with the Office for Civil Rights, call an attorney, and the news media may also be contacted.

Develop an external communications plan.

Your business associates and patients are your two primary external audiences. Keep the practice's management informed of any communications efforts so that they can support you as you implement key messages. Your approach to business associates will be different than the messages you send to patients.

What to do:

Regularly communicate with your business associates about privacy, breach notification, and security issues.

How to do it:

- Your privacy official will talk to each business associate about the privacy and security regulations and also obtain signatures on business associate agreements. (Business associate agreements must be in place by April 14, 2003, unless you already have a confidentiality agreement in place. In that case, your agreement must be signed by April 14, 2004, or on the current agreement's renewal, amendment, or modification date, whichever comes first.)
- Make a list of questions to discuss with vendors, and then determine who should take those questions to the vendor. For example, a good list of questions to ask transactions vendors is included in Chapter 2. A good list of security questions is in Chapter 4.

  The privacy official should also talk to the staff about the privacy and security safeguards you expect from the business associates. In most cases, business associates want to do business with medical offices, and so your participation in this relationship should be trustful and present yourself with good business ethics.
- Expect business associates to have some questions. HIPAA is a very big law, and you may not know the answer. Don't guess. Unless you have been trained to answer specific content, refer questions to the privacy official.

- Include business associates in some of your internal e-mail reminders. Ask them if they'd like to submit questions or comments that are not promotional to your communications effort.

What to do:
Regularly communicate with your patients.

How to do it:

- Establish a patient advisory board. Ask select patients to participate in your HIPAA implementation efforts by giving you feedback on what you're doing. Request a signed confidentiality statement before they participate, and be cautious about what issues are brought to the patient advisory board.
- Conduct a survey about patient satisfaction. Include a few questions about privacy and security safeguards.
- When presenting the Notice of Privacy Practices (NPP), be positive and expect that there will only be a few questions that relate to the NPP's content, but be prepared with appropriate answers.
- Develop a cheat sheet of questions and answers from typical patient questions. You can extract some Q&As from the list presented earlier in this chapter.
- Post wall charts or hang posters informing patients of their rights . . . no kidding. This is an excellent pre-emptive strategy. It says we know your rights, do you?
- A one-page patient newsletter from the medical practice goes a long way in building patient-physician relationships. If you are sending your newsletter electronically, ask if patients would like to sign up to be on your newsletter list. Postage is costly, but you could place printed copies of your newsletter in the waiting room. When selecting topics, take a poll of the most common questions patients ask and put those comments into an easy-to-read format. Be sure to include one column on privacy or security topics.
- If you are communicating with patients via e-mail or you provide content on the Internet, consult Chapter 4 on security requirements, such as whether encryption is addressable or required for your system.

CRITICAL POINT
Be sure you have authorizations in place before exchanging health information through secure patient portals. Do NOT send protected health information to an unsecure e-mail address. If a patient sends an e-mail message to you, ask the patient to call the office or register with your patient portal.

HIPAA gives medical offices an excellent opportunity to promote themselves. More than ever before, physicians should take the lead on privacy issues and retain their position as a trusted resource.

What to do:
When your communications committee has implemented its internal communications plan, ask them to excerpt news clips or articles that could also be used for external audiences.

How to do it:

- Identify the topics of greatest interest. Typically those topics are:
  - ☐ Care or treatment of illnesses or conditions common to your specialty
  - ☐ Privacy
  - ☐ Billing questions
  - ☐ Who's new in the office?
  - ☐ Ask the doctor column
  - ☐ What to do in emergencies
  - ☐ Email communications between patient and physician.

HIPAA CRISIS COMMUNICATIONS MANAGEMENT

If the HHS Office for Civil Rights calls or if a reporter calls wanting to follow up on a notification that a tablet containing protected health information has been stolen, most people's immediate reaction is to hang up the phone and throw up. There's a better way to handle what appears to be a crisis situation.

In theory, any communications crisis can be managed using the following strategy.

Step 1: Get the facts.

What to do:

Evaluate what is happening and remain calm. Do NOT assume that anyone is guilty. Establish a level of trust by asking questions, not by making judgments or accusations or statement of guilt.

How to do it:

- Ask what happened? Ask others if they also know what happened. Disregard answers that include "it wasn't my fault" until later.
- Examine the damage. Did we do something to create an investigation? Has a patient taken a complaint to the state's attorney general? Are we going to be sued (longer response time) or will we be on the 5 o'clock news (shorter response time)?
- Find out if anyone was hurt—emotionally or physically. Immediately inquire about their condition or state of mind.
- Buy time to gather your thoughts; don't shoot from the hip. If this is a reporter, ask if you can call back in 15 minutes—and then call back! If this is the Department of Justice or the Office for Civil Rights calling, get the facts, ask if you can have a small amount of time to conduct a quick internal review, and schedule an appointment to meet with the caller.
- Ask for the focus of the investigation or story.
- Stay calm. The temperature of most crises escalates within the first 3 to 5 hours. People like to draw conclusions about what will likely happen next and the fear factor can kick in. Depending on how the leadership handles the crisis, one of four things can happen:

1. Employees will start to blame one another, which cripples morale.
2. Management responds with a knee-jerk reaction and loses critical data. This forces employees into hiding.
3. Management loses focus on the big picture and focuses on the problem, resulting in lost cash flow and disloyal customers, and that compromises the organization's public image.
4. Management keeps it together, stays calm, evaluates this crisis in comparison with other crises, and then calls together a team of advisors to determine next steps.

Step 2: Call together your team of advisors.

What to do:
Your advisors' job is to develop a game plan.

How to do it:

- The worst thing to do is do nothing.
- Your advisory team is made up of trusted decision makers, and in most cases your attorney of record. Team members may be a colleague, an office manager, a practice management consultant, or others with whom you have great confidence.
- Briefly tell the advisors what happened as best you know it, without adding any interpretations or conclusions. Those opinions should be left to your advisors.
- Your advisors should give you directions on the following:

  —How should we handle this situation?

  —What do we legally bound to do, and what are we ethically bound to do?

  —What are our key messages? ("No comment" is not a key message; it is an admission of guilt.) This includes:

  - ☐ What we should tell our employees—count on the message getting out, unless you tell employees to keep it absolutely confidential, and then you can depend on it getting out.
  - ☐ What should we tell the public?
  - ☐ Who is our spokesperson? This is one person who is influential with the public, but is also knowledgeable about the situation.

Step 3: Prepare the spokesperson.

What to do:
Show no mercy by grilling the spokesperson.

How to do it:

- Ask the spokesperson three questions that you hope you'll never be asked. At least one of them will come up in the investigation.

- Think about questions the caller is likely to ask. Questions from OCR and the Department of Justice are more likely to be focused on your policies and HIPAA implementation. Questions from a reporter will likely to have a consumer angle, such as "How did this happen?' or "Could you have prevented this?" or "Could this happen somewhere else?"
- Coach the spokesperson by giving feedback on the messages.
- Directly connect the answers to the question. Do not give more information than is asked.
- Practice allowing silence to happen. Reporters and federal investigators like to use silence to their advantage hoping you'll fill the void with chatter. Don't do it.

Step 4: Do your homework. Know to whom you are speaking.

- Find out who the caller is. If you are uncertain, get the caller's office switchboard telephone number and call back to verify identity. If a journalist, research the writing style (combative, argumentative, soft news) and whether the journalist gets first page assignments. A quick search on the Internet can pull that up for you. If it's a federal agent, go to the federal government's Office for Personnel Management and conduct a search for that person's name. You may only learn the person's title and region, but it's a start.
- If this is a journalist, send an e-mail to friends inquiring whether any of them have had an experience with this person.

About journalists:

- They are the gatekeepers of information to consumers.
- Few local journalists are informed about HIPAA. They usually cover several beats, and health information management is just one of them.
- Most journalists are financially rewarded for writing a good story.
- Many are parents, they attend church or synagogues; they believe in family and are members of the community.

Step 5: Make the call back.

What to do:

Take the lead on the call back.

How to do it:

- Keep your promise to call back when you said you would.
- Place a cheat sheet beside you on your desk.
- Speak slowly, and think before you speak. If you're to be quoted, make sure you articulate so that the interviewer understands what you are saying. Don't make jokes, and don't compare yourself to your competition. This gives the interviewer a reason to call the competition to see if they want to say something about you.
- Respond to the questions while you're on the phone or set up an in-person interview. With reporters, we prefer an in-person interview so that you can

size up each other and build a relationship. OCR and DOJ will have their own processes, but most government agencies will prefer the phone interview first.

- Be honest. Do not lie. Nothing causes a six-part, team coverage investigative series faster than a lie.
- Ask if you can record the conversation.

CRITICAL POINT

Ask someone else to sit in and listen to the conversation.

- Answer the questions, but don't be a slave to the questions. Provide the key message several times so that the caller understands what you're trying to say.
- When the interview is done, ask the interviewer if you can provide answers to questions not asked. This usually throws the interviewer off, but it's your turn to say what your advisory team wants said.
- If this is a print interview, ask if you can preview your quotes before it goes to press. Most journalists will let you conduct this preview.
- When you're done with the interview, hang up. Do not call back with just one more thing unless you made an incorrect statement and need to clarify.

Step 6: Prepare differently if this is a TV interview.

What to do:

Prepare for the visual story.

How to do it:

- A television story is 85% visual and 15% content, just the opposite of a written news story or federal investigation.
- Present your business card to the interviewer and also to the cameraman. Don't forget the camera operator. This is the person responsible for making you look good.
- Television news is a show. It generates the highest advertising dollars. If you think you're providing news, think again. Television news anchors are actors, except on the national television news. Then they are very smart journalists *and* actors.
- Viewers will determine whether to believe you based on whether they like you. They will believe your body language over what you say.
- Be confident. Smile, even when asked a mean-spirited question. Remember you're conveying believable body language.
- Don't slouch. Slouching says "victim."
- Pull your coat down over your posterior and sit on it so that your jacket doesn't bunch up around your shoulders.
- Speak directly to the interviewer. Do not speak to the camera. Viewers think you can see them, and that will make you appear to be a voyeur.

- Wear clothes that draw attention to your face. Men usually wear red or blue ties. Women should wear a scarf or blouse that highlights their face. Don't wear dangling earrings.
- If this is a live story, keep your answers very short—15 seconds or less. If this is a taped interview and you stumble, ask if you can do that answer again.
- Do not repeat a negative. Such as, "No, we don't breach a patient's privacy." In the edit room, that could be cut into "We breach patient's privacy."

On-Camera Performance Techniques

Interview Do's	Interview Don'ts
Use good posture.	Slouch.
Maintain eye contact.	Look away from reporter.
Keep notes, refer to them.	Speak off the cuff.
Use key messages.	Be a slave to the reporter's questions.
Ask for clarification.	Argue with reporter.
Ask to see quotes.	Ask to preview article.
Follow up with a note.	Accuse reporter.

Step 7: Plan for a communications crisis.

CRITICAL POINT

The number of crises you'll experience is inversely proportional to the amount of time you spend planning for contingencies and training on scenarios. The more time spent planning, the less time you'll spend managing crises.

What to do:

Develop a plan so that you can use it if you need it. All the better if you never need it. But communications plans are usually three times as expensive when you need them and don't have one.

How to do it:

Develop a high level, trusted strategic team, including an attorney and spokesperson.

If you think you might be featured in a television news spot, get media trained before you go on camera. It's not at all the same as speaking to a live audience.

Establish a spokesperson policy and stick to it. In doing a story, TV media will talk to anyone on the street, capture the story, then get it on the evening news. Your policy should be that no one speaks to the media except for the designated spokesperson.

Practice, practice, practice.

Remember that crises happen all the time. It's how you manage them that determine whether it's a crisis or not.

Ask for help if you need it.

HIPAA Forms

Table of Contents

Business Associate Agreements Tracking Form

Business Associate	Contact Info	Signed Prior BA Agreement	Needs New BA Agreement	Status
Company	Contact name, address, e-mail, phone number	Yes/No	Yes/No	**C**=completed **R**=in review **NB**=no longer in business

PRIVACY OFFICIAL JOB RESPONSIBILITIES

General duties: Be the advocate that maintains the privacy of patients' protected health information (PHI) and oversee activities that keep our practice in compliance with rules that govern the privacy of protected health information in oral, written, and electronic form.

Specific duties: The privacy official has the following specific duties:

Management Advisor

Work with the medical practice's management team and lawyers to comply with federal and state laws governing the privacy of individually identifiable health information. Stay current on privacy laws and updates in privacy technology. Immediately notify medical management of requested investigations and reviews by HHS or other governing agency.

Human Resources and Training

Develop, or serve as team leader in the development of, the practice's privacy policies and procedures. Integrate those policies into the practice's day-to-day activities and provide training, either as on-the-spot refresher courses or planned courses. Oversee sanctions according to our policies and procedures and bring them to the attention of the practice's leadership committee.

Risk Management

Collaborate with the security official to ensure privacy and security risks are analyzed and policies and procedures are developed, updated, and enforced to prevent unauthorized disclosures of PHI.

Business Associates

Lead the practice in updating business associate contracts and, with our lawyers, developing and executing business associate agreements in accordance with the HITECH, HIPAA, and Breach Notification Rules.

Patient Rights

Oversee patient requests to the practice and help the practice's employees understand how to address patient questions about the practice's privacy initiatives. Develop an effective internal and external communications effort to help patients and workforce understand how to practice protects patient rights.

Complaint Management

Implement and manage complaints regarding the practice's standards and protocols, including documenting and investigating and, if necessary, mitigating those complaints. Educate workforce on the practice's policies and procedures on complaints and prohibited retaliatory actions against individuals who exercise their patient rights.

Qualifications

Be familiar with medical and administrative functions of the practice. Have excellent communication, problem solving, and research skills. Have an interest in privacy laws and regulations; be recognized as having high integrity, detail oriented. Have strong organizational skills and work well with management and staff.

Workforce Training Session Attendee List

Name of Trainer: ______________________________

Trainer's Company Affiliation: ______________________________

Date of Training: ______________ Hours in Training: ______________

Topics Included in Training (or attach outline): ______________________________

____

____

Attendee List

Print Name	Signature	Date

Notice of Privacy Practices Receipt

Our Notice of Privacy Practices provides information on how our practice may use and/or disclose protected health information about you for treatment, payment, and health care operations. A copy of our NPP can be found ________ on our Web site; ________ at the check-in desk.

I acknowledge that I have received a copy of ____________________ (name of practice) ___________ Notice of Privacy Practices.

Patient's Name: ____
(print)

Patient's Signature: ____
(signature)

Today's Date: ____

Patient's Date of Birth: ____

If signed by a personal representative:

Name of Personal Representative: ________________________________
(print)

Signature of Personal Representative: ________________________________
(signature)

Relationship to Patient: ________________________________

Driver's License Number: ______________________ State: __________

Today's Date: ________________________________

- -

For practice use only:

Patient's ID/Chart Number: ________________________________

Signature of Employee: ______________________ **Date:** __________

Sample Authorization Form

Patient Name: ______________________________

Patient's Date of Birth: ______________ Patient's ID/Chart No: ____________

I hereby authorize the use and disclosure of individually identifiable health information relating to me as described below:

Specific Description of Information to be Used or Disclosed

Purpose for Disclosure

____

____

____

I authorize the following person(s) to use or disclose the above health information.

____

____

Person(s) receiving my authorized information include:

____

____

____

Check all that apply:

☐ I understand that I may revoke this authorization at any time by notifying ______ ______________________________ (Name of Practice) in writing. If I choose to do so, my revocation will not affect any actions taken by ____________ (Name of Practice) before receiving my revocation.

☐ I understand that I may refuse to sign this authorization; and that my refusal to sign in no way affects my treatment, payment, enrollment in a health plan, or eligibility for benefits.

This authorization expires on ______________________________.

Signature of Patient or Patient's Personal Representative

____

Date: ______________________________

If personal representative, print:

Name: ______________________________

Signature: ______________________________

Relationship to Patient: ______________________________

Driver's License Number: ______________________ State: ____________

For internal use only

Patient Chart/ID Number: ____________

Date: ____________ Physician: ____________

Sample Verification Form/Patient Certification

Please provide us with the following information.

General Information

Name: ____________

Address: ____________

City: ____________ State: ____________ Zip: ____________

Date of Birth: ____________ SS#: ____________

Driver's License Number: ____________ State: ____________

Insurance Information

Name of Subscriber: ____________

Relationship to Subscriber: ____________

Group No: ____________ Individual No: ____________

Responsible Party

Who is responsible for your charges today?

Name: ____________

Address: ____________

City: ____________ State: ____________ Zip: ____________

I certify that the above information is correct.

Signature of Patient: ____________ Date: ____________

Personal Representative

Name of Personal Representative: ____________

Relationship to Patient: ____________

Driver's License Number: ____________ State: ____________

Sample Consent to Disclose PHI for Treatment, Payment, and Health Care Operations

This form must be completed by the individual whose protected health information is to be disclosed, or by a parent or guardian if the person is a minor under state law.

Name: ____

Date of Birth: ______________________________ (for identification purposes)

I hereby authorize <physician practice> to release the following personal health information for (check all that apply)

☐ Medical services claims information

☐ Prescription, diagnostic, treatment, and/or care management services

☐ Reviews required by HHS or HIPAA-compliant health care operations.

The above information may be released by:

☐ Phone ☐ Fax ☐ Mail ☐ Friend or Relative ____________

My Consent:

Effective: Today's Date: ____________________________________

I want this consent to:

☐ Continue indefinitely ☐ Effective only until ____________ (date).

I understand that consent may be revoked by me at any time. I understand why I have been asked to disclose this information and am aware that my patient rights are identified in the practice's Notice of Privacy Practices.

Signature of Patient: ______________________ Date: ______________

Or Personal Representative: __________________ Date: ______________

Sample Marketing Authorization Form

Dear <Patient>

<Insert description of marketing activity>

The immediate benefit to our practice is that we will receive a financial incentive of up to <$XX.00> for each individual within our practice who signs up for this program. The immediate benefit to you is <xxxxx>.

Our goal is to safeguard your protected health information, and we will NOT provide information about you to this company without your authority.

If you have an interest in a representative from <company> contacting you about this marketing endeavor, please respond below with your authorization. You are under no obligation to respond, and we will continue to provide the highest quality of care regardless of your decision.

<Name, address, phone number>

Authorization to Market

I hereby authorize <physician practice> to provide only my name, address, and phone number to <company> for the purposes of reviewing a discount on my medical fees.

Print Patient Name: ______________________________

Date of Birth: ______________________ (for identification purposes, not to be disclosed to <company>.)

Patient's Signature: ______________________ Date: ______________

Personal Representative

Name of Personal Representative: ______________________________

Relationship to Patient: ______________________ Date: ______________

Driver's License Number: ______________________ State: ______________

Personal Representative Signature: ______________________________

Request to Access Records

Submitted to <Privacy Official, Contact Information>

Patient's Name: ______________________________
(print)

Describe records requested and approximate dates of records you wish to review.

____

____

What would you like for us to do for you?

☐ I wish to inspect the requested records.

☐ I wish to obtain a copy of the requested records.

☐ I wish to inspect and copy the requested records.

Fees:

Our practice charges a reasonable fee to copy the records and also for postage to mail your requested records.

Questions?

Please contact our privacy official listed at the top of this page if you have any questions about your request to inspect or copy records.

Patient information

Patient Signature: ______________________ Date: __________

Date of Birth: ______________________ (for identification purposes)

For the personal representatives of the patient:

Print the name of the personal representative: ______________________

Relationship to Patient: ______________________ Date: __________

Driver's License Number: ______________________ State: __________

I certify that I have the legal authority under federal and state laws to make this request on behalf of the patient identified above.

Signature of Personal Representative: ______________________

Response to Request to Access Records

Patient Name: ____

Address: ____

Access Request Date:

Dear ________________ (Patient):

In response to your request to access records, please see our response below.

Access is

☐ Granted

Our practice grants you access to medical records specified below. Please contact ___________________________, our privacy official, to arrange a convenient time for you to inspect and copy your requested records. You also may request that we send this information to you via US Postal Service. Our practice may charge a reasonable fee to cover the cost of copying and postage.

☐ Denied

Our practice denies your request to access records in whole or in part for the following reasons:

☐ Partially granted, partially denied

Review of Denial

You may request that our practice have the denial reviewed by a licensed health care professional who did not participate in the original decision to deny access. To request a review, please contact our practice's privacy official.

Access Denial Log

<Name of Practice>

Patient Name	Chart ID Number	Date of Review	Reason for Denial	Date Patient Notified

Request to Amend Records

Directions: Please use this form to make a request that our practice amend or make corrections to information maintained about you. If mailing, please return this form to the privacy official listed on the bottom of this form.

Patient information

Name of Patient (Print Name): ____________________

Signature of Patient: ____________________

Date: ____________ Patient's Date of Birth: ____________

For Personal Representatives of the Patient

Your Name: ____________________

Relationship to Patient: ____________________

Your Driver's License Number: ____________ State: ____________

I hereby certify that I have legal authority under applicable law to make this request on behalf of the patient identified above.

Signature of Personal Representative: ____________________

Date: ____________________

Requested Amendment

Please describe in detail how you want your records amended.

Reason for Requested Amendment

Contact Person

Please contact our practice's privacy official if you have any questions relating to your request to amend records.

Signature

Patient: ____________________

Date: ____________________

Response to Request to Amend Records

Patient Name: ______________________________

Patient Chart/ID Number: ______________________________

Date of Amendment Request: ______________________________

Dear <Patient>:

On <date>, you requested our practice amend certain information stored in our records about you. Your request has been:

☐ Granted

☐ Denied

☐ Partially Granted

If granted, our practice has made the following amendment to your records:

____

____

____

If denied, our practice denies your amendment request for the following specific reasons:

_____ The protected health information was not created by our practice.

_____ The PHI is not part of the designated record set maintained by our practice.

_____ The PHI is not available for inspection under the HIPAA Privacy Rule.

_____ The PHI is accurate and complete.

You have a right to submit a written statement disagreeing with our denial to the practice's privacy official. You also have a right to submit a complaint denying this request to our privacy official and/or to the Secretary of the US Department of Health and Human Services at www.hhs.gov/ocr within 180 days of any alleged violation. Your complaint must describe the acts or omissions that you believe are in violation of the HIPAA Privacy Rule.

Please contact me if you have any questions regarding your amendment request.

Sincerely

<Name>

Privacy Official

Signature: ______________________________ Date: ______________________________

Request for Accounting of Disclosures

To our patient: You have requested an accounting of disclosures of protected health information that our practice has made during a specified time period. Use this form to complete your request.

Print Patient Name: ______________________________

Date of Birth: ______________________ (for identification purposes)

Specified Time Frame for Accounting

Start Date: ____________________ End Date: ____________________

Please specify if you wish to limit our accounting to:

_____ Certain types of disclosures _____ Disclosures to a specific entity[1]

Please provide details of the scope of disclosures for this request:

____

____

____

Patient Signature: ____________________ Today's Date: __________

For Personal Representative of the Patient

Print Name: ______________________________

Relationship to Patient: ______________________________

Driver's License: ____________________ State: __________

Note 1. Our practice is not required to keep disclosures for the following: to the patient, incidental disclosures; pursuant to a HIPAA-compliant authorization, for a facility directory, to persons involved in the patient's care, for national security or intelligence, to correctional institutions or law enforcement officials having custody of patient, in compliant limited data set disclosures, prior to April 14, 2003.

Response to Request for Accounting of Disclosures

Patient Name: ____________________

Address: ____________________

____

Chart/ID Number: ____________________

Request Date: ____________________

To our patient:

In response to your request for an accounting of disclosures of protected health information about you during the timeframe you requested, the following includes all disclosures we are required to make to you, according to the HIPAA Privacy Rule and our policies.

Time Period:

From: ____________________ To: ____________________

Date of Disclosure	Name and Address of Entity Receiving Disclosure	Description of PHI Disclosed	Purpose of Disclosure

Please contact me if you have any questions regarding your accounting of disclosures.

Privacy Official: ____________________

Signature: ____________________

Date: ____________________

Request to Restrict Disclosure

In the presence of my physician, ______________________________ , I am requesting that the medical practice withhold submitting health information to the health plan _____________________________ for purposes of payment or health care operations relating to the following items or services:

____

____

____

In return, I have paid in full out-of-pocket for the items and services itemized above.

_________________________________ ____________________

Patient Signature Date

Patient's Date of Birth: ____________________

_________________________________ ____________________

Physician or Administrator's Signature Date

Request to Terminate Restrictions

Patient Name: ______________________________

Patient Date of Birth: ______________________________ (for identification purposes)

Today's Date: ______________________________

I hereby consent to terminate additional restrictions on the use and disclosure of protected health information that were previously agreed to by the practice's privacy official on the date identified below. I understand the practice will continue to protect my PHI according to the HIPAA Privacy Rule, Breach Notification Rule, and the HITECH Rule.

Date of Agreed Restriction: ______________________________

(Attach previously agreed restriction)

Patient Agreement to Terminate Restriction:

____

____

Patient Signature: ______________________________

Date: ______________________________

For Personal Representative of Patient

Name: ______________________________

Relationship to Patient: ______________________________

Driver's License Number: ______________________________ State: ______________

Signature of Personal Representative: ______________________________

Date: ______________________________

Disclosure Log[1]

Patient Name	Chart/ID Number	Date of Disclosure	Name/ Entity Receiving Disclosure	Description of PHI Disclosed	Purpose of Disclosure

Note 1. You are not required to keep disclosures for the following: to the patient, incidental disclosures; pursuant to a HIPAA-compliant authorization, for a facility directory, to persons involved in the patient's care, for national security or intelligence, to correctional institutions or law enforcement officials having custody of patient, in compliant limited data set disclosures, prior to April 14, 2003.

Request for Alternative Communications

Note to patient: Use this form to request that our practice communicate with you other than at your primary phone number. Fill out this request in its entirety.

Patient Name: ______________________________
(print)

Alternative communication request (Please describe your request to be contacted at an alternative location or by alternative means.)

____

____

____

Payment Information

Your request to be contacted at an alternative location may affect our normal billing and payment procedure. Please specify your alternative method for handling payment.

____

____

____

Alternative Address or Alternative Means of Contact:

____

____

Our Contact Person

If you have any questions about this request, you may contact our privacy official provided at the top of this page.

Patient Information

Signature of Patient: ______________________ Date: __________

Date of Birth: ______________________________

For personal representatives of the patient:

Print name of Personal Representative: ______________________

Relationship to Patient: ______________________

Driver's License Number: ______________________ Date: __________

Sample Complaint Form

Note to patient: We will follow up on your complaints, whether they are submitted to us in oral or written form. You are not required to complete a written report, but your comments are helpful to us as we continue to provide excellent service to our patients.

Date: ______________________________

Name of Complainant: ______________________________

Address: ______________________________

____

Phone: ______________________________

Description of Complaint

Signature of Complainant: ______________________________

What would you like to happen?

_____ I want someone from the office to contact me by ____ phone ____ mail.

_____ I don't want to be contacted.

Other: ______________________________

____

For Internal Use Only

Date Reviewed: ______________________________

Reviewer: ______________________________

Details and Findings: ______________________________

____

____

Follow up

_______ Phone _______ Mail _______ Both Phone and Mail

Minimum Necessary Checklist

Our practice has assigned access to the following PHI.

Name	Billing	Medical/ Clinical	Administrative Access	Scheduling
(Physician)				
(Physician)				
(Physician)				
(Nurse Practitioner)				
(Physician Assistant)				
(Medical Assistant)				
(Medical Assistant)				
(Receptionist)				

De-Identification Check List

To meet the requirements of a limited data set, our privacy official will eliminate the following identifiers from the record.

(a) Names;

(b) Postal address information, other than town or city, state and zip code;

(c) Telephone numbers;

(d) Fax numbers;

(e) Electronic mail addresses:

(f) Social Security numbers;

(g) Medical record numbers;

(h) Health plan beneficiary numbers;

(i) Account numbers;

(j) Certificate/license numbers;

(k) Vehicle identifiers and serial numbers, including license plate numbers;

(l) Device identifiers and serial numbers;

(m) Web Universal Resource Locators (URLs);

(n) Internet Protocol (IP) address numbers;

(o) Biometric identifiers, including finger and voice prints;

(p) Full face photographic images and any comparable images.

Security-Related Repair Form

Use this form to maintain a log of repairs that are made to ensure your physical location is secure.

Name of Practice: ______________________________

Facility Address: ______________________________

City: ____________________ State: __________ Zip: __________

Description of Repair	Date Scheduled	Date Repaired	Contractor		Cost	Approval[1]
			Name, Address	Phone		

Note 1. Security official or appointed representative should initial when the repair has been completed.

Emergency Access Log

Use this form to maintain a log of emergency access activities. Identify when emergency access involved emergency responders, such as the fire department, law enforcement, or emergency rescue. Also, log events that were the result of a workforce member's abusive activity and the sanctions imposed.

Name of Practice: ________________________

Facility Address: ________________________

City: ____________ State: ________ Zip: ________

Describe Incident		**Who Initiated Access?**[1]	**Emergency Involved**		**Abusive Activity**		**Official**[2]
Description	**Date**		**Yes/ No**	**Dept.**[3]	**Describe**	**Sanctions**	

Notes

1. Identify the person who initiated emergency access procedures.
2. Security official or delegated representative acting on the S/O's behalf.
3. Indicate the emergency responder.

Electronic Media and Hardware Movement Log

Use this form to check out and track the location of electronic media such as portable computers, laptops, and backup disks.

Name of Practice: ______________________________

Facility Address: ______________________________

City: ______________ State: __________ Zip: __________

Workstation	Static IP Address	Assigned User		Check Out		Initials
		Name	Location	Out	In	

Acknowledgement of Responsibilities Regarding Access to Practice's Electronic Systems Containing Electronic Protected Health Information

Use this form for workforce to acknowledge their responsibilities when accessing the practice's electronic systems that contain protected health information.

Name of Practice: ______________________________

Facility Address: ______________________________

City: ____________________ State: __________ Zip: __________

Acknowledgement

I, ______________________________, have read and
(print workforce member's name)

understand that my job assignment grants me clearance to access protected health information (PHI) about individuals and/or their personal representatives. I also have read and understand our practice's policies and procedures on safeguarding PHI, including sanctions that may be imposed against me, regarding the electronic use and disclosure of protected health information.

I further understand that any questions about the security and privacy of protected health information should be addressed to our privacy and/or security official for guidance.

____

Signature of Employee

____

Signature of Security Official

Date: ______________________________

Consequences of Unauthorized Access to the Practice's Electronic Protected Health Information

Use this form to acknowledge receipt of the workforce member's consequences for abusing privileges to access electronic protected health information.

Name of Practice: ______________________________

Facility Address: ______________________________

City: ______________ State: __________ Zip: __________

Acknowledgement

I, ______________________________, have read and
(Print workforce member's name)

understand our policies and procedures and sanctions may be applied to me if I abuse the clearance assigned to me.

I also understand that my job responsibilities may change, eliminating my access to protected health information, and if I abuse my privileges and access PHI, even though access has changed, that the practice has the authority to terminate immediately my employment.

I also understand that if I lose or misplace electronic devices, or if I disable the encryption software safeguarding PHI, and thereby enable an unauthorized user to access protected health information, that I may be subject to legal action taken against me as an individual.

____

Signature of Employee

____

Signature of Security Official

Date: ______________________________

Workforce Member Exit Interview Checklist

Use this checklist to close out a workforce member's access to protected health information upon exiting the practice. Use this checklist irrespective of whether the workforce member left voluntarily or involuntarily.

Name of Practice: ______________________________

Facility Address: ______________________________

City: ____________ State: ________ Zip: ________

Employee: ____________________ Employee ID: ________

Departure Effective Date: ______________________

_____ Disable immediately user ID and passwords to practice management system

_____ Disable immediately user ID and password access to electronic health records

_____ Disable access to practice-hosted e-mail and e-mail server

_____ Credit cards returned; cancel online purchasing authority

_____ Retrieve any portable electronic devices

_____ Cancel telephone voice mail

_____ Retrieve keys, cancel card-key or biometric access privileges to facility

_____ Handbooks, including policies and procedures returned

Human Resources List

_____ Letter of resignation received; or notice of termination delivered

_____ Final timesheet and/or activity report delivered

_____ Final check sent to address provided by workforce member

_____ Forwarding address on file

_____ Benefits (health, retirement contributions, sick leave/vacation leave) discussed

Workforce Member Acknowledgement of Awareness and Understanding of Practice's Exit Interview

Use this form in an exit interview for the workforce member to acknowledge termination of a workforce member, irrespective of whether the workforce member is terminated voluntarily or involuntarily.

Name of Practice: ______________________________

Facility Address: ______________________________

City: ________________ State: __________ Zip: __________

I, ______________________________, understand
(Print workforce member's name)

that in terminating my employment, whether voluntarily or involuntarily, that the practice will take the following actions: (Workforce initials each of the following.)

_____ My access to electronic protected health information is terminated and all authentication and authorization credentials for access are invalidated and, as appropriate, are removed.

_____ Keys, card-keys, and/or biometric access will be retrieved or canceled.

_____ The practice will refer any unauthorized attempts at access to the practice's electronic protected health information to appropriate authorities.

_____ A representative of the practice has completed an exit interview and I have provided a forwarding address.

____

Signature of Terminated Employee

____

Signature of Security Official

Date: ______________________________

OTHERWISE PERMITTED USES AND DISCLOSURES (45 CFR 164.512)

Expanded from Step 2F, Chapter 3.

1. **Public Health Activities**[1] Our practice may disclose protected health information without the individual's authorization for public health activities and purposes as follows:
   a. **Public Health Reporting.** Our practice may disclose protected health information without the individual's authorization to a public health authority that is authorized by law to collect or receive such information for the purposes of preventing or controlling disease, injury, or disability, including but not limited to the reporting of disease, injury, vital events such as birth or death, and the conduct of public health surveillance, public health investigations, and public health interventions; or, at the direction of a public health authority, to an official of a foreign government agency that is acting in collaboration with a public health authority;
   b. **Child Abuse or Neglect.** Our practice may disclose protected health information without the individual's authorization to a public health authority or other appropriate government authority authorized by law to receive reports of child abuse or neglect;
   c. **Food and Drug Administration (FDA).** Our practice may disclose protected health information without the individual's authorization about a person subject to the jurisdiction of the FDA with respect to an FDA-regulated product or activity for which that person has responsibility, for the purpose of activities related to the quality, safety, or effectiveness of such FDA-regulated product or activity;
   d. **Communicable Disease.** Our practice may disclose protected health information without the individual's authorization to a person who may have been exposed to a communicable disease or may otherwise be at risk of contracting or spreading a disease or condition, if the covered entity or public health authority is authorized by law to notify such person as necessary in the conduct of a public health intervention or investigation.
2. **Abuse, Neglect, or Domestic Violence**[2]
   a. **If disclosure is required by law.** In cases that do not involve reports of child abuse or neglect (see above), our practice shall not require an individual's authorization to disclose protected health information about an individual whom we reasonably believe to be a victim of abuse, neglect, or domestic violence to a government

---

1. 45 C.F.R. § 164.512(b)
2. 45 C.F.R. § 164.512(c)

authority, including a social service or protective services agency, authorized by law to receive reports of such abuse, neglect, or domestic violence to the extent the disclosure is required by law and the disclosure complies with and is limited to the relevant requirements of such law.

b. **If disclosure is not required by law.** If disclosure is not required by law, and in our professional judgment we believe the disclosure is necessary to prevent serious harm to the individual or other potential victim, we will consult legal counsel to determine whether the disclosure is expressly authorized by statute or regulation and to determine if any other legal requirements have been met.

c. **Informing the individual.** If our practice makes such a permitted disclosure of abuse, neglect, or domestic violence, whether or not the individual agreed to the disclosure, we shall promptly inform the individual that such a report has been or will be made, except if:

   i. In the exercise of professional judgment, we believe informing the individual would place the individual at risk of serious harm, or

   ii. We would be informing a personal representative, and we reasonably believe the personal representative is responsible for the abuse, neglect, or other injury, and that informing such person would not be in the best interests of the individual as we determine in the exercise of professional judgment.

3. **Government Health Oversight Activities.**[3] If our practice receives a request for disclosure from a health oversight agency in connection with an activity such as an audit, investigation, inspection, licensure or disciplinary action, civil, administrative, or criminal proceeding or action, we shall contact legal counsel to determine how to respond and whether we must obtain authorization from the appropriate individual(s) prior to disclosing any requested protected health information. Examples of such activities include:

   a. Oversight of the health care system
   b. Government benefit programs such as Medicare and Medicaid
   c. Government regulatory programs
   d. Determining compliance with civil rights laws
   e. Investigation of an individual related to the receipt of health care, a claim for public benefits related to health, or qualification for public benefits or services when a patient's health is integral to his or her claim for public benefits or services.

---

3. 45 C.F.R. § 164.512(d)

4. **Judicial and administrative proceedings.**[4] If our practice receives an order of a court or administrative tribunal or a subpoena, discovery request, or other lawful process, we shall contact our legal counsel to determine:
   a. How to respond
   b. Whether we must obtain authorization from the appropriate individual(s) prior to disclosing any requested protected health information
   c. Whether we must receive "satisfactory assurances" from the party seeking the information
   d. Whether a "qualified protective order" is required
   e. Whether we must give the individual notice of the request or obtain the individual's authorization prior to disclosing protected health information.
5. **Law Enforcement Official**[5]
   a. **Request.** Our practice shall promptly contact legal counsel if we receive a request for information for law enforcement purposes from a law enforcement official, including any of the following:
      i. A court order or court-ordered warrant, or a subpoena or summons issued by a judicial officer
      ii. A grand jury subpoena
      iii. An administrative request, including an administrative subpoena or summons, or a civil or an authorized investigative demand, or similar process authorized under law
      iv. A request for information about an individual who is or is suspected to be a victim of a crime.
   b. **Response.** Before our practice responds to a request for a law enforcement purpose to a law enforcement official, we shall determine in consultation with our legal counsel how to respond, what information must be disclosed, whether any additional items (such as samples of body fluids or tissue must be disclosed), and whether we require authorization from the individual prior to disclosure.
   c. **Decedent.** If an individual has died and we suspect that the death may have resulted from criminal conduct, our practice may disclose protected health information to a law enforcement official about the individual for the purpose of alerting law enforcement of the death.
   d. **Crime on premises.** We may disclose to a law enforcement official protected health information that we believe in good faith constitutes evidence of criminal conduct that occurred on our premises.

4. 45 C.F.R. § 164.512(e)

5. 45 C.F.R. § 164.512(f)

e. **Reporting crime in emergency.** If we provide emergency health care in response to a medical emergency (other than a medical emergency on our premises), we may disclose protected health information to a law enforcement official if the disclosure appears necessary to alert law enforcement to:
   i. The commission and nature of a crime
   ii. The location of the crime or the victim(s) of the crime, and
   iii. The identity, description, and location of the perpetrator of the crime.

However, if we believe the medical emergency is the result of abuse, neglect, or domestic violence of the individual who needed emergency health care, our practice must follow the procedure in Point 2, "Abuse, Neglect, and Domestic Violence."

6. **Coroners, Medical Examiners, and Funeral Directors.**[6] We may disclose protected health information to a coroner or medical examiner for the purpose of identifying a deceased person, determining a cause of death, or other duties as authorized by law. We may disclose protected health information to funeral directors, consistent with applicable law, as necessary to carry out their duties with respect to the decedent. If necessary for funeral directors to carry out their duties, we may disclose the protected health information prior to, and in reasonable anticipation, of the individual's death.
7. **Organ and Tissue Donation.**[7] We may use or disclose protected health information to organ procurement organizations or other entities engaged in the procurement, banking, or transplantation of cadaveric organs, eyes, or tissue for donation or transplantation.
8. **Research.**[8] Our dental practice shall not use or disclose protected health information for research purposes without consulting legal counsel to make sure all necessary requirements have been met. Examples of such requirements include approval by an Institutional Review Board or privacy board, reviews preparatory to research, review and approval procedures, and required signatures.
9. **Averting a Serious Threat to Health or Safety.**[9] Our practice will consult our legal counsel to determine whether HIPAA and other applicable law permit us to disclose protected health information if we believe in good faith that such disclosure is necessary:
   a. To prevent or lessen a serious and imminent threat to the health or safety of a person or the public

6. 45 C.F.R. § 164.512(g)
7. 45 C.F.R. § 164.512(h)
8. 45 C.F.R. § 164.512(i)
9. 45 C.F.R. § 164.512(j)

b. For law enforcement authorities to identify or apprehend an individual where it appears from all the circumstances that the individual has escaped from a correctional institution or from lawful custody
c. For law enforcement authorities to identify or apprehend an individual because of a statement by an individual admitting participation in a violent crime that we reasonably believe may have caused serious physical harm to the victim.

10. **Specialized Government Functions.**[10] Our practice shall consult legal counsel to determine whether HIPAA and other applicable law permit us to disclose protected health information involving:
    a. Military and veterans activities
    b. National security and intelligence activities
    c. Protective services for the President and others
    d. Correctional institutions and other law enforcement custodial situations.
11. **Workers' Compensation.**[11] Our practice may disclose protected health information as authorized by and to the extent necessary to comply with laws relating to workers' compensation or other similar programs, established by law, that provide benefits for work-related injuries or illness without regard to fault.

Since 2003 when HIPAA Privacy Rules became enforceable, health care providers have exercised great caution not to disclose PHI. However, significant disasters, including earthquakes, hurricanes, and terrorist activities, have caused confusion as to what to disclose and what not to disclose. As a result, the HHS Office for Civil Rights (OCR) issued, and continues to issue, guidances such as the Communicating with Friends and Family, FAQs for Family Members, and the Emergency and Disaster Disclosure Decision Tree, which are included in this appendix.

COMMUNICATING WITH A PATIENT'S FAMILY, FRIENDS, OR OTHERS INVOLVED IN THE PATIENT'S CARE

U.S. Department of Health and Human Services • Office for Civil Rights

This guide explains when a health care provider is allowed to share a patient's health information with the patient's family members, friends, or others identified by the patient as involved in the patient's care under the Health Insurance Portability and Accountability Act of 1996 (HIPAA)

10. 45 C.F.R. § 164.512(k)

11. 45 C.F.R. § 164.512(l)

Privacy Rule. HIPAA is a Federal law that sets national standards for how health plans, health care clearinghouses, and most health care providers are to protect the privacy of a patient's health information.[12]

Even though HIPAA requires health care providers to protect patient privacy, providers are permitted, in most circumstances, to communicate with the patient's family, friends, or others involved in their care or payment for care. This guide is intended to clarify these HIPAA requirements so that health care providers do not unnecessarily withhold a patient's health information from these persons. This guide includes common questions and a table that summarizes the relevant requirements.[13]

Common Questions About HIPAA

1. **If the patient is present and has the capacity to make health care decisions, when does HIPAA allow a health care provider to discuss the patient's health information with the patient's family, friends, or others involved in the patient's care or payment for care?**

   If the patient is present and has the capacity to make health care decisions, a health care provider may discuss the patient's health information with a family member, friend, or other person if the patient agrees or, when given the opportunity, does not object. A health care provider also may share information with these persons if, using professional judgment, he or she decides that the patient does not object. In either case, the health care provider may share or discuss only the information that the person involved needs to know about the patient's care or payment for care.

   Here are some examples:

   - An emergency room doctor may discuss a patient's treatment in front of the patient's friend if the patient asks that her friend come into the treatment room.
   - A doctor's office may discuss a patient's bill with the patient's adult daughter who is with the patient at the patient's medical appointment and has questions about the charges.

---

12. The HIPAA Privacy Rule applies to those health care providers that transmit any health information in electronic form in connection with certain standard transactions, such as health care claims. See the definitions of "covered entity," "health care provider," and "transaction" at 45 C.F.R. §160.103.

13. The full text of these requirements can be found at 45 C.F.R. §164.510(b). Note that this guide does not apply to a health care provider's disclosure of psychotherapy notes, which generally requires a patient's written authorization. See 45 C.F.R. § 164.508(a)(2).

- A doctor may discuss the drugs a patient needs to take with the patient's health aide who has accompanied the patient to a medical appointment.
- A doctor may give information about a patient's mobility limitations to the patient's sister who is driving the patient home from the hospital.
- A nurse may discuss a patient's health status with the patient's brother if she informs the patient she is going to do so and the patient does not object.

BUT:

- A nurse may <u>not</u> discuss a patient's condition with the patient's brother after the patient has stated she does not want her family to know about her condition.

2. If the patient is not present or is incapacitated, may a health care provider still share the patient's health information with family, friends, or others involved in the patient's care or payment for care?

Yes. If the patient is not present or is incapacitated, a health care provider may share the patient's information with family, friends, or others as long as the health care provider determines, based on professional judgment, that it is in the best interest of the patient. When someone other than a friend or family member is involved, the health care provider must be reasonably sure that the patient asked the person to be involved in his or her care or payment for care. The health care provider may discuss only the information that the person involved needs to know about the patient's care or payment.

Here are some examples:

- A surgeon who did emergency surgery on a patient may tell the patient's spouse about the patient's condition while the patient is unconscious.
- A pharmacist may give a prescription to a patient's friend who the patient has sent to pick up the prescription.
- A hospital may discuss a patient's bill with her adult son who calls the hospital with questions about charges to his mother's account.
- A health care provider may give information regarding a patient's drug dosage to the patient's health aide who calls the provider with questions about the particular prescription.

BUT:

- A nurse may <u>not</u> tell a patient's friend about a past medical problem that is unrelated to the patient's current condition.

- A health care provider is not required by HIPAA to share a patient's information when the patient is not present or is incapacitated, and can choose to wait until the patient has an opportunity to agree to the disclosure.

3. **Does HIPAA require that a health care provider document a patient's decision to allow the provider to share his or her health information with a family member, friend, or other person involved in the patient's care or payment for care?**

   No. HIPAA does not require that a health care provider document the patient's agreement or lack of objection. However, a health care provider is free to obtain or document the patient's agreement, or lack of objection, in writing, if he or she prefers. For example, a provider may choose to document a patient's agreement to share information with a family member with a note in the patient's medical file.

4. **May a health care provider discuss a patient's health information over the phone with the patient's family, friends, or others involved in the patient's care or payment for care?**

   Yes. Where a health care provider is allowed to share a patient's health information with a person, information may be shared face-to-face, over the phone, or in writing.

5. **If a patient's family member, friend, or other person involved in the patient's care or payment for care calls a health care provider to ask about the patient's condition, does HIPAA require the health care provider to obtain proof of who the person is before speaking with them?**

   No. If the caller states that he or she is a family member or friend of the patient, or is involved in the patient's care or payment for care, then HIPAA doesn't require proof of identity in this case. However, a health care provider may establish his or her own rules for verifying who is on the phone. In addition, when someone other than a friend or family member is involved, the health care provider must be reasonably sure that the patient asked the person to be involved in his or her care or payment for care.

6. **Can a patient have a family member, friend, or other person pick up a filled prescription, medical supplies, X-rays, or other similar forms of patient information, for the patient?**

   Yes. HIPAA allows health care providers to use professional judgment and experience to decide if it is in the patient's best interest to allow another person to pick up a prescription, medical supplies, X-rays, or other similar forms of information for the patient.

For example, the fact that a relative or friend arrives at a pharmacy and asks to pick up a specific prescription for a patient effectively verifies that he or she is involved in the patient's care. HIPAA allows the pharmacist to give the filled prescription to the relative or friend. The patient does not need to provide the pharmacist with their names in advance.

7. **May a health care provider share a patient's health information with an interpreter to communicate with the patient or with the patient's family, friends, or others involved in the patient's care or payment for care?**

Yes. HIPAA allows covered health care providers to share a patient's health information with an interpreter without the patient's written authorization under the following circumstances:

- A health care provider may share information with an interpreter who works for the provider (e.g., a bilingual employee, a contract interpreter on staff, or a volunteer).

For example, an emergency room doctor may share information about an incapacitated patient's condition with an interpreter on staff who relays the information to the patient's family.

- A health care provider may share information with an interpreter who is acting on its behalf (but is not a member of the provider's workforce) if the health care provider has a written contract or other agreement with the interpreter that meets HIPAA's business associate contract requirements.

For example, many providers are required under Title VI of the Civil Rights Act of 1964 to take reasonable steps to provide meaningful access to persons with limited English proficiency. These providers often have contracts with private companies, community-based organizations, or telephone interpreter service lines to provide language interpreter services. These arrangements must comply with the HIPAA business associate agreement requirements at 45 C.F.R. 164.504(e).

- A health care provider may share information with an interpreter who is the patient's family member, friend, or other person identified by the patient as his or her interpreter, if the patient agrees, or does not object, or the health care provider determines, using his or her professional judgment, that the patient does not object.

For example, health care providers sometimes see patients who speak a certain language and the provider has no employee, volunteer, or contractor who can competently interpret that language. If the provider is aware of a telephone interpreter service that can help, the provider may have that interpreter tell the patient that the service is available. If the provider decides, based on professional judgment, that the patient has chosen to continue using the interpreter, the provider may talk to the patient using the interpreter.

8. Where can I find additional information about HIPAA?

The Office for Civil Rights, part of the Department of Health and Human Services, has more information about HIPAA on its Web site. Visit http://www.hhs.gov/ocr/hipaa for a wide range of helpful information, including the full text of the Privacy Rule, a HIPAA Privacy Rule Summary, fact sheets, over 200 Frequently Asked Questions, as well as many other resources to help health care providers and others understand the law.

HIPAA Privacy Rule Disclosures to a Patient's Family, Friends, or Others Involved in the Patient's Care or Payment for Care

	Family Member or Friend	Other Persons
Patient is present and has the capacity to make health care decisions	Provider may disclose relevant information if the provider does one of the following: (1) obtains the patient's agreement (2) gives the patient an opportunity to object and the patient does not object (3) decides from the circumstances, based on professional judgment, that the patient does not object Disclosure may be made in person, over the phone, or in writing.	Provider may disclose relevant information if the provider does one of the following: (1) obtains the patient's agreement (2) gives the patient the opportunity to object and the patient does not object (3) decides from the circumstances, based on professional judgment, that the patient does not object Disclosure may be made in person, over the phone, or in writing.
Patient is not present or is incapacitated	Provider may disclose relevant information if, based on professional judgment, the disclosure is in the patient's best interest. Disclosure may be made in person, over the phone, or in writing. Provider may use professional judgment and experience to decide if it is in the patient's best interest to allow someone to pick up filled prescriptions, medical supplies, X-rays, or other similar forms of health information for the patient.	Provider may disclose relevant information if the provider is reasonably sure that the patient has involved the person in the patient's care and in his or her professional judgment, the provider believes the disclosure to be in the patient's best interest. Disclosure may be made in person, over the phone, or in writing. Provider may use professional judgment and experience to decide if it is in the patient's best interest to allow someone to pick up filled prescriptions, medical supplies, X-rays, or other similar forms of health information for the patient.

Emergency and Disaster Disclosure Decision Tree

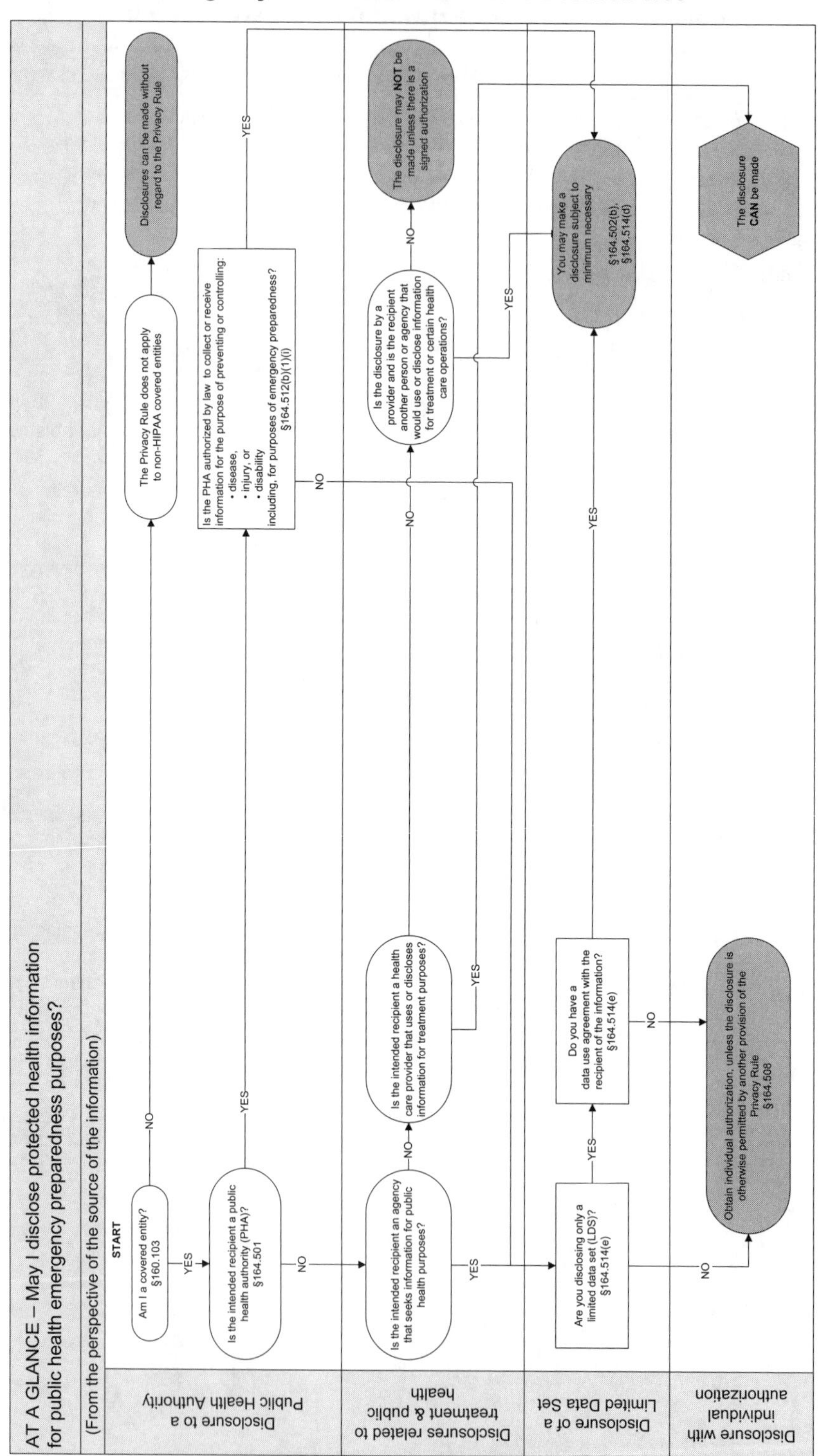

appendix B

Sample 12-Month Privacy and Security Refresher Training Sessions

Prerequisites to Monthly Training:

- Privacy and security officials have reviewed Chapters 1 through 4.
- Practice has implemented HIPAA's Privacy Rule and is using these training sessions to build on current best practices.

First Month (45 minutes)	Second Month (15 minutes)	Third Month (12 minutes)	Fourth Month (10–15 minutes)
Topic: What's New with HIPAA?	**Topic:** Accounting of Disclosures and Restrictions	**Topic:** Password Management	**Topic:** Managing Patient Complaints
Resource: Chapter 1	Resource: Chapter 3	Resource: Chapters 3 and 4	Resource: Chapter 3
Ask workforce members to bring in a news story about a stolen laptop or device containing confidential information. Make a list of favorite reporters and what affect it would have on the practice if the reporter completed a news story on your missing laptop. Inform workforce members about new HIPAA and Breach Notification requirements established by the HITECH Act. Include a discussion about enhanced enforcement and internal sanctions.	Discuss the six Patient Rights under HIPAA and the role of your privacy official. Remind staff of your policies and procedures on patient requests. Train staff on the new electronic accounting of disclosures and patient rights to restrict disclosures in the event the patient pays in full out-of-pocket for treatment. Demonstrate (if possible) how the system conducts audit monitoring, user access, and audit controls.	Provide a safe place for workforce to store passwords if they cannot remember them. For example, free or low-cost software is available online; more expensive solutions include a biometric authentication system that authenticates finger images and connects them to automatically stored passwords.	If you plan to participate in meaningful use reimbursements, you cannot have any open complaints filed with OCR or your state's attorney general. Discuss the complaint process and train workforce on how to manage complaints presented orally or in an e-mail or letter.

Fifth Month (10–15 minutes)	**Sixth Month (10 minutes)**	**Seventh Month (20 minutes)**	**Eighth Month (10 minutes)**
Topic: Permissions for Use and Disclosure	**Topic:** Managing Business Associates	**Topic:** When to Share PHI with the Patient's Friends and Family	**Topic:** Security Settings
Resource: Chapter 3 There are 11 Permissions and 9 Special Requirements in HIPAA Privacy. Assign a Permission or Special Requirement to each staff person and ask him or her to explain how it has been (or will be) used in your office. Remind staff of your practice's HIPAA policies and procedures and where they are located.	Resource: Chapters 1, 3, and 4 Refresher for staff on business associate obligations to secure protected health information. Discuss possible business associate breaches and what you would do to resolve the incident.	Resource: Chapter 3 and Appendix C Present policies and procedures on how to verify a caller or person requesting information and guidance on dealing with friends and family. Ask how the practice manages inquiries from friends and family.	Resource: Chapters 1, 3, and 4 Present policies and procedures on administrative, physical, and technical safeguards. Include discussion about use of e-mail, USB drives, security and encryption of portable computers, and/or accessing the Internet.

Ninth Month (15 minutes)	Tenth Month (60 minutes)	Eleventh Month (20 minutes)	Twelfth Month (1 hour)
Topic: Disclosures to Officials	**Topic:** Disaster Recovery	**Topic:** Valid Authorizations	**Topic:** Year-end Evaluation
Resource: Chapter 3	Resource: Chapter 4	Resource: Chapters 3 and 4	Resource: Chapters 1, 3, and 4
Discuss procedures to follow when a public official requests information about a patient. Discuss confidentiality, patients' right to request restrictions on use and disclosure, and patients' right to request an accounting of disclosures.	Conduct a planned fire drill when patients are not scheduled. Most fire departments will assist in this drill. Upon returning to the practice, imagine everything has been damaged or destroyed. What would you need to continue doing business? Make a list of small and large items, then modify your disaster recovery plan, if necessary, in light of what you learn from the drill. Build a Downtime Cabinet.[1]	Discuss content that defines a "valid authorization." Include guidance on where to store authorizations in the patient's record, how to withdraw an authorization, and what happens if authorized processes are already in place. Include de-identified sample authorizations for marketing, insurance, long-term care, and so forth. Leverage authorizations into a discussion of documentation and HIPAA logs. -How are we doing on documentation? -Schedule an audit of documentation processes. -Assign teams to review policies and procedures to determine what needs to be updated.	Report findings of internal audit. Report findings of notice of privacy practices, business associate, and policies and procedures teams. Report findings of forms and logs team. Evaluate training needs, particularly with new staff or staff with new responsibilities.

[1] A Downtime Cabinet contains essentials you are likely to need if your system goes down for more than 2–3 hours. These items may include paper pads, pens, a checkbook, a tamper-proof prescription pad, a list of local pharmacies, a billing encounter sheet with updated billing codes, dental referrals, and system contacts information.

appendix C

Additional Resources

The additional resources presented in this appendix are either American Medical Association's HIPAA resources or third-party HIPAA-related resources, which you may find useful in your quest to further achieve compliance with HIPAA and the HITECH Act. Please note that some of the dates and content may have changed since these resources were published. It is advisable to check the AMA, CMS, and HHS web sites for the latest updates.

To download a PDF of the *New HIPAA Breach Notification Rule*, go to *www.ama-assn.org/ama1/pub/upload/mm/368/hipaa-breach.pdf.*

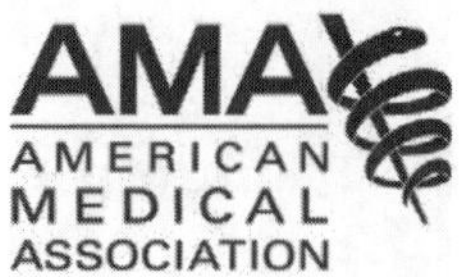

WHAT YOU NEED TO KNOW ABOUT THE NEW HIPAA BREACH NOTIFICATION RULE[1]

New regulations effective September 23, 2009 require all physicians who are covered by HIPAA to notify patients if there are breaches of security involving their medical information. The following summarizes these new requirements. These requirements apply in addition to any notification obligations imposed by state law. These requirements also supplement the obligations imposed by the HIPAA Privacy and Security Rules.

HIPAA covered entities (ie, health plans, health care clearinghouses, physicians, and other health care providers who transmit any health information electronically in connection with a HIPAA standard transaction) must comply with the new breach notification requirements specified in interim final regulations promulgated pursuant to the "American Recovery and Reinvestment Act of 2009" that was signed into law on February 17, 2009. Following the discovery of a breach of unsecured protected health information (PHI), physicians must provide notification to affected individuals, to the Secretary of the Department of Health and Human Services (HHS), and in some cases, to the media.

The breach notification provisions are effective, and compliance is required for breaches occurring on or after September 23, 2009. However, HHS will use its discretion not to enforce the new breach notice requirements and will not impose sanctions or financial penalties for breaches discovered before February 22, 2010. After the breach notification rule takes effect, but before HHS imposes sanctions, HHS expects compliance with the breach notification requirements. Accordingly, we recommend that physicians (and their business associates) plan immediately to comply with these new breach notification requirements.

This new HIPAA Breach Notification Rule only concerns the unauthorized acquisition, access, use or disclosure of unsecured patient health information as a result of a security breach. This Rule does not replace the existing HIPAA Privacy Rule that permits a covered entity (i.e., physician)

1. Disclaimer: The information provided in this document does not constitute, and is no substitute for, legal or other professional advice. Users should consult their own legal or other professional advisors for individualized guidance regarding the application of the law to their particular situations, and in connection with other compliance-related concerns. Prepared September 21, 2009 based on available information.

to use and disclose patient health information, within certain limits and protections, for treatment, payment, and health care operations activities.

Breach Notification Requirements

What Constitutes a Breach

A breach is defined as the acquisition, access, use, or disclosure of unsecured PHI which is not permitted by the HIPAA Privacy Rules and compromises the security or privacy of the PHI. In order to determine whether a breach of unsecured PHI has occurred, the Rule calls for physicians to perform risk assessments to establish whether a significant risk of financial, reputational, or other harm to the affected individual(s) exists. If the physician performs a risk assessment and determines that there is significant risk of harm to the affected individual(s) as a result of the unauthorized use or disclosure of unsecured PHI, then breach notification(s) are required. For example, a stolen laptop containing patient health records that is not encrypted would constitute a breach and trigger notification requirements, unless the laptop was returned and a forensic analysis demonstrates that the PHI was not accessed or otherwise compromised.

What Constitutes Unsecured PHI

Unsecured PHI is any patient health information that is not secured through a technology or methodology, specified by HHS, that renders the PHI unusable, unreadable, or indecipherable to unauthorized individuals. Unsecured PHI (ie, patient's full name, patient's address, social security number, diagnosis) can be in any form or medium including electronic, paper, or in oral form.

Exceptions to the Breach Notification Requirements

The law identifies the following circumstances when a breach notification is NOT required:

- Any ***unintentional*** acquisition, access, or use of the PHI by a workforce member (ie, employees, volunteers, trainees, and other persons whose conduct is under the direct control of a covered entity, whether or not they are paid by the covered entity) or an individual, acting upon the authority of the HIPAA covered entity or a business associate (BA), who acquired, accessed, or used the PHI in good faith and within the normal scope of his/her authority, and if that PHI is not further used or disclosed. For example, breach notification would not be required where a billing employee receives and opens an e-mail containing PHI about a patient which a nurse mistakenly sent to the billing employee but, upon noticing that he/she is not the intended recipient, the billing employee alerts the nurse of the misdirected e-mail, and then deletes it;

- Any ***inadvertent*** disclosure by a person who is authorized to access PHI at a covered entity or BA to another person authorized to access PHI at the same covered entity, BA, or organized health care arrangement[2] in which the covered entity participates, and the PHI is not further used or disclosed in violation of the HIPAA Privacy Rules;
- A disclosure of PHI where a covered entity or BA has a ***good faith belief*** that an unauthorized person to whom the disclosure was made would not reasonably have been able to retain such information (ie, a laptop is lost or stolen and then recovered, and a forensic analysis of the computer shows that information was not opened, altered, transferred, or otherwise compromised);
- If law enforcement determines that notification would impede a criminal investigation or cause damage to national security, covered entities are allowed to delay notification, ***but only for up to 30 days as orally directed by the law enforcement agency, or for such longer period as the law enforcement agency specifies in writing;*** and
- Encryption and destruction are deemed as the technologies and methods for securing PHI. Covered entities that have thus secured their PHI through appropriate encryption or destruction methods are relieved of the notification obligation (unless otherwise required by federal or state law or necessary to mitigate the harmful effect of the breach). The encryption must be an algorithmic process with a confidential process or encryption key, and the decryption tools are stored at a location separate from the encrypted data. With regard to destruction, paper copies of PHI must be shredded or destroyed and electronic media copies of PHI must be cleared, purged, or destroyed such that PHI cannot be retrieved.

Breach Notification

HIPAA covered entities (ie, physicians) are required to notify the affected individuals of any unauthorized acquisition, access, use, or disclosure of unsecured PHI without unreasonable delay but not later than 60 calendar days after discovery. Thus if the physician has compiled all of the necessary information to provide notification of a breach of unsecured PHI to affected individual(s) by day 10 (10 days from the day the breach was discovered) but waits until day 60 to send notifications, this would constitute an unreasonable delay.

BAs who have access to PHI are required to notify the covered entity of any such breach, including the name of any individual whose unsecured PHI has been released. Physicians should make sure that their agreements with

---

2. An organized health care arrangement is a clinically integrated care setting in which individuals typically receive health care from more than one health care provider such as a hospital and the health care providers who have staff privileges at the hospital.

BAs address these new breach notification requirements, including the timing of BA notification to a physician following a breach and responsibility for paying costs resulting from a breach. While HHS has indicated that the parties to BA agreements have flexibility in this regard, it has encouraged the parties to ensure that individuals do not receive notification from both the BA and the covered entity, as this could be confusing.

Discovery of Breaches

Breaches are treated as discovered as of the first day on which the breach is known or should have been known to the physician (or where the BA is acting as their agent, their BA).

How to Provide Notice

Physicians should send written notification via first class mail to each affected individual (or if deceased, the individual's next of kin) at the last known address, unless the individual has indicated a preference for e-mail. In situations where a physician deems possible imminent misuse of unsecured PHI, the physician may provide other forms of notice, such as by telephone or e-mail, in addition to the written notice.

If the address is unknown for fewer than 10 individuals, then a substitute notice must be provided by other means reasonably calculated to reach the affected individual, such as by telephone. If the address is unknown for 10 or more individuals, then a substitute notice must be provided by either a conspicuous posting on the entity's Web Homepage for a specified period of time (period of time proposed by HHS is 90 days) or a conspicuous publication in major print or broadcast media in the geographic areas where the individuals affected by the breach likely reside. The substitute notice must include a toll-free number that remains active for at least 90 days.

Notice to 500+ Affected Individuals

If the breach of unsecured PHI affects 500 or more individuals, then the notice must also be provided to major media outlets serving the relevant state or jurisdiction. The notice to the media must contain the same information as the written notice to individuals, and must similarly be provided without unreasonable delay, but in no case later than 60 calendar days after discovery of the breach.

Notice to HHS

Additionally, the physician must notify HHS, in the manner specified on the HHS website, contemporaneously with the notice sent to the individuals. The HHS web site will have a list that identifies the covered entities involved in a breach in which 500 or more individuals are affected. If less than 500 individuals are affected, then the covered entity may maintain a log of the breaches and must submit this log annually to HHS (within 60 days after the end of each calendar year).

Contents of the Written Notice

The written notice must contain the following content:

1. Notification must be written in plain language;
2. A brief description of what happened, including the date of the breach and the date of the discovery of the breach to the extent these dates are known;
3. A description of the types of unsecured PHI that were disclosed in the breach (ie, full name, Social Security number, date of birth, home address, account number, diagnosis, disability code, etc.);
4. Steps that the patients should take to protect themselves from potential harm resulting from the breach of unsecured PHI (such as contacting their credit card companies);
5. A brief description of the actions taken by the physician to investigate the breach, mitigate harm to individuals, and to protect against any further breaches; and
6. Contact procedures for individuals to ask questions or learn additional information, including a toll-free number, an e-mail address, website, or postal address.

Compliance with Federal and State Laws on Breach Notifications

The new HIPAA breach notification requirements override any conflicting state laws. However, physicians must comply with both federal and state breach notification laws if the state law does not conflict with these new HIPAA breach notification requirements (ie, a state law requires the covered entity to send a notice of a breach of unsecured PHI to the affected individual(s) in 30 calendar days (not 60 days), and the physician has all of the necessary information to comply with the state's 30 day requirement. Issuing the notice by day 30 does not conflict with federal law.)

These requirements similarly do not override obligations imposed by other federal laws, such as requirements imposed by Title VI of the Civil Rights Act to take reasonable steps to ensure meaningful access to the notice by those with Limited English Proficiency, and requirements imposed by the Americans with Disabilities Act to ensure effective communication of the notice to individuals with disabilities.

Additional Requirements

In addition to the breach notification requirements, the federal regulations impose additional compliance obligations on physician practices consistent with those imposed by other HIPAA obligations, including the requirement to:

1) Revise the practice's policies and procedures and Notice of Privacy Practices to reflect the HIPAA Breach Notification Rule. For example, physicians should make sure that their practice's HIPAA compliance program, including record retention practices, address risk assessments for determining whether a breach of unsecured PHI has occurred;
2) Train their workforce members on the practice's policies and procedures with respect to the notification requirements;
3) Allow individuals to complain about those policies and procedures, or whether the notification requirements have been violated;
4) Sanction workforce members who violate the notification requirements; and
5) Refrain from retaliating against those who exercise their rights.

Visit *www.ama-assn.org/go/hipaa* for additional information.

To download a PDF of *What you need to know about the new health privacy and security requirements*, go to *www.ama-assn.org/ama1/pub/upload/mm/368/hipaa-guidance.pdf.*

PRACTICE MANAGEMENT CENTER

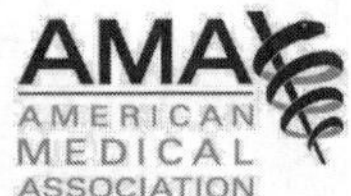

WHAT YOU NEED TO KNOW ABOUT THE NEW HEALTH PRIVACY AND SECURITY REQUIREMENTS

Currently, privacy standards under the Health Insurance Portability and Accountability Act of 1996 (HIPAA) require physicians to protect the privacy of patients' medical information. Physicians are required to control the ways in which they use and disclose patients' protected health information. In addition, physicians are required to offer patients certain rights with respect to their information, such as the right to access and copy this information, the right to request amendments and the right to request an accounting of disclosures. Physicians are also required to have certain administrative protections in place (eg, staff training and implementation of appropriate policies and procedures) to further protect the privacy of patients' information. The American Recovery and Reinvestment Act of 2009 (ARRA), which was signed into law on Feb. 17, 2009, maintains and expands the current HIPAA patient health information privacy and security protections, especially as patient health information is transferred electronically.

Compliance Deadlines

Following is a summary of the new requirements that physicians should plan to comply with immediately.

Effective date—Sept. 23, 2009

- HIPAA-covered entities—including physicians—must comply with the new breach notification requirements effective Sept. 23, 2009. However, the Department of Health and Human Services (HHS) will use its discretion not to enforce the new breach notice requirements and will not impose sanctions or financial penalties for breaches discovered before Feb. 22, 2010. Physicians should review and revise their business associate agreements to include breach notification requirements. Visit the AMA's web site at *www.ama-assn.org/go/hipaa* for more guidance on the new breach notification requirements. You can also visit *www.hhs.gov/ocr/privacy/hipaa/administrative/* and select "Breach Notification Rule" from the left navigation menu to view information from HHS.

Effective date—Feb. 17, 2010

- HIPAA-covered entities—including physicians—and their business associates are required to honor a patient's request to not disclose certain protected health information to a commercial health plan if the information solely concerns a health care item or service that the patient has paid for in full out-of-pocket (ie, patient pays in full for a service upon delivery of that service and requests that his/her physician not submit the bill to his/her commercial health plan).
- HIPAA-covered entities—including physicians—should use a limited data set of identifiable patient information to meet the minimum necessary standard, if such use is practicable, until HHS issues guidance on what exactly constitutes the minimum necessary standard.[1]

To be a "limited data set," the health information must not include any of the following identifiers of the individual and any relatives, employers or household members of the individual: (a) names; (b) all geographic subdivisions smaller than a State, including street address or precinct, other than town or city and zip code; (c) telephone numbers; (d) fax numbers; (e) electronic mail addresses; (f) social security numbers; (g) medical record numbers; (h) health plan beneficiary numbers; (i) account numbers; (j) certificate/license numbers; (k) vehicle identifiers and serial numbers, including license plate numbers; (l) device identifiers and serial numbers; (m) Web Universal Resource Locators (URLs); (n) Internet Protocol (IP) address numbers; (o) biometric identifiers, including finger and voice prints; (p) full face photographic images and any comparable images; and (q) any other unique identifying number, characteristic, or code, except as permitted by the regulation (45 C.F.R. §164.514(c)) to allow the data to be re-identified by the sender.
(45 C.F.R. §164.512(e))

- HIPAA-covered entities—including physicians—using electronic health records are required to honor a patient's request for an electronic copy of his/her medical record, which must be transmitted directly to an entity or person specified by the patient, as long as that directive is clear, conspicuous and specific. HIPAA requires that such requests be honored within 30 days of notice. Any fee charged for the record must be reasonable and must also comply with applicable state law.

1. When using or disclosing protected health information, or when requesting protected health information from others, in general, a physician must make reasonable efforts to limit use or disclosure to "the minimum necessary to accomplish the intended purpose of the use, disclosure, or request."

- If a HIPAA-covered entity—including a physician—is paid by an outside entity to send a communication to a patient, the communication is deemed to be marketing material, and therefore requires prior written authorization from the patient. There are limited exceptions to this requirement. Physicians must also give patients an opportunity to opt out of receiving fundraising communications.
- Business associates of HIPAA-covered entities are required to directly comply with HIPAA requirements.

Effective date—Jan. 1, 2011

- HIPAA-covered entities—including physicians—using electronic health records are required to honor a patient's request for an accounting of disclosures, including disclosures for treatment, payment and health care operations. HHS will be adopting a technical standard so that electronic health records have the capability to account for disclosures for treatment, payment and health care operations.
- **Exception:** Physicians who adopt electronic health records on or after Jan. 1, 2009 must comply by Jan. 1, 2011 or by the date they acquire the electronic health record, whichever is later.[2]
- **Exception:** Physicians who adopted electronic health records by Jan. 1, 2009 must comply by Jan. 1, 2014.

Additional Resources

Visit ***www.hhs.gov/ocr/privacy/hipaa/understanding/*** and select "For Covered Entities" from the left navigation menu for more information from HHS about the HIPAA privacy and security requirements.

For more information about the HIPAA enforcement rules, including increased civil monetary penalties for violations, visit the American Medical Association's web site at ***www.ama-assn.org/go/hipaa*** and select "HIPAA Violations and Enforcement."

HHS also provides information about HIPAA violations and their enforcement. Visit ***www.hhs.gov/ocr/privacy/hipaa/administrative/*** and select "Enforcement Rule" from the left navigation menu to access this information.

2. HHS has discretion to extend these compliance deadlines.

In addition to the new privacy and security requirements specified above, the federal regulations impose additional compliance obligations on physician practices consistent with those imposed by other HIPAA obligations, including the following requirements:

1. Review and revise the practice's policies and procedures to reflect the HIPAA Breach Notification Rule. For example, physicians should make sure that their practice's HIPAA compliance program, including record retention practices, address risk assessments for determining whether a breach of unsecured protected health information has occurred.
2. Train their workforce members on the practice's policies and procedures with respect to the notification requirements.
3. Allow individuals to complain about those policies and procedures and any violations of the notification requirements.
4. Sanction workforce members who violate the notification requirements.
5. Refrain from retaliating against those who exercise their rights.

Questions or concerns about practice management issues?

AMA members and their practice staff may e-mail the AMA Practice Management Center at **practicemanagementcenter@ama-assn.org** for assistance.

For additional information and resources, there are three easy ways to contact the AMA Practice Management Center:

- Call **(800) 621-8335** and ask for the AMA Practice Management Center.
- Fax information to **(312) 464-5541**.
- Visit *www.ama-assn.org/go/pmc* to access the AMA Practice Management Center web site.

Physicians and their practice staff can also visit *www.ama-assn.org/go/pmalerts* to sign up for free Practice Management Alerts from the AMA Practice Management Center.

The Practice Management Center is a resource of the AMA Private Sector Advocacy unit.

To download a PDF of *HIPAA Security Rule: Frequently asked questions regarding encryption of personal health information*, go to *www.ama-assn.org/ama1/pub/upload/mm/368/hipaa-phi-encryption.pdf.*

PRACTICE MANAGEMENT CENTER

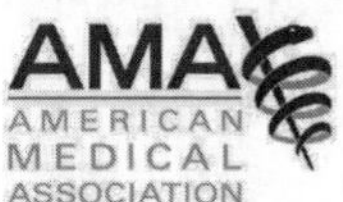

HIPAA SECURITY RULE: FREQUENTLY ASKED QUESTIONS REGARDING ENCRYPTION OF PERSONAL HEALTH INFORMATION

Please note that some of the links below may take you off the AMA web site. The AMA is not responsible for the content of other Web sites.

The Health Information Technology for Economic and Clinical Health (HITECH) Act, part of the American Recovery and Reinvestment Act of 2009, has made several important changes to the HIPAA Security Rule. These changes have raised a number of questions among physicians and other health care professionals as well as other HIPAA-covered entities and business associates.* This resource addresses the most common of these questions.

1. **I manage a small practice. Why should I care about the changes to the HIPAA Security Rule?**

   Perhaps the most significant of the changes to the HIPAA Security Rule is the requirement for HIPAA-covered entities and their business associates to provide notification in the event of a breach of "unsecured protected health information [PHI]." This means, for example, that if a hacker were able to gain access to a physician practice's computer system that contained patient information, the physician practice would have to inform all patients and the Department of Health and Human Services (HHS) of the breach. In some cases, the physician practice would also need to notify the media.

   The one and only exception to this new requirement is encryption technology: **If the electronic PHI (or *e*PHI) is stored and transmitted in encrypted form, then you do not need to notify patients, even if there is a security breach.** The National Institute of Standards and Technology (NIST) has issued Special Publication 800-66-Revision 1, "**An Introductory Resource Guide for Implementing the HIPAA Security Rule**," which is intended to describe the technologies and methodologies that physicians and

* Visit *www.cms.hhs.gov/HIPAAGenInfo/06_AreYouaCoveredEntity.asp* to learn more about who is considered a HIPAA-covered entity.

other HIPAA-covered entities and their business associates can use to render ePHI unusable, unreadable or indecipherable to unauthorized individuals. While HIPAA-covered entities and their business associates are not required to follow this guidance, if your practice does follow the specified technologies and methodologies, you will avoid having to comply with the extensive notification requirements otherwise required by the HITECH Act in the event of a security breach.

2. **What is encryption exactly?**

   Encryption is a technique for transforming information in such a way that it becomes unreadable. This means that even if a hacker is able to gain access to a computer that contains PHI, he or she will not be able to read or interpret that information. The patient's privacy will still be protected.

FIGURE 1

Encrypted data

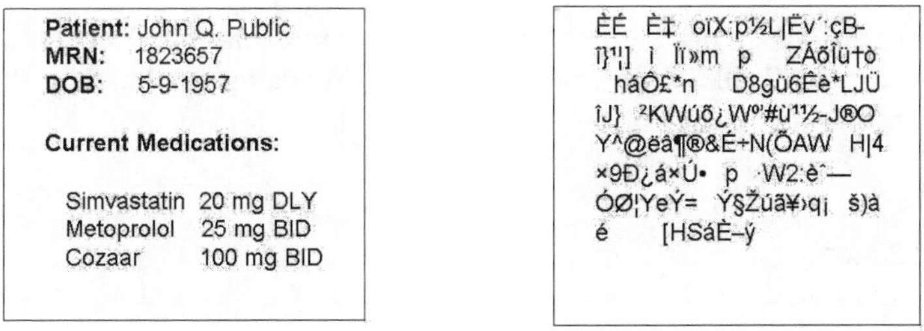

Patient: John Q. Public
MRN: 1823657
DOB: 5-9-1957

Current Medications:

Simvastatin	20 mg DLY
Metoprolol	25 mg BID
Cozaar	100 mg BID

Unencrypted data ("plaintext")

ÈÉ È‡ oïX:p½L|Ëv´:çB-
ñ}'¦] ì Ïï»m p ZÁõÎü†ò
háÔ£*n D8gü6Êè*LJÜ
îJ} ²KWúõ¿W°'#ù¹½-J®O
Y^@ëâ¶®&É÷N(ÕAW H|4
×9Ð¿á×Ú• p ·W2:è˜—
ÓØ¦YeÝ= Ý§Žúã¥›q¡ š)à
é [HSáÈ–ý

Encrypted data ("ciphertext")

3. **How does encryption work?**

   Encryption is done either by computer programs or by specially designed computer hardware devices. These programs or devices apply a mathematical algorithm (ie, a recipe for producing encrypted data) to the information. The output is a scrambled form of the original data. When a legitimate user needs to access the data, the scrambling process is reversed, and the data is restored to its original form. Only those who are in possession of the "key" can unscramble (ie, "decrypt") the data.

4. **What is a "key?"**

   A key is a piece of data that an encryption algorithm uses to determine exactly how to unscramble the protected information. It is called a key because it "unlocks" the encryption formula to unscramble the encrypted data.

5. **I keep seeing abbreviations such as "RSA" and "AES." What do these abbreviations mean?**

   These abbreviations are the names of specific mathematical algorithms. Algorithms are like recipes. Algorithms specify the ingredients (the key and the "plaintext" data to be protected) and the specific steps that need to be taken to produce the output (the "ciphertext," or encrypted data) from the information that is inputted. "RSA" gets its name from its inventors—Ron Rivest, Idi Shamir and Leonard Adelman—and "AES" stands for "advanced encryption standard." Other encryption algorithm names include "DES," "Triple-DES" (or "3DES"), "Rijndael," "Twofish," "MARS" and "Serpent."

6. **People talk about "public" and "private" keys. What is the difference?**

   Actually, there are three types of keys: "secret," "public" and "private." Different encryption algorithms use different types of keys. The more traditional encryption schemes use secret keys to both encrypt and decrypt data. Newer methods of encryption, known as "public-key" algorithms, use a public key to encrypt a piece of information and its corresponding private key to decrypt the information. (This kind of encryption is like a post office box. Anyone can put a letter in the box, but only the owner of the box can take the letter out.)

FIGURE 2

Types of keys

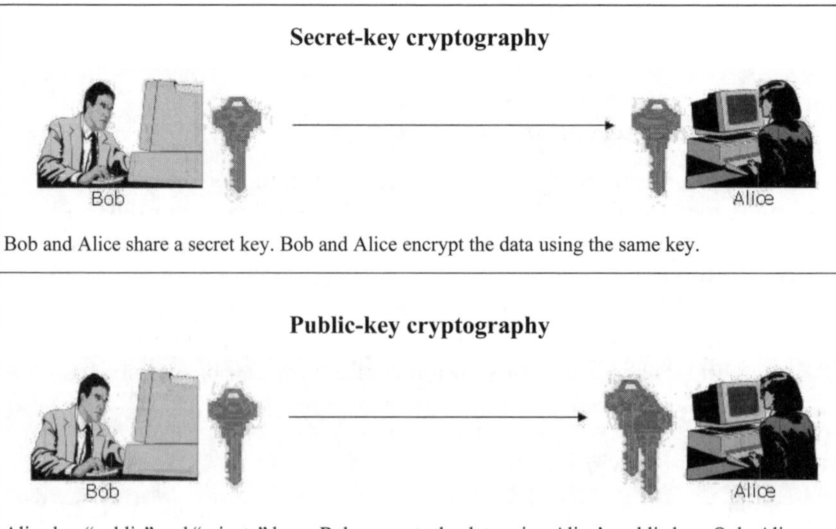

Secret-key cryptography
Bob
Alice
Bob and Alice share a secret key. Bob and Alice encrypt the data using the same key.
Public-key cryptography
Bob
Alice
Alice has "public" and "private" keys. Bob encrypts the data using Alice's public key. Only Alice can decrypt the data because only she has the private key.

7. **Which types of data can be encrypted?**

   Any kind of data can be encrypted. You can encrypt plaintext files, PDF documents, spreadsheets, images and any other form of information in your computer. You can even encrypt database information and information on back-up media.

8. **Which data should a physician practice typically encrypt?**

   You should encrypt any systems and individual files containing *e*PHI. Data you should encrypt includes your practice management system; electronic medical records; documents containing *e*PHI, such as claims payment appeals; scanned images, such as copies of remittance advices; e-mails containing *e*PHI; and *e*PHI that you transmit, such as the claims sent to a clearinghouse.

9. **Do e-mails containing *e*PHI have to be encrypted?**

   Yes, e-mails containing *e*PHI must be encrypted. E-mail is not like mailing a sealed letter or package. It is more like sending a postcard. People are not supposed to read it while it is in transit, but it passes through many hands, and one can never be sure that someone is not reading it illegally. Fortunately, there are many tools available for encrypting e-mail.

10. **Does *e*PHI that is accessed via the Internet need to be encrypted?**

    Yes, data that is published on the Internet is available to the public. The only way to protect health information that is made available on a Web site is to use a technology known as "secure sockets layer" (SSL). You are probably already using this encryption method, whether you are aware of it or not. Any Web site that has a URL (ie, an Internet address) beginning with "https" is using SSL or a similar encryption method. When you are on these Web sites, you may notice a small padlock icon on your browser. Double-clicking this icon usually gives you more information about how that browsing session is protected.

FIGURE 3

SSL protection

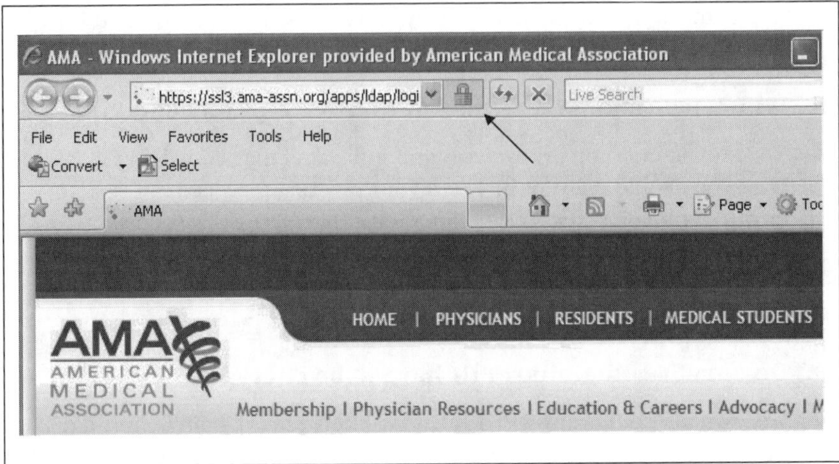

11. Is it difficult to encrypt data?

The difficulties involved in encrypting sensitive information depend on the method you choose. There are many possible approaches to implementing data encryption practices. Typically, a system administrator will make an initial investment of time and effort to install and configure the encryption products. Physician practices that do not employ a full-time system administrator may need to work with a contractor to accomplish the necessary set-up tasks. In many cases, you will need to work with your electronic medical transcription or practice management system vendor to have them implement the appropriate encryption technology on your system and to configure it properly.

After initial implementation, the process of encrypting and decrypting data should be virtually automatic—the most user involvement encryption may require is minimal effort to specify which data items should be encrypted. If the installation and set-up are completed properly, you should not experience any impact at all on workflow or normal operations.

12. How can I encrypt the data on my computers?

You have several choices. There are built-in encryption programs, such as Microsoft® Encrypting File System (EFS), which you can use simply by changing the properties of the folder in which the sensitive data is kept (if you use a computer with Microsoft Windows®). Most of the popular database technologies, such as Microsoft SQLServer®, MySQL®, Oracle®, and Sybase®, include an encryption option you can use. There are also several encryption products, such as Pretty Good Privacy® (PGP®), that you can purchase and install on your computer.

13. Is encryption expensive?

Encryption can be expensive, but it doesn't have to be. Some encryption programs are available at no cost. Microsoft EFS, for example, is shipped as part of the Windows operating system. Microsoft also provides whole-disk encryption on Windows 7 systems with a program called BitLocker™ Drive Encryption. Other programs, such as TrueCrypt®, may be downloaded and installed for free. At the other extreme, encryption devices known as hardware security modules (HSMs) can be quite expensive. The choice you make depends on many factors, including encryption strength, speed, available technical support and ease of use.

14. What is the best encryption technology to use?

In 2000, NIST sponsored a competition to identify the best available encryption algorithm. The Rijndael algorithm won the competition hands down. This algorithm has been designated as the current advanced encryption standard (AES). AES is a good choice for protecting *e*PHI.

FIGURE 4

Sample encryption program

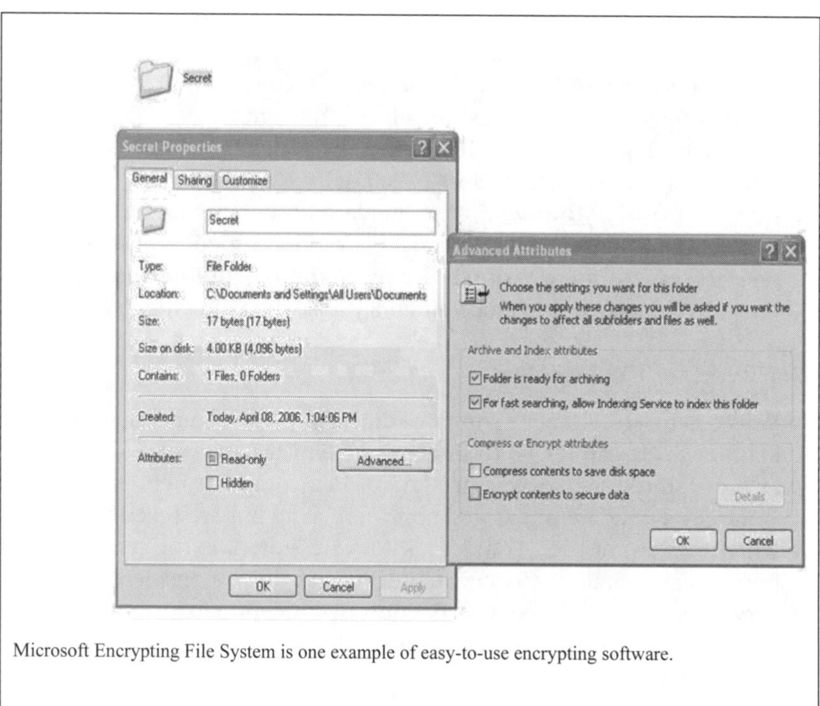

Microsoft Encrypting File System is one example of easy-to-use encrypting software.

The most widely used public-key algorithm is RSA. But this algorithm is not a good choice for protecting *e*PHI because it is much slower than AES. However, RSA is an excellent choice for encrypting electronic signatures and exchanging keys. A newer public-key algorithm is known as "elliptic curve cryptography" (ECC). NIST has specified a preference for ECC over RSA in future government procurement because ECC is believed to be stronger and faster than RSA.

The HHS Office for Civil Rights (OCR) has published guidance on choosing an encryption method on its **Web site**. The OCR guidance identifies ways to avoid the breach notification requirement—including recommended processes by NIST—and provides information on the new HIPAA breach notification requirements that HIPAA-covered entities must comply with. Following are several NIST publications that you may find useful:

- NIST Special Publication 800-111, "**Guide to Storage Encryption Technologies for End-User Devices**," provides extensive information on encrypting data on laptops
- NIST Special Publication 800-52, "**Guidelines for the Selection and Use of Transport Layer Security (TLS) Implementations**," includes detailed information on technologies that are used to protect sensitive Web site information
- NIST Special Publications 800-77, "**Guide to IPsec VPNs**," and **800-113**, "**Guide to SSL VPNs**," provide guidance on selecting the appropriate technology for establishing virtual private networks

Visit ***www.csrc.nist.gov/publications/PubsSPs.html*** to download all NIST Special Publications titles free of charge.

The OCR guidance also references the Federal Information Processing Standard (FIPS) 140-2, "**Security Requirements for Cryptographic Modules**." This standard describes a rating system that is used to evaluate commercial encryption products and assign a security level to them. Visit ***www.csrc.nist.gov/publications/PubsFIPS.html*** to download all FIPS publications free of charge.

15. Where are the keys kept?

Keys can be stored in a number of different places. Sometimes keys are kept on smart cards, USB flash drives or similar devices. Sometimes keys are stored on "key server" devices in a computer network. Sometimes keys are not stored anywhere at all but are regenerated when they are needed. Sometimes keys are stored on the same computers that contain the encrypted data—but this is considered to be a very insecure arrangement. HHS notes that an entity is **not** exempt from the breach notification requirements if the entity keeps the keys on the same device as the encrypted data.

For this reason, it is important that you know where your keys are kept. If the location of the key storage is not made clear in the product documentation, then you should ask your vendor before selecting a product for your practice. A number of encryption products allow you to choose where the keys are kept as an option during installation or configuration. Microsoft EFS, for example, allows you to decide whether the keys are kept on the same system as the encrypted data, on a floppy disk that you can remove from the system and store separately, or not stored at all but rather regenerated from a user-supplied password when needed.

Some people find it helpful to keep their key on an encrypted USB flash drive that they keep on their key chain with their car keys. To unencrypt their data, they just insert the flash drive and type in their password. For added security, it is even possible to get a flash drive with a thumb-print reader that is programmed to recognize only the user's thumb print.

16. What if a hacker finds the key?

If a hacker finds the key, the encrypted data to which that key provides access is no longer safe. That is why it is never a good idea to keep the key on the same device as the encrypted data. Visit ***www.ama-assn.org/go/pmc*** to access "**Steps physicians should take if in danger of identity theft**" for more information about protecting data that is no longer safe.

17. Why are people concerned about key size?

Key size can indicate how weak or strong the encryption is. As a general rule, the greater the key size, the better the data is protected (eg, a 256-bit key generally provides better protection than a 128-bit key). However, this is not always true. For example, data encrypted with the RSA algorithm using a 256-bit key is not as safe as data encrypted using the AES algorithm using a 128-bit key.

Most encryption products allow you to choose which encryption algorithm and which key size you will use. You are usually given a chance to make these decisions as an option during installation or configuration. While a larger key size generally provides greater protection, it can also result in slower performance. You will need to decide whether the slower performance is an acceptable trade-off for the greater security.

18. Can anything else go wrong?

One possible problem would be losing the encryption key and not being able to retrieve the encrypted information when you need it. **Make sure you have a back up of the key in a safe place.** Another problem would be using an old encryption algorithm, such as the "data encryption standard" (DES), that is no longer considered secure. Hackers have figured out how to break these out-of-date encryption standards and have even published their findings on the Internet. Yet another problem is not sufficiently protecting encryption keys. Using the strongest possible encryption method does not protect patient information if a hacker can find a way to break the security used to protect the keys.

19. I'm convinced that I need to encrypt my sensitive data. What should I do?

First, you need to tend to the most pressing problem areas. Refer to NIST Special Publication 800-66-Revision 1, "**An Introductory Resource Guide for Implementing the HIPAA Security Rule**," for guidance in addressing these areas.

- Encrypt any back-up media that leave your building.

  If you send back-up media to a vault, disaster recovery site or any other location, then any one of these items going astray would trigger a breach notification situation. This means that the back-up program that you use must include an encryption step. Fortunately, there are many back-up products that include this capability. Perform an Internet search on "back-up encryption software" to obtain a list of products that might fit your needs.

- Encrypt any e-mail that contains *e*PHI.

  If you currently correspond with patients, health insurers or other health care professionals via e-mail and those e-mails contain *e*PHI, then you could be accused of failing to protect *e*PHI for which you are responsible. There are two basic approaches to encrypting e-mail: PGP and S/MIME. PGP is a technology that was pioneered by the PGP Corporation, and S/MIME is the e-mail encryption capability that is built into Microsoft Outlook®. But these two are not the only e-mail encryption product vendors. Perform an Internet search on "e-mail encryption software" to get a more complete list of your options.

- Encrypt any laptops that contain *e*PHI.

  Even laptops that are protected with strong "boot passwords" are vulnerable. This is because a hacker can remove the hard drive from a stolen laptop and install it in a system that he or she controls. Only encryption can protect PHI on a laptop. Microsoft EFS, which is installed by default on all Windows systems, offers some protection, but "whole disk encryption" technology is a more secure solution. Perform an Internet search on "whole disk encryption software" to get an idea of products to consider.

- If *e*PHI is accessed via the Internet, encrypt these sessions.

  Check with your Web designer or Web services provider to ensure that any PHI that travels across the Internet is protected by SSL, TLS or similar technology.

- Encrypt any other remote access sessions.

  If you have situations in which physicians or staff from your practice connect to the home office remotely, such as physicians attending conferences who connect to read e-mail or access other resources containing *e*PHI, then this access may constitute a vulnerability to unauthorized snooping. It is important that these sessions be conducted using encrypted "tunnels," known as "virtual private networks" (VPNs). You have many options for implementing VPNs in your environment. Perform an Internet search on "virtual private networks" for more information. (Note that VPN technology usually requires experienced professional help to install and configure.)

Once you have addressed these areas, you can then consider the pros and cons of encrypting "data at rest" (data that never leaves your facility, such as data kept in your practice management system or other electronic medical record databases). Some people choose to encrypt all *e*PHI so that they have a "safety net" in the event that a hacker manages to penetrate their network defenses. Other people encrypt only that portion of the *e*PHI that actually leaves their facility. You should consider the recommendations of the OCR guidance as well as the cost/benefit tradeoffs before making a decision for your practice.

20. Where can I learn more?

The quickest and easiest way to obtain some good information is to perform an Internet search on "HIPAA PHI encryption." Many companies that sell HIPAA compliance solutions offer training and consulting advice in this area. Vendors who provide encryption hardware and software provide information in the form of "white papers" that are available through their Web sites. Technical support services, such as Microsoft TechNet, provide detailed information on configuring and using specific encryption products.

Following is a brief list of online resources if you wish to explore this subject further:

- RSA Laboratories Cryptography frequently asked questions (*www.rsasecurity.com/rsalabs/node.asp?id=2152*)
- The PKI Pages (*www.pki-page.org/*)
- History of Cryptography (*http://world.std.com/~cme/html/timeline.html*)

- List of Encryption Products (*www.timberlinetechnologies.com/products/encryption.html*)

Visit the HHS web site at *www.hhs.gov/ocr/privacy/* for updated guidance on encryption technology.

To download a PDF of *Understanding the HIPAA standard transactions: The HIPAA Transactions and Code Set rule*, go to *www.ama-assn.org/ama1/pub/upload/mm/368/hipaa-tcs.pdf.*

PRACTICE MANAGEMENT CENTER

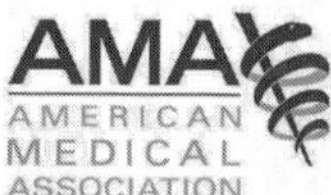

UNDERSTANDING THE HIPAA STANDARD TRANSACTIONS: THE HIPAA TRANSACTIONS AND CODE SET RULE

Many physician practices recognize the Health Information Portability and Accountability Act (HIPAA) as both a patient information privacy law and electronic patient information *security* law. However, HIPAA actually encompasses a number of regulations. As such, the federal government has published several "rules" that instruct the health care industry on how to comply with the law. HIPAA began as a bipartisan effort to provide portability of health insurance benefits to individuals who left the employment of a company that provided group health insurance (that is why HIPAA is the "Health Information Portability and Accountability Act").

In response to this initiative and the additional expense of billing individuals for continuation of coverage, the health insurance industry requested standardization and promotion of electronic health care transactions. The health insurance industry argued that electronic health care transactions would reduce administrative cost and justify the new costs associated with premium billing and administration that portability would create. The health insurance industry's request became the "administrative simplification" component, called "Health Insurance Reform: Standards for Electronic Transactions." These standards include both the form and format of electronic transactions as well as their content—such as the Current Procedural Terminology (CPT®)* and the International Classification of Diseases-9th Edition-Clinical Modification (ICD-9-CM) codes. This document refers to this part of HIPAA as the "Transaction and Code Set rule" (HIPAA TCS rule).

> Note: The Department of Health and Human Services (HHS) published two HIPAA final rules on January 16, 2009. One of these rules adopted version 005010. See the section "Upgrading to newer standards" for more information.

* CPT is a registered trademark of the American Medical Association.
The AMA Practice Management Center is a resource of the AMA Private Sector Advocacy unit.

The HIPAA standard transactions are designed to improve your claims management revenue cycle

The push for administrative simplification originated in the health insurance industry as a way to standardize the claims processing and payment cycle, the eligibility and enrollment cycle, and even health insurers' premium billing. However, use of the HIPAA standard transactions holds tremendous promise for physicians as a way to reduce their costs and overhead expenses associated with billing, collections, referral authorization, eligibility and other related components of the claims management revenue cycle. Physician practices that use the HIPAA standard electronic transactions are saving **thousands of dollars annually** by using the standard transactions. Visit the American Medical Association (AMA) Practice Management Center's web site to access the resource "**Follow that Claim**" for more information on these savings.

How is the HIPAA TCS rule related to the HIPAA Privacy and Security rules?

At the time HIPAA was enacted, the Internet was fast becoming a standard method of commerce and communication in its own right. Many people were concerned that promoting electronic health care transactions, especially over the Internet, would expose sensitive and confidential patient information to hackers and other entities that did not have authorized access. Thus, the HIPAA Privacy rule was developed as an attempt to establish a federal standard for protecting individually identifiable health information. During the development of the HIPAA Privacy rule, it became apparent that patient information was created, maintained and stored in electronic formats on computers and not just as paper records or oral communications. This realization resulted in the HIPAA Security rule, which deals with the administrative, physical and technical requirements that safeguard electronic protected health information that is maintained on computers and similar devices.

It is important to note that HIPAA does not require physicians to conduct transactions electronically, but if a physician practice conducts any of the transactions named under HIPAA, the physician practice must submit these transactions according to the HIPAA standards. Furthermore, under a separate but related law known as the Administrative Simplification Compliance Act (ASCA), most physician practices are required to submit their claims to Medicare electronically and in accordance with the HIPAA standards (physician practices that contain fewer than 10 full-time equivalents are exempt).

What are the Standard Transactions?

TABLE 1

Electronic transactions considered standard under HIPAA: Between a physician practice and health insurer

Common Name of Transaction	Formal Name of Transaction	Transaction Function
Claims	ASC* X12 837 Health Care Claim: Professional	Submitting claims to the health insurer
EOB/RA	ASC X12 835 Health Care Claim Payment/Remittance Advice	Receiving payment and/or remittance information from the health insurer for claims
Claim status	ASC X12 276 Heath Care Claim Status Request	Contacting the health insurer about the status of a claim
Claim status response	ASC X12 277 Health Care Claim Status Response	Receiving information about the status of a claim from the health insurer
Patient eligibility	ASC X12 270 Health Care Eligibility Benefit Inquiry	Contacting the health insurer about the eligibility and benefits of a patient
Patient eligibility response	ASC X12 271 Response	Receiving information from the health insurer about the eligibility and benefits of a patient
Referrals	ASC X12 278 Health Care Services Review Information	Sending or receiving referrals or authorizations
Coordination of benefits	ASC X12 837 Health Care Claim: Professional	Determining payment responsibilities of the health insurer
Claims attachments†	ASC X12 275 Additional Information to Support a Health Care Claim or Encounter	Submitting claims attachments to the health insurer
First report of injury†	ASC X12 148 First Report of Injury, Illness or Incident	First report of injury to the health insurer

* Accredited Standards Committee

† Note: Standards for claims attachments and first report of injury have not yet been adopted.

TABLE 2

Electronic transactions considered standard under HIPAA: Between an insurance purchaser and a health insurer or between health insurers

Common Name of Transaction	Formal Name of Transaction	Transaction Function
Membership enrollment	ASC X12 834 Benefit Enrollment and Maintenance	Enrolling members in the health plan
Premium payments	ASC X12 820 Payment Order and Remittance Advice	Making premium payments for the health insurance coverage
Coordination of benefits	ASC X12 837 Health Care Claim: Professional	Coordination of benefits

What is X12?

Health care industry groups develop standards, which the government then adopts. The HIPAA TCS rule adopts the standards for the transactions included in **Table 1: Electronic transactions considered standard under HIPAA: Between a physician practice and a health insurer** and **Table 2: Electronic transactions considered standard under HIPAA: Between an insurance purchaser and a health insurer or between health insurers**, as defined by the Accredited Standards Committee (ASC) X12. Recognized by the Department of Health and Human Services (HHS), ASC X12 is a standards development organization that focuses on developing standards for electronic information exchanges. ASC X12 has subcommittees that focus on different industries, such as finance, government, transportation and insurance. The AMA is a member of ASC X12 and participates on the Insurance Subcommittee (X12N), which has a task group focused on health care (TG2). X12N TG2 develops and maintains standards related to the health care insurance industry, such as the standards in **Table 1** and **Table 2**.

What is an Implementation Guide?

The X12N subcommittee has documented the specific details of each HIPAA standard transaction in an implementation guide. The implementation guide is a very detailed document that defines:

- The electronic format of the transaction
- The details of the necessary data and where to place them in the electronic file
- The details of the various code sets that are used and how to use them
- The kind of electronic "envelopes" each transaction requires (these are sometimes known as the headers and control documents)
- References for the different code sets used in that transaction

The implementation guides are complex documents. For example, the X12 837 professional version for health care claims is 768 pages in length. The primary entities that use these guides are: (1) health insurers (to program their software to process claims); (2) clearinghouses (to ensure that claims conform to the implementation guides); and (3) physician practice management software vendors (to program their software to capture information and transmit a compliant standard transaction or receive and process a standard transaction). The first version of the guides that the government adopted is known as version 004010.

Upgrading to Newer Standards

Similar to upgrading software programs for computers to meet new market needs, ASC X12 continues to update the HIPAA transactions to better meet health care business needs. While there are multiple versions of X12 health care transactions, the version that the government first adopted under HIPAA was version 004010. These guides were followed by an addendum; thus, the current implementation guides are 004010A1. The latest completed version of the X12 HIPAA transactions, version 005010, was recommended to HHS for adoption under HIPAA and has been adopted for implementation in January 2012. The 005010 version resolves many practical issues that were identified in version 004010, especially related to the use of situational codes (codes that are used only when a specific situation is in place), and adds and deleted certain code sets that are difficult to use or have been deemed unnecessary.

For example, the current version of the remittance advice (the X12 835 transaction) does not require health insurers to specify when they received a claim from a physician practice. Without this information, it may be difficult for the physician practice to calculate interest due on untimely payments. The 005010 version requires Claim Received Date as a specific data element.

The 005010 version has recently been named in regulation, and all HIPAA-covered entities (health insurers, physicians and clearinghouses) are required to adopt the 005010 version by January 1, 2012. Implementing the version 005010 transactions will require changes to practice management systems, changes to some data reporting requirements, potential changes to work flow processes and staff training. This transition period also provides physician practices with the opportunity to implement other HIPAA transactions they are not currently using, such as checking a patient's eligibility or the status of a claim.

Another recent regulation will also require the replacement of the ICD-9-CM code sets with International Classification of Diseases-10th Edition-Clinical Modification (ICD-10-CM) on October 1, 2013. Because the 004010 version of the HIPAA transactions does not accommodate the format of the ICD-10-CM codes, implementation of the 005010 transactions is required in order to move to the ICD-10-CM code set.

What are Companion Guides?

The health care industry has provided a method of communicating how an individual "trading partner" will implement an X12 standard; the collection of this implementation information is known as a "companion guide." (A trading partner is a vendor with which a physician practice exchanges patient data or protected health information electronically in the course of its operations.) The X12 implementation guides provide some flexibility in terms of data elements that can be used. The complexity of these transactions also sometimes requires health insurers to implement these transactions in phases as they update their internal software or business processes.

Health insurers publish companion guides that provide detailed information about their specific implementation of a HIPAA standard transaction and any pertinent requirements. These guides are usually available for review on health insurers' Web sites. Health insurers may change and modify their companion guides whenever they make a change to their implementation of a HIPAA standard transaction. For example, a health insurer might begin to use situational codes (many health insurers did not require situational codes when they first implemented HIPAA standard transactions). The materials in the implementation and health insurers' companion guides contain important information for physician practices' software vendors. These vendors are frequently the ones that ensure physician practices are able to send their claims and other transactions according to the X12N standards and the health insurer requirements.

Companion guides in real life

When a health insurer changes its companion guide, a change is reflected in its implementation of the HIPAA standard transactions. Some of these changes could result in claims processing delays or denials. For example, if your practice management system does not currently use one of the HIPAA-required designated situational codes (such as birth weight), and a health insurer decides to place a claim edit on this field, the claim will be denied.

How will you know whether a companion guide change is going to affect you and suddenly result in a claim rejection? It is virtually impossible for most physician practices to audit the companion guides of each contracted health insurer and then remain on top of the constant changes. There are more than 1200 companion guides, and each one can be hundreds of pages in length.

A practical solution is to choose a practice management software, billing service or a clearinghouse that can assure you it can perform this function. You may also need to continue to update and modify your practice management software to ensure compliance with the health insurers' claim submission requirements.

Determine whether your vendor will be staying up to date on health insurer claim submission requirements. If not, or if you are a small physician practice, consider a claims clearinghouse approach, in which the clearinghouse commits to remaining current. You can also implement a system of routine review of companion guides, at least for the health insurers with which you submit the most claims.

How is the HIPAA TCS Rule Enforced?

October 16, 2003 was the deadline for HIPAA-covered entities (health insurers, physicians and clearinghouses) to comply with HIPAA's electronic transaction and code set provisions, and January 1, 2012 will be the adoption date for use of the updated transactions, version 005010. However, some health insurers still have not adopted all of the standard transactions or implemented the code set edits and rules. For example, some health insurers may accept an electronic claim (X12 837) but do not create an electronic remittance advice (X12 835) or do not provide an electronic claims status transaction (X12 277). This inconsistency creates a burden for physician practices.

As a best practice, you should be able to check eligibility electronically (X12 270/271) with every health insurer. By implementing this best practice, you will receive written documentation of patient eligibility and avoid excessive telephone wait times. Consider how using these electronic transactions would improve your practice efficiency.

The AMA strongly encourages health insurers to use the HIPAA standard transactions. The HIPAA regulation states, "If an entity requests a health plan to conduct a transaction as a standard transaction the health plan must do so." 45 CFR §162.925

Non-compliance by a health insurer

Health insurers and self-insured employer-sponsored health insurers are covered entities under HIPAA. As such, they must comply with all applicable HIPAA regulations, including the HIPAA TCS rule. A health insurer that does not accept a standard transaction or produce one of the transactions for which it is responsible (such as the electronic remittance advice) is in violation of the law.

The AMA urges physicians to ask health insurers with which they work to comply with HIPAA. If the health insurers do not comply, you can file a complaint using the AMA HIPAA complaint form.

The Centers for Medicare & Medicaid Services (CMS) has stated it will focus on voluntary and complaint-driven enforcement. If you are ready to use the standard transactions and you have a health insurer that is not cooperating, consider filing a complaint.

What are the typical areas in which health insurers are not compliant, and how does this noncompliance increase physician practice costs?

The health insurer does not accept X12 837 Health Care Claim. As a result, your practice's clearinghouse must convert your electronic claim to paper and send that paper claim to the health insurer. Both of these steps cost you time and money in getting the claim paid.

The health insurer does not offer Health Care Claim Payment/ Remittance Advice X12 835. If your practice management software supports this feature, the health insurer's non-compliance will prevent you from automatically posting the payment. It will also prevent you from using electronic denial management and other electronic payment reconciliation tools that dramatically improve payment recovery.

The health insurer does not accept the Health Care Eligibility Verification Benefit Inquiry X12 270 or provide the Response X12 271. When the only option is the health insurer's Web portal, your practice will not realize the full cost savings of direct electronic transactions and will incur additional expense by manually re-entering eligibility request information on multiple health insurers' Web sites and verifying eligibility through phone calls.

The health insurer does not accept Health Care Services Review Information (referral authorization) X12 278. If your practice performs these two functions manually by phone or fax or through the health insurer's Web portal, your practice will not achieve the cost savings possible through performing these functions electronically.

The health insurer does not accept the Health Care Claims Status Request X12 276 or provide the Response X12 277. Avoiding the follow-up time of manually tracking claims will reduce administrative time and expense for your practice.

Health insurer Web portals

Using health insurer Web portals is not as cost efficient as using the HIPAA standard transactions. Using a Web portal requires your practice to re-key data that is already in your practice management system and visit different Web portals for each health insurer. In addition, you have to re-key the response data received from the Web portal, such as referral authorization numbers, which could otherwise be posted electronically in your practice management system.

Your state may mandate the use of HIPAA standard transactions

States may begin to help in the enforcement effort by mandating that any health insurer doing business in their state use the HIPAA standard transactions. For example, Minnesota passed legislation that became effective in 2009 that requires health insurers and health care providers to use the standard transactions. This law requires the exchange of eligibility, claim, and payment and remittance advice information electronically. Other states are considering similar legislation. The push at the state level for adoption of the HIPAA standard transactions is aimed at reducing administrative costs associated with the claims management revenue cycle.

What are the HIPAA Transaction Code Sets?

The HIPAA TCS are a major component of each standard transaction. In many cases, the code sets are familiar to most physician practices (for example, CPT codes or ICD-9-CM codes). Code sets may also be ones that you do not actively choose during a patient encounter but are instead behind the scenes. Two examples of such code sets are Place of Service codes and relationship codes (the relationship of the patient to the insurance guarantor).

There are also many new codes that have been developed for the X12 transactions. For example, the X12 835 remittance now has standardized claims adjustment reason and remark codes. Using standardized codes for X12 835 remittance advice may provide a practice management system with the logic it needs to automatically and correctly post a payment.

When the code set is part of a transaction you submit, such as the electronic claim, eligibility request or claim status, it is important that you understand how the codes within the code set are used, and you should also have a way of entering these codes into your practice management software. When a code is contained in a transaction you receive, such as the electronic remittance advice, being familiar with the meaning of the code is helpful. But not every health insurer uses the code sets the same way. Some health insurers will use a very specific adjustment reason code and related remark code for each line item they adjudicate, while other health insurers may use more generalized codes. This inconsistency makes your efforts to process an electronic remittance advice and determine the accuracy of the payment more difficult.

AMA Practice Management Center tip

Visit *www.ama-assn.org/go/pmc* to learn more about the inconsistency in use of the reason and remark codes with the AMA's **National Health Insurer Report Card**.

A number of different organizations maintain the code sets. The various X12 subcommittees maintain some of these code sets, and other organizations maintain other code sets. For example, the AMA maintains the CPT® codes, the National Uniform Claim Committee maintains the Health Care Provider Taxonomy code set and CMS maintains the Place of Service code set.

How can physicians improve practice efficiencies by using HIPAA standard transactions?

Steps you can take to improve practice efficiency

Using the HIPAA standard transactions can bring efficiency and cost savings to physician practices. If you are not sure how these transactions will help your practice or what you may need to do in preparation, a good place to start is conducting a brief internal assessment.

The **first step** of an internal assessment is to determine whether you are currently submitting or receiving any of the following transactions:

- X12 837 Electronic Claims
- X12 835 Remittance Advice
- X12 270/271 Eligibility Benefit Inquiry and Response
- X12 276/277 Claim Status Inquiry and Response

The requirement for the claims attachment standard transaction has not yet been adopted, but you should keep this future standard transaction in mind when evaluating your practice management system.

The **second step** of an internal assessment is to understand some basic information about your claims management revenue cycle process by answering the following questions:

- Do you use a billing service?
- Do you maintain your own billing software?
- If you create electronic claims, are they HIPAA-compliant standard transactions? Many older versions of practice management software that physician practices and billing services use do not create a standard transaction but instead rely on a clearinghouse to take the paper claims' print image or other format and convert those to electronic claims. This method is only a temporary solution.
- Do you use a clearinghouse? Does the clearinghouse offer any other transactions in addition to claims?
- Are you a specialty physician practice that might be impacted by the situational fields and new code sets?
- How much time and cost does your practice spend to manually verify eligibility, check claims status or manage referral authorizations?
- How much time does your practice spend posting manual remittance advice?

The **third step** of an internal assessment is to understand how well your practice management system vendor, billing service and/or clearinghouse supports the HIPAA standard transactions.

Practice Management Software and Billing Service Vendor Readiness

It is imperative to understand how your practice management software and billing vendors are complying with the HIPAA TCS rule. First, determine how many vendors are involved. For example, you might have one vendor for your billing and claims generation and another vendor for electronic eligibility or referral authorizations. Survey each vendor by asking them to complete the **AMA vendor survey tool** (PDF, 79KB).

Clearinghouse Readiness

If you currently use a clearinghouse, you should determine the clearinghouse's ability to provide standard transactions and the costs associated with providing those transactions. For example, some clearinghouses charge per physician and others per transaction. You should know how the clearinghouse(s) you are considering will charge your practice for services prior to selecting a clearinghouse as a solution. You should be aware that some clearinghouses that perform HIPAA standard transactions may also convert to paper any electronic claims that they cannot process. In some cases, the clearinghouse performs this conversion because it has not tested its HIPAA standard transactions with the health insurer. Sometimes it is more efficient to use the clearinghouse as a portal for standard transactions other than claims. Competent clearinghouses should provide a mechanism to receive the electronic remittance advice, submit an eligibility and benefits verification request, receive a response, and review the claim's status.

Questions or concerns about practice management issues?

AMA members and their practice staff may e-mail the AMA Practice Management Center at ***practicemanagementcenter@ama-assn.org*** for assistance.

For additional information and resources, there are three easy ways to contact the AMA Practice Management Center:

- Call **(800) 621-8335** and ask for the AMA Practice Management Center.
- Fax information to **(312) 464-5541**.
- Visit *www.ama-assn.org/go/pmc* to access the AMA Practice Management Center Web site.

Physicians and their practice staff can also visit *www.ama-assn.org/go/pmalerts* to sign up for free Practice Management Alerts, which help you stay up to date on unfair payer practices, ways to counter these practices, and practice management resources and tools.

The AMA Practice Management Center is a resource of the AMA Private Sector Advocacy unit.

This informational resource was developed through a cooperative effort between the American Medical Association and PrivaPlan Associates, Inc.
The AMA Practice Management Center is a resource of the AMA Private Sector Advocacy unit.

To download a PDF of *Health Insurance Portability and Accountability Act (HIPAA) Transaction Code Set Vendor survey*, visit *www.ama-assn.org/ama1/x-ama/upload/mm/368/tcs-vendor-survey.pdf.*

PRACTICE MANAGEMENT CENTER

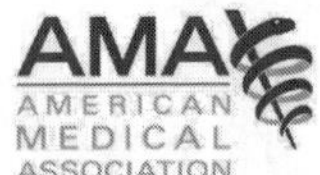

American Medical Association (AMA) Health Insurance Portability and Accountability Act (HIPAA) Transaction Code Set Vendor survey

You can submit the following questions to your vendor(s), or you can ask your sales or support representative to answer them. We recommend that you request the answers in writing.

If selecting a new billing or practice management software/system, please visit *www.ama-assn.org/go/pmc* and view the resource under "Health Information Technology" "How to select a billing software vendor for the physician practice" (PDF, 106KB) for a billing software/system vendor comparison checklist.

This informational resource was developed through a cooperative effort between the American Medical Association and PrivaPlan Associates, Inc.
The AMA Practice Management Center is a resource of the AMA Private Sector Advocacy unit.

Vendor survey: This version can be used as a reference for the physician practice.

Please list the name and current version number of your practice management software/system: ______________________________

Question	Comments	Responses
1) Please list the HIPAA standard transactions your software/system creates or receives.	The list can include: • X12 270 Health Care Eligibility and Benefit Inquiry • X12 271 Health Care Eligibility Benefit Inquiry and Response • X12 276 Health Care Claims Status Inquiry • X12 277 Health Care Claim Status Response • X12 278 Referral Certification and Authorization • X12 835 Health Care Claim Payment and Remittance Advice • X12 837 Health Care Claim or Encounter: Professional • X12 997 Functional Acknowledgement	
2) Please describe how you test your software/system's compliance with the HIPAA standard transactions.	Vendors should have a formal mechanism to determine whether its transactions are indeed compliant with HIPAA standard transactions. Vendors can use third-party certification firms or an internal process to test their compliance with HIPAA standard transactions.	
3) Does your software/system perform direct sending (X12 837 Health Care Claim or Encounter: Professional) or receiving (X12 835 Health Care Claim Payment and Remittance Advice) of electronic transactions with any health insurers?	Some vendors rely on clearinghouses to send electronic claims. This usually is an indication that the vendor has not updated its software/system adequately for the HIPAA standard transactions. This reliance also limits use of the other standard transactions.	

This informational resource was developed through a cooperative effort between the American Medical Association and PrivaPlan Associates, Inc.
The Practice Management Center is a resource of the AMA Private Sector Advocacy unit.

Question	Comments	Responses
4) If you are using a clearinghouse approach, will you keep your software/system updated to provide clients the ability to enter new required HIPAA transaction code sets?	Some vendors have decided not to upgrade their software/system to generate the new HIPAA standard transaction code sets but have instead employed a clearinghouse to perform the "translation." This may be a concern when HIPAA transaction code sets are revised or updated with new standards.	
5) Does your software/system log the date a claim was received? If so, does it rely on the X12 997 Functional Acknowledgment? If your software/system does not use the X12 997 Functional Acknowledgment, what other method does your software/system use to determine whether the health insurer received the electronic claim?	If the software/system can directly send electronic claims to a health insurer, it is important that the software/system be able to record that the claims were received and acknowledged. If a clearinghouse is used for claims submission, you are encouraged to verify that the clearinghouse makes the record that the claims were received and acknowledged.	
6) Does your software/system automatically post the payments from an X12 835 Health Care Claim Payment and Remittance Advice?	One of the primary advantages to receiving an electronic X12 835 Health Care Claim Payment and Remittance Advice is the ability to post uncomplicated payments directly to the patient's account.	
7) Does your software/system automatically send eligibility requests (X12 270 Healthcare Eligibility and Benefit Inquiry transactions) from the appointment scheduler?	The vendor ability to send eligibility requests automatically from the appointment scheduler can simplify the eligibility verification process and demonstrates that the vendor can create an X12 270 Health Care Eligibility and Benefit Inquiry transaction.	

This informational resource was developed through a cooperative effort between the American Medical Association and PrivaPlan Associates, Inc.
The Practice Management Center is a resource of the AMA Private Sector Advocacy unit.

Question	Comments	Responses
8) What are your plans for upgrading to the version 005010 X12 transactions? Will there be a separate upgrade fee in addition to your annual maintenance and support fee? How soon will the upgraded software be available for installation?	Recent regulation requires the use of the version 005010 transactions beginning January 1, 2012. System upgrades must be completed prior to the compliance date. The regulation also allows the use of the 005010 transactions prior to the compliance date, which will provide an opportunity to identify any issues and resolve them prior to the compliance deadline.	
9) What are your plans for upgrading the software/ system to ICD-10? Will there be a separate upgrade fee in addition to your annual maintenance and support fee? How soon will the upgraded software be available for installation?	ICD-10 may be the most profound standards change since the National Provider Identifier was implemented. Recent regulation will require the use of the ICD-10 code sets beginning October 1, 2013. System upgrades must be completed prior to the compliance date.	
10) Please describe how your organization stays up to date with changes to the HIPAA transactions and code sets and the HIPAA implementation guides.	Your vendor should help you stay up to date on changes to the HIPAA transaction code sets.	
11) Will your organization sign the Council for Affordable Quality Healthcare (CAQH) Committee on Operating Rules for Information Exchange (CORE) pledge and become CORE Phase II certified? Visit *www.caqh .org* for more information.	The CAQH CORE has developed a series of operating rules that expand the X12 270/271 Healthcare Eligibility Benefit Inquiry and Response Transactions. An organization that obtains Phase II certification will have the most current implementation of this transaction.	

This informational resource was developed through a cooperative effort between the American Medical Association and PrivaPlan Associates, Inc.
The Practice Management Center is a resource of the AMA Private Sector Advocacy unit.

Vendor survey: This version can be completed by the vendor.

Please list the name and current version number of your practice management software/system: ______________________________

Question	Responses
1) Please list the HIPAA standard transactions your software/system creates or receives.	
2) Please describe how you test your software/system's compliance with the HIPAA standard transactions.	
3) Does your software/system perform direct sending (X12 837 Health Care Claim or Encounter: Professional) or receiving (X12 835 Health Care Claim Payment and Remittance Advice) of electronic transactions with any health insurers?	
4) If you are using a clearinghouse approach, will you keep your software/system updated to provide clients the ability to enter new required HIPAA transaction code sets?	
5) Does your software/system log the date a claim was received? If so, does it rely on the X12 997 Functional Acknowledgment? If your software/system does not use the X12 997 Functional Acknowledgment, what other method does your software/system use to determine that the health insurer received the electronic claim?	
6) Does your software/system automatically post the payments from an X12 835 Health Care Claim Payment and Remittance Advice?	
7) Does your software/system automatically send eligibility requests (X12 270 Healthcare Eligibility and Benefit Inquiry transactions) from the appointment scheduler?	

Question	Responses
8) What are your plans for upgrading to the version 005010 X12 transactions? Will there be a separate upgrade fee in addition to your annual maintenance and support fee? How soon will the upgraded software be available for installation?	
9) What are your plans for upgrading the software/system to ICD-10? Will there be a separate upgrade fee in addition to your annual maintenance and support fee? How soon will the upgraded software be available for installation?	
10) Please describe how your organization stays up to date on changes to the HIPAA transactions and code sets and the HIPAA Implementation Guides.	
11) Will your organization sign the Council for Affordable Quality Healthcare (CAQH) Committee on Operating Rules for Information Exchange (CORE) pledge and become CORE Phase II certified? Visit *www.caqh.org* for more information.	

This informational resource was developed through a cooperative effort between the American Medical Association and PrivaPlan Associates, Inc.
The Practice Management Center is a resource of the AMA Private Sector Advocacy unit.

For additional information on HIPAA and HIPAA-related topics, visit:

- *www.ama-assn.org/go/hipaa*
- *www.ama-assn.org/go/5010*
- *www.ama-assn.org/go/icd-10.*

glossary

Definitions[1]

Except as otherwise provided, the following definitions apply to subpart sections as noted:

Access means the ability or the means necessary to read, write, modify, or communicate data/information or otherwise use any system resource. (This definition applies to "access" as used in this subpart, not as used in subparts D or E of this part.) **§ 164.304**

Act means the Social Security Act. **§ 160.103**

Administrative safeguards are administrative actions, and policies and procedures, to manage the selection, development, implementation, and maintenance of security measures to protect electronic protected health information and to manage the conduct of the covered entity's workforce in relation to the protection of that information. **§ 164.304**

Administrative simplification provision means any requirement or prohibition established by:

(1) 42 U.S.C. 1320d—1320d-4, 1320d-7, and 1320d-8;

(2) Section 264 of Pub. L. 104-191; or

(3) This subchapter. **§ 160.302**

ALJ means Administrative Law Judge. **§ 160.302**

ANSI stands for the American National Standards Institute. **§ 160.103**

---

1. The HIPAA Administrative Simplification definitions in this section are from the *electronic Code of Federal Regulations* (eCFR), which is available at http://ecfr.gpoaccess.gov. The definitions are current as of August 17, 2010. They are from Title 45 (Public Welfare), Subtitle A (Department of Health and Human Services), Subchapter C (Administrative Data Standards and Related Requirements), Parts 160 (General Administrative Requirements), 162 (Administrative Requirements), and 164 (Security and Privacy). At the end of each definition, in bold, is the location designator of the part and subpart section where the definition is located. For example, the definition, *Administrative safeguards*, is located in **§ 164.304:** The Security and Privacy part (164) and Security Standards for the Protection of Electronic Protected Health Information subpart (C) Definitions section (304).

Authentication means the corroboration that a person is the one claimed. **§ 164.304**

Availability means the property that data or information is accessible and useable upon demand by an authorized person. **§ 164.304**

Board means the members of the HHS Departmental Appeals Board, in the Office of the Secretary, who issue decisions in panels of three. **§ 160.502**

Breach means the acquisition, access, use, or disclosure of protected health information in a manner not permitted under subpart E of this part which compromises the security or privacy of the protected health information.

(1) (i) For purposes of this definition, *compromises the security or privacy of the protected health information* means poses a significant risk of financial, reputational, or other harm to the individual.

(ii) A use or disclosure of protected health information that does not include the identifiers listed at §164.514(e)(2), date of birth, and zip code does not compromise the security or privacy of the protected health information.

(2) Breach excludes:

(i) Any unintentional acquisition, access, or use of protected health information by a workforce member or person acting under the authority of a covered entity or a business associate, if such acquisition, access, or use was made in good faith and within the scope of authority and does not result in further use or disclosure in a manner not permitted under subpart E of this part.

(ii) Any inadvertent disclosure by a person who is authorized to access protected health information at a covered entity or business associate to another person authorized to access protected health information at the same covered entity or business associate, or organized health care arrangement in which the covered entity participates, and the information received as a result of such disclosure is not further used or disclosed in a manner not permitted under subpart E of this part.

(iii) A disclosure of protected health information where a covered entity or business associate has a good faith belief that an unauthorized person to whom the disclosure was made would not reasonably have been able to retain such information. **§ 164.402**

Business associate: (1) Except as provided in paragraph (2) of this definition, *business associate* means, with respect to a covered entity, a person who:

(i) On behalf of such covered entity or of an organized health care arrangement (as defined in §164.501 of this subchapter) in which the covered entity participates, but other than in the capacity of a member of the workforce of such covered entity or arrangement, performs, or assists in the performance of:

(A) A function or activity involving the use or disclosure of individually identifiable health information, including claims processing or administration, data analysis, processing or administration, utilization review, quality assurance, billing, benefit management, practice management, and repricing; or

(B) Any other function or activity regulated by this subchapter; or

(ii) Provides, other than in the capacity of a member of the workforce of such covered entity, legal, actuarial, accounting, consulting, data aggregation (as defined in §164.501 of this subchapter), management, administrative, accreditation, or financial services to or for such covered entity, or to or for an organized health care arrangement in which the covered entity participates, where the provision of the service involves the disclosure of individually identifiable health information from such covered entity or arrangement, or from another business associate of such covered entity or arrangement, to the person.

(2) A covered entity participating in an organized health care arrangement that performs a function or activity as described by paragraph (1)(i) of this definition for or on behalf of such organized health care arrangement, or that provides a service as described in paragraph (1)(ii) of this definition to or for such organized health care arrangement, does not, simply through the performance of such function or activity or the provision of such service, become a business associate of other covered entities participating in such organized health care arrangement.

(3) A covered entity may be a business associate of another covered entity. **§ 160.103**

Civil money penalty or ***penalty*** means the amount determined under §160.404 of this part and includes the plural of these terms. **§ 160.302**

CMS stands for Centers for Medicare & Medicaid Services within the Department of Health and Human Services. **§ 160.103**

Code set means any set of codes used to encode data elements, such as tables of terms, medical concepts, medical diagnostic codes, or medical procedure codes. A code set includes the codes and the descriptors of the codes. **§ 162.103**

Code set maintaining organization means an organization that creates and maintains the code sets adopted by the Secretary for use in the transactions for which standards are adopted in this part. **§ 162.103**

Common control exists if an entity has the power, directly or indirectly, significantly to influence or direct the actions or policies of another entity. **§ 164.103**

Common ownership exists if an entity or entities possess an ownership or equity interest of 5 percent or more in another entity. **§ 164.103**

Compliance date means the date by which a covered entity must comply with a standard, implementation specification, requirement, or modification adopted under this subchapter. **§ 160.103**

Confidentiality means the property that data or information is not made available or disclosed to unauthorized persons or processes. **§ 164.304**

Contrary, when used to compare a provision of state law to a standard, requirement, or implementation specification adopted under this subchapter, means:

(1) A covered entity would find it impossible to comply with both the state and federal requirements; or

(2) The provision of state law stands as an obstacle to the accomplishment and execution of the full purposes and objectives of part C of title XI of the Act, section 264 of Public Law 104–191, or section 13402 of Public Law 111–5, as applicable. **§ 160.202**

Correctional institution means any penal or correctional facility, jail, reformatory, detention center, work farm, halfway house, or residential community program center operated by, or under contract to, the United States, a state, a territory, a political subdivision of a state or territory, or an Indian tribe, for the confinement or rehabilitation of persons charged with or convicted of a criminal offense or other persons held in lawful custody. *Other persons* held in lawful custody includes juvenile offenders adjudicated delinquent, aliens detained awaiting deportation, persons committed to mental institutions through the criminal justice system, witnesses, or others awaiting charges or trial. **§ 164.501**

Covered entity means:

(1) A health plan.

(2) A health care clearinghouse.

(3) A health care provider who transmits any health information in electronic form in connection with a transaction covered by this subchapter. **§ 160.103**

Covered functions means those functions of a covered entity the performance of which makes the entity a health plan, health care provider, or health care clearinghouse. **§ 164.103**

Covered health care provider means a health care provider that meets the definition at paragraph (3) of the definition of "covered entity" at §160.103 of this subchapter. **§ 162.402**

Data aggregation means, with respect to protected health information created or received by a business associate in its capacity as the business associate of a covered entity, the combining of such protected health information by the business associate with the protected health information received by the business associate in its capacity as a business associate of another covered entity, to permit data analyses that relate to the health care operations of the respective covered entities. **§ 164.501**

Data condition means the rule that describes the circumstances under which a covered entity must use a particular data element or segment. **§ 162.103**

Data content means all the data elements and code sets inherent to a transaction, and not related to the format of the transaction. Data elements that are related to the format are not data content. **§ 162.103**

Data element means the smallest named unit of information in a transaction. **§ 162.103**

Data set means a semantically meaningful unit of information exchanged between two parties to a transaction. **§ 162.103**

Descriptor means the text defining a code. **§ 162.103**

Designated record set means:

(1) A group of records maintained by or for a covered entity that is:
   (i) The medical records and billing records about individuals maintained by or for a covered health care provider;
   (ii) The enrollment, payment, claims adjudication, and case or medical management record systems maintained by or for a health plan; or
   (iii) Used, in whole or in part, by or for the covered entity to make decisions about individuals.

(2) For purposes of this paragraph, the term *record* means any item, collection, or grouping of information that includes protected health information and is maintained, collected, used, or disseminated by or for a covered entity. **§ 164.501**

Designated standard maintenance organization (DSMO) means an organization designated by the Secretary under §162.910(a). **§ 162.103**

Direct treatment relationship means a treatment relationship between an individual and a health care provider that is not an indirect treatment relationship. **§ 164.501**

Direct data entry means the direct entry of data (for example, using dumb terminals or Web browsers) that is immediately transmitted into a health plan's computer. **§ 162.103**

Disclosure means the release, transfer, provision of, access to, or divulging in any other manner of information outside the entity holding the information. **§ 160.103**

EIN stands for the employer identification number assigned by the Internal Revenue Service, U.S. Department of the Treasury. The EIN is the taxpayer identifying number of an individual or other entity (whether or not an employer) assigned under one of the following:

(1) 26 U.S.C. 6011(b), which is the portion of the Internal Revenue Code dealing with identifying the taxpayer in tax returns and statements, or corresponding provisions of prior law.

(2) 26 U.S.C. 6109, which is the portion of the Internal Revenue Code dealing with identifying numbers in tax returns, statements, and other required documents. **§ 160.103**

Electronic media means:

(1) Electronic storage media including memory devices in computers (hard drives) and any removable/transportable digital memory medium, such as magnetic tape or disk, optical disk, or digital memory card; or

(2) Transmission media used to exchange information already in electronic storage media. Transmission media include, for example, the Internet (wide-open), extranet (using Internet technology to link a business with information accessible only to collaborating parties), leased lines, dial-up lines, private networks, and the physical movement of removable/transportable electronic storage media. Certain transmissions, including of paper, via facsimile, and of voice, via telephone, are not considered to be transmissions via electronic media, because the information being exchanged did not exist in electronic form before the transmission. **§ 160.103**

Electronic protected health information means information that comes within paragraphs (1)(i) or (1)(ii) of the definition of *protected health information* as specified in this section. **§ 160.103**

Employer is defined as it is in 26 U.S.C. 3401(d). **§ 160.103**

Encryption means the use of an algorithmic process to transform data into a form in which there is a low probability of assigning meaning without use of a confidential process or key. **§ 164.304**

Facility means the physical premises and the interior and exterior of a building(s). **§ 164.304**

Format refers to those data elements that provide or control the enveloping or hierarchical structure, or assist in identifying data content of, a transaction. **§ 162.103**

Group health plan (also see definition of *health plan* in this section) means an employee welfare benefit plan (as defined in section 3(1) of the Employee Retirement Income and Security Act of 1974 (ERISA), 29 U.S.C. 1002(1)), including insured and self-insured plans, to the extent that the plan provides medical care (as defined in section 2791(a)(2) of the Public Health Service Act (PHS Act), 42 U.S.C. 300gg-91(a)(2)), including items and services paid for as medical care, to employees or their dependents directly or through insurance, reimbursement, or otherwise, that:

(1) Has 50 or more participants (as defined in section 3(7) of ERISA, 29 U.S.C. 1002(7)); or

(2) Is administered by an entity other than the employer that established and maintains the plan. **§ 160.103**

HCPCS stands for the Health [Care Financing Administration] Common Procedure Coding System. **§ 162.103**

HHS stands for the Department of Health and Human Services. **§ 160.103**

Health care means care, services, or supplies related to the health of an individual. *Health care* includes, but is not limited to, the following:

(1) Preventive, diagnostic, therapeutic, rehabilitative, maintenance, or palliative care, and counseling, service, assessment, or procedure with respect to the physical or mental condition, or functional status, of an individual or that affects the structure or function of the body; and

(2) Sale or dispensing of a drug, device, equipment, or other item in accordance with a prescription. **§ 160.103**

Health care clearinghouse means a public or private entity, including a billing service, repricing company, community health management information system or community health information system, and "value-added" networks and switches, that does either of the following functions:

(1) Processes or facilitates the processing of health information received from another entity in a nonstandard format or containing nonstandard data content into standard data elements or a standard transaction.

(2) Receives a standard transaction from another entity and processes or facilitates the processing of health information into nonstandard format or nonstandard data content for the receiving entity. **§ 160.103**

Health care component means a component or combination of components of a hybrid entity designated by the hybrid entity in accordance with §164.105(a)(2)(iii)(C). **§ 164.103**

Health care operations means any of the following activities of the covered entity to the extent that the activities are related to covered functions:

(1) Conducting quality assessment and improvement activities, including outcomes evaluation and development of clinical guidelines, provided that the obtaining of generalizable knowledge is not the primary purpose of any studies resulting from such activities; population-based activities relating to improving health or reducing health care costs, protocol development, case management and care coordination, contacting of health care providers and patients with information about treatment alternatives; and related functions that do not include treatment;

(2) Reviewing the competence or qualifications of health care professionals, evaluating practitioner and provider performance, health plan performance, conducting training programs in which students, trainees, or practitioners in areas of health care learn under supervision to practice or improve their skills as health care providers, training of non-health care professionals, accreditation, certification, licensing, or credentialing activities;

(3) Underwriting, premium rating, and other activities relating to the creation, renewal or replacement of a contract of health insurance or health benefits, and ceding, securing, or placing a contract for reinsurance of risk relating to claims for health care (including stop-loss

insurance and excess of loss insurance), provided that the requirements of §164.514(g) are met, if applicable;

(4) Conducting or arranging for medical review, legal services, and auditing functions, including fraud and abuse detection and compliance programs;

(5) Business planning and development, such as conducting cost-management and planning-related analyses related to managing and operating the entity, including formulary development and administration, development or improvement of methods of payment or coverage policies; and

(6) Business management and general administrative activities of the entity, including, but not limited to:

    (i) Management activities relating to implementation of and compliance with the requirements of this subchapter;

    (ii) Customer service, including the provision of data analyses for policy holders, plan sponsors, or other customers, provided that protected health information is not disclosed to such policy holder, plan sponsor, or customer.

    (iii) Resolution of internal grievances;

    (iv) The sale, transfer, merger, or consolidation of all or part of the covered entity with another covered entity, or an entity that following such activity will become a covered entity and due diligence related to such activity; and

    (v) Consistent with the applicable requirements of §164.514, creating de-identified health information or a limited data set, and fundraising for the benefit of the covered entity. **§ 164.501**

Health care provider means a provider of services (as defined in section 1861(u) of the Act, 42 U.S.C. 1395x(u)), a provider of medical or health services (as defined in section 1861(s) of the Act, 42 U.S.C. 1395x(s)), and any other person or organization who furnishes, bills, or is paid for health care in the normal course of business. **§ 160.103**

Health information means any information, whether oral or recorded in any form or medium, that:

(1) Is created or received by a health care provider, health plan, public health authority, employer, life insurer, school or university, or health care clearinghouse; and

(2) Relates to the past, present, or future physical or mental health or condition of an individual; the provision of health care to an individual; or the past, present, or future payment for the provision of health care to an individual. **§ 160.103**

Health insurance issuer (as defined in section 2791(b)(2) of the PHS Act, 42 U.S.C. 300gg-91(b)(2) and used in the definition of *health plan* in this section) means an insurance company, insurance service, or insurance organization (including an HMO) that is licensed to engage in the business of insurance in a state and is subject to state law that regulates insurance. Such term does not include a group health plan. **§ 160.103**

Health maintenance organization (HMO) (as defined in section 2791(b)(3) of the PHS Act, 42 U.S.C. 300gg-91(b)(3) and used in the definition of *health plan* in this section) means a federally qualified HMO, an organization recognized as an HMO under state law, or a similar organization regulated for solvency under state law in the same manner and to the same extent as such an HMO. **§ 160.103**

Health oversight agency means an agency or authority of the United States, a state, a territory, a political subdivision of a state or territory, or an Indian tribe, or a person or entity acting under a grant of authority from or contract with such public agency, including the employees or agents of such public agency or its contractors or persons or entities to whom it has granted authority, that is authorized by law to oversee the health care system (whether public or private) or government programs in which health information is necessary to determine eligibility or compliance, or to enforce civil rights laws for which health information is relevant. **§ 164.501**

Health plan means an individual or group plan that provides, or pays the cost of, medical care (as defined in section 2791(a)(2) of the PHS Act, 42 U.S.C. 300gg-91(a)(2)).

(1) ***Health plan*** includes the following, singly or in combination:

- (i) A group health plan, as defined in this section.
- (ii) A health insurance issuer, as defined in this section.
- (iii) An HMO, as defined in this section.
- (iv) Part A or Part B of the Medicare program under title XVIII of the Act.
- (v) The Medicaid program under title XIX of the Act, 42 U.S.C. 1396, *et seq*.
- (vi) An issuer of a Medicare supplemental policy (as defined in section 1882(g)(1) of the Act, 42 U.S.C. 1395ss(g)(1)).
- (vii) An issuer of a long-term care policy, excluding a nursing home fixed-indemnity policy.
- (viii) An employee welfare benefit plan or any other arrangement that is established or maintained for the purpose of offering or providing health benefits to the employees of two or more employers.
- (ix) The health care program for active military personnel under title 10 of the United States Code.
- (x) The veterans health care program under 38 U.S.C. chapter 17.
- (xi) The Civilian Health and Medical Program of the Uniformed Services (CHAMPUS) (as defined in 10 U.S.C. 1072(4)).
- (xii) The Indian Health Service program under the Indian Health Care Improvement Act, 25 U.S.C. 1601, *et seq*.
- (xiii) The Federal Employees Health Benefits Program under 5 U.S.C. 8902, *et seq*.

(xiv) An approved state child health plan under title XXI of the Act, providing benefits for child health assistance that meet the requirements of section 2103 of the Act, 42 U.S.C. 1397, *et seq.*

(xv) The Medicare+Choice program under Part C of title XVIII of the Act, 42 U.S.C. 1395w-21 through 1395w-28.

(xvi) A high risk pool that is a mechanism established under state law to provide health insurance coverage or comparable coverage to eligible individuals.

(xvii) Any other individual or group plan, or combination of individual or group plans, that provides or pays for the cost of medical care (as defined in section 2791(a)(2) of the PHS Act, 42 U.S.C. 300gg-91(a)(2)).

(2) ***Health plan*** excludes:

(i) Any policy, plan, or program to the extent that it provides, or pays for the cost of, excepted benefits that are listed in section 2791(c)(1) of the PHS Act, 42 U.S.C. 300gg-91(c)(1); and

(ii) A government-funded program (other than one listed in paragraph (1)(i)-(xvi) of this definition):

(A) Whose principal purpose is other than providing, or paying the cost of, health care; or

(B) Whose principal activity is:

(1) The direct provision of health care to persons; or

(2) The making of grants to fund the direct provision of health care to persons. **§ 160.103**

Hybrid entity means a single legal entity:

(1) That is a covered entity;

(2) Whose business activities include both covered and non-covered functions; and

(3) That designates health care components in accordance with paragraph §164.105(a)(2)(iii)(C). **§ 164.103**

Implementation specification means specific requirements or instructions for implementing a standard. **§ 160.103**

Indirect treatment relationship means a relationship between an individual and a health care provider in which:

(1) The health care provider delivers health care to the individual based on the orders of another health care provider; and

(2) The health care provider typically provides services or products, or reports the diagnosis or results associated with the health care, directly to another health care provider, who provides the services or products or reports to the individual. **§ 164.501**

Individual means the person who is the subject of protected health information. **§ 160.103**

Individually identifiable health information is information that is a subset of health information, including demographic information collected from an individual, and:

(1) Is created or received by a health care provider, health plan, employer, or health care clearinghouse; and

(2) Relates to the past, present, or future physical or mental health or condition of an individual; the provision of health care to an individual; or the past, present, or future payment for the provision of health care to an individual; and

  (i) That identifies the individual; or

  (ii) With respect to which there is a reasonable basis to believe the information can be used to identify the individual. **§ 160.103**

Information system means an interconnected set of information resources under the same direct management control that shares common functionality. A system normally includes hardware, software, information, data, applications, communications, and people. **§ 164.304**

Inmate means a person incarcerated in or otherwise confined to a correctional institution. **§ 164.501**

Integrity means the property that data or information have not been altered or destroyed in an unauthorized manner. **§ 164.304**

Law enforcement official means an officer or employee of any agency or authority of the United States, a state, a territory, a political subdivision of a state or territory, or an Indian tribe, who is empowered by law to:

(1) Investigate or conduct an official inquiry into a potential violation of law; or

(2) Prosecute or otherwise conduct a criminal, civil, or administrative proceeding arising from an alleged violation of law. **§ 164.103 & § 164.501**

Maintain or ***maintenance*** refers to activities necessary to support the use of a standard adopted by the Secretary, including technical corrections to an implementation specification, and enhancements or expansion of a code set. This term excludes the activities related to the adoption of a new standard or implementation specification, or modification to an adopted standard or implementation specification. **§ 162.103**

Malicious software means software, for example, a virus, designed to damage or disrupt a system. **§ 164.304**

Marketing means:

(1) To make a communication about a product or service that encourages recipients of the communication to purchase or use the product or service, unless the communication is made:

  (i) To describe a health-related product or service (or payment for such product or service) that is provided by, or included in a plan of benefits of, the covered entity making the communication, including communications about: the entities participating in a health care provider network or health plan network; replacement of, or enhancements to, a health plan; and health-related products or services available only to a health plan enrollee that add value to, but are not part of, a plan of benefits.

(ii) For treatment of the individual; or

(iii) For case management or care coordination for the individual, or to direct or recommend alternative treatments, therapies, health care providers, or settings of care to the individual.

(2) An arrangement between a covered entity and any other entity whereby the covered entity discloses protected health information to the other entity, in exchange for direct or indirect remuneration, for the other entity or its affiliate to make a communication about its own product or service that encourages recipients of the communication to purchase or use that product or service. **§ 164.501**

Maximum defined data set means all of the required data elements for a particular standard based on a specific implementation specification. **§ 162.103**

Modify or ***modification*** refers to a change adopted by the Secretary, through regulation, to a standard or an implementation specification. **§ 160.103**

More stringent means, in the context of a comparison of a provision of state law and a standard, requirement, or implementation specification adopted under subpart E of part 164 of this subchapter, a state law that meets one or more of the following criteria:

(1) With respect to a use or disclosure, the law prohibits or restricts a use or disclosure in circumstances under which such use or disclosure otherwise would be permitted under this subchapter, except if the disclosure is:

(i) Required by the Secretary in connection with determining whether a covered entity is in compliance with this subchapter; or

(ii) To the individual who is the subject of the individually identifiable health information.

(2) With respect to the rights of an individual, who is the subject of the individually identifiable health information, regarding access to or amendment of individually identifiable health information, permits greater rights of access or amendment, as applicable.

(3) With respect to information to be provided to an individual who is the subject of the individually identifiable health information about a use, a disclosure, rights, and remedies, provides the greater amount of information.

(4) With respect to the form, substance, or the need for express legal permission from an individual, who is the subject of the individually

identifiable health information, for use or disclosure of individually identifiable health information, provides requirements that narrow the scope or duration, increase the privacy protections afforded (such as by expanding the criteria for), or reduce the coercive effect of the circumstances surrounding the express legal permission, as applicable.

(5) With respect to recordkeeping or requirements relating to accounting of disclosures, provides for the retention or reporting of more detailed information or for a longer duration.

(6) With respect to any other matter, provides greater privacy protection for the individual who is the subject of the individually identifiable health information. **§ 160.202**

Organized health care arrangement means:

(1) A clinically integrated care setting in which individuals typically receive health care from more than one health care provider;

(2) An organized system of health care in which more than one covered entity participates and in which the participating covered entities:

  (i) Hold themselves out to the public as participating in a joint arrangement; and

  (ii) Participate in joint activities that include at least one of the following:

    (A) Utilization review, in which health care decisions by participating covered entities are reviewed by other participating covered entities or by a third party on their behalf;

    (B) Quality assessment and improvement activities, in which treatment provided by participating covered entities is assessed by other participating covered entities or by a third party on their behalf; or

    (C) Payment activities, if the financial risk for delivering health care is shared, in part or in whole, by participating covered entities through the joint arrangement and if protected health information created or received by a covered entity is reviewed by other participating covered entities or by a third party on their behalf for the purpose of administering the sharing of financial risk.

(3) A group health plan and a health insurance issuer or HMO with respect to such group health plan, but only with respect to protected health information created or received by such health insurance issuer or HMO that relates to individuals who are or who have been participants or beneficiaries in such group health plan;

(4) A group health plan and one or more other group health plans each of which are maintained by the same plan sponsor; or

(5) The group health plans described in paragraph (4) of this definition and health insurance issuers or HMOs with respect to such group

health plans, but only with respect to protected health information created or received by such health insurance issuers or HMOs that relates to individuals who are or have been participants or beneficiaries in any of such group health plans. **§ 160.103**

Password means confidential authentication information composed of a string of characters. **§ 164.304**

Payment means:

(1) The activities undertaken by:

   (i) A health plan to obtain premiums or to determine or fulfill its responsibility for coverage and provision of benefits under the health plan; or

   (ii) A health care provider or health plan to obtain or provide reimbursement for the provision of health care; and

(2) The activities in paragraph (1) of this definition relate to the individual to whom health care is provided and include, but are not limited to:

   (i) Determinations of eligibility or coverage (including coordination of benefits or the determination of cost sharing amounts), and adjudication or subrogation of health benefit claims;

   (ii) Risk adjusting amounts due based on enrollee health status and demographic characteristics;

   (iii) Billing, claims management, collection activities, obtaining payment under a contract for reinsurance (including stop-loss insurance and excess of loss insurance), and related health care data processing;

   (iv) Review of health care services with respect to medical necessity, coverage under a health plan, appropriateness of care, or justification of charges;

   (v) Utilization review activities, including precertification and preauthorization of services, concurrent and retrospective review of services; and

   (vi) Disclosure to consumer reporting agencies of any of the following protected health information relating to collection of premiums or reimbursement:

      (A) Name and address;

      (B) Date of birth;

      (C) Social Security number;

      (D) Payment history;

      (E) Account number; and

      (F) Name and address of the health care provider and/or health plan. **§ 164.501**

Person means a natural person, trust or estate, partnership, corporation, professional association or corporation, or other entity, public or private. **§ 160.103**

Physical safeguards are physical measures, policies, and procedures to protect a covered entity's electronic information systems and related buildings and equipment, from natural and environmental hazards, and unauthorized intrusion. **§ 164.304**

Plan sponsor is defined as at section 3(16)(B) of ERISA, 29 U.S.C. 1002(16)(B). **§ 164.103**

Protected health information means individually identifiable health information:

(1) Except as provided in paragraph (2) of this definition, that is:
   (i) Transmitted by electronic media;
   (ii) Maintained in electronic media; or
   (iii) Transmitted or maintained in any other form or medium.

(2) ***Protected health information*** excludes individually identifiable health information in:
   (i) Education records covered by the Family Educational Rights and Privacy Act, as amended, 20 U.S.C. 1232g;
   (ii) Records described at 20 U.S.C. 1232g(a)(4)(B)(iv); and
   (iii) Employment records held by a covered entity in its role as employer. **§ 160.103**

Psychotherapy notes means notes recorded (in any medium) by a health care provider who is a mental health professional documenting or analyzing the contents of conversation during a private counseling session or a group, joint, or family counseling session and that are separated from the rest of the individual's medical record. *Psychotherapy notes* excludes medication prescription and monitoring, counseling session start and stop times, the modalities and frequencies of treatment furnished, results of clinical tests, and any summary of the following items: Diagnosis, functional status, the treatment plan, symptoms, prognosis, and progress to date. **§ 164.501**

Public health authority means an agency or authority of the United States, a state, a territory, a political subdivision of a state or territory, or an Indian tribe, or a person or entity acting under a grant of authority from or contract with such public agency, including the employees or agents of such public agency or its contractors or persons or entities to whom it has granted authority, that is responsible for public health matters as part of its official mandate. **§ 164.501**

Relates to the privacy of individually identifiable health information means, with respect to a state law, that the state law has the specific purpose of protecting the privacy of health information or affects the privacy of health information in a direct, clear, and substantial way. **§ 160.202**

Required by law means a mandate contained in law that compels an entity to make a use or disclosure of protected health information and that is enforceable in a court of law. *Required by law* includes, but is not limited to, court orders and court-ordered warrants; subpoenas or summons issued by a court, grand jury, a governmental or tribal inspector general, or an administrative body authorized to require the production of information; a civil or an authorized investigative demand; Medicare conditions of participation with respect to health care providers participating in the program; and statutes or regulations that require the production of information, including statutes or regulations that require such information if payment is sought under a government program providing public benefits. **§ 164.103**

Research means a systematic investigation, including research development, testing, and evaluation, designed to develop or contribute to generalizable knowledge. **§ 164.501**

Respondent means a covered entity upon which the Secretary has imposed, or proposes to impose, a civil money penalty. **§ 160.302**

Secretary means the Secretary of Health and Human Services or any other officer or employee of HHS to whom the authority involved has been delegated. **§ 160.103**

Security or ***Security measures*** encompass all of the administrative, physical, and technical safeguards in an information system. **§ 164.304**

Security incident means the attempted or successful unauthorized access, use, disclosure, modification, or destruction of information or interference with system operations in an information system. **§ 164.304**

Segment means a group of related data elements in a transaction. **§ 162.103**

Small health plan means a health plan with annual receipts of $5 million or less. **§ 160.103**

Standard means a rule, condition, or requirement:

(1) Describing the following information for products, systems, services or practices:

  (i) Classification of components.

  (ii) Specification of materials, performance, or operations; or

  (iii) Delineation of procedures; or

(2) With respect to the privacy of individually identifiable health information. **§ 160.103**

Standard setting organization (SSO) means an organization accredited by the American National Standards Institute that develops and maintains standards for information transactions or data elements, or any other standard that is necessary for, or will facilitate the implementation of, this part. **§ 160.103**

Standard transaction means a transaction that complies with an applicable standard adopted under this part. **§ 162.103**

State refers to one of the following:

(1) For a health plan established or regulated by federal law, state has the meaning set forth in the applicable section of the United States Code for such health plan.

(2) For all other purposes, *state* means any of the several states, the District of Columbia, the Commonwealth of Puerto Rico, the Virgin Islands, and Guam. **§ 160.103**

State law means a constitution, statute, regulation, rule, common law, or other state action having the force and effect of law. **§ 160.202**

Technical safeguards means the technology and the policy and procedures for its use that protect electronic protected health information and control access to it. **§ 164.304**

Trading partner agreement means an agreement related to the exchange of information in electronic transactions, whether the agreement is distinct or part of a larger agreement, between each party to the agreement. (For example, a trading partner agreement may specify, among other things, the duties and responsibilities of each party to the agreement in conducting a standard transaction.) **§ 160.103**

Transaction means the transmission of information between two parties to carry out financial or administrative activities related to health care. It includes the following types of information transmissions:

(1) Health care claims or equivalent encounter information.

(2) Health care payment and remittance advice.

(3) Coordination of benefits.

(4) Health care claim status.

(5) Enrollment and disenrollment in a health plan.

(6) Eligibility for a health plan.

(7) Health plan premium payments.

(8) Referral certification and authorization.

(9) First report of injury.

(10) Health claims attachments.

(11) Other transactions that the Secretary may prescribe by regulation. **§ 160.103**

Treatment means the provision, coordination, or management of health care and related services by one or more health care providers, including the coordination or management of health care by a health care provider with a third party; consultation between health care providers relating to a patient; or the referral of a patient for health care from one health care provider to another. **§ 164.501**

Unsecured protected health information means protected health information that is not rendered unusable, unreadable, or indecipherable to unauthorized individuals through the use of a technology or methodology specified by the Secretary in the guidance issued under section 13402(h)(2) of Public Law 111-5 on the HHS Web site. **§ 164.402**

Use means, with respect to individually identifiable health information, the sharing, employment, application, utilization, examination, or analysis of such information within an entity that maintains such information. **§ 160.103**

User means a person or entity with authorized access. **§ 164.304**

Violation or ***violate*** means, as the context may require, failure to comply with an administrative simplification provision. **§ 160.302**

Workforce means employees, volunteers, trainees, and other persons whose conduct, in the performance of work for a covered entity, is under the direct control of such entity, whether or not they are paid by the covered entity. **§ 160.103**

Workstation means an electronic computing device, for example, a laptop or desktop computer, or any other device that performs similar functions, and electronic media stored in its immediate environment. **§ 164.304**

index

A

D

Q

R

S